Realizing the Right to Health

Andrew Clapham and Mary Robinson
Claire Mahon and Scott Jerbi

Swiss Human Rights Book Vol. 3

Edited by the Chair of Political Philosophy
of the University of Zurich, Switzerland
On request of the Political Division IV,
Human Security, DFA, Berne
www.swisshumanrightsbook.com

Druck: bod

ISBN 978-3-907625-45-3

Contents

Universal Declaration of Human Rights [Art. 25]

1. Everyone has the right to a standard of living adequate for the health and well-being of himself and of his family, including food, clothing, housing and medical care and necessary social services, and the right to security in the event of unemployment, sickness, disability, widowhood, old age or other lack of livelihood in circumstances beyond his control.

2. Motherhood and childhood are entitled to special care and assistance. All children, whether born in or out of wedlock, shall enjoy the same social protection.

International Covenant on Economic, Social and Cultural Rights [Art. 12]

1. The States Parties to the present Covenant recognize the right of everyone to the enjoyment of the highest attainable standard of physical and mental health.

2. The steps to be taken by the States Parties to the present Covenant to achieve the full realization of this right shall include those necessary for:

a) The provision for the reduction of the stillbirth-rate and of infant mortality and for the healthy development of the child;

b) The improvement of all aspects of environmental and industrial hygiene;

c) The prevention, treatment and control of epidemic, endemic, occupational and other diseases;

d) The creation of conditions which would assure to all medical service and medical attention in the event of sickness.

Preface

The purpose of the Swiss Human Rights Book series is to highlight a specific human rights topic and to consider it from a variety of different perspectives. Launched in 2006, the first volume of the series was entitled Realizing Property Rights; it was followed by the second volume in 2007 dedicated to the rights of the child.

The right to health is both a practical and a political issue. For millions of people in the world, the full enjoyment of the right to health is still elusive, especially for those living in poverty. The cost of health care remains unaffordable for many, even in wealthy countries, despite the adoption of health policies and programmes. Realizing the right to health is an opportunity and a challenge, and the bulk of the work to achieve this right for all is still to be done.

Health is a fundamental human right, indispensable to the enjoyment of other human rights. It is to be understood as the right of everyone to the highest attainable standard of physical and mental health as it is defined in the relevant international conventions. It is not confined to the right to health care but embraces a wide range of socio-economic factors that create the conditions in which people can lead healthy lives, and it extends to the underlying determinants of health, including food and nutrition, housing, access to safe drinking water and adequate sanitation, safe and healthy working conditions, and a healthy environment.

In spite of the indivisible nature of all human rights, economic, social and cultural rights have not always received adequate treatment at the international level. The development of those rights is a priority of Swiss foreign policy, and this publication contributes to furthering the renewed interest in economic, social and cultural rights. It is a contribution of an interministerial approach of the Swiss government towards the promotion of a global health policy.

I am very pleased that the Political Philosophy Department of Zurich University, headed by Professor Georg Kohler, together with the editors Mary Robinson, former United Nations High Commissioner for Human Rights, and Andrew Clapham, Director of the Geneva Academy of International Humanitarian Law and Human Rights, together with Rüffer & Rub Publishers are presenting the third volume of the Swiss Human Rights Book. I thank the experts who made it possible. As authors, they explore and map the right to health from various thematic and geographic perspectives, offering a comprehensive picture of this challenging issue. Their contributions are available to interested readers at: www.swisshumanrightsbook.com.

Ambassador Thomas Greminger
Head of Political Affairs Division IV
(Human Security)
Federal Department of Foreign Affairs

Foreword: The Right to Health as an Example

Georg Kohler*

1. Ask any serious philosopher whether there is a conclusive reasoning for the logical validity of human rights and the honest answer will be: No, there is no such conclusive argument but there are many good reasons for acknowledging human rights and, above all – the philosopher will continue – their binding force is currently no longer dependent on any theories and philosophical reflections but the expression of the will of the community of nations and of a world-encompassing experience, which humanity has learned from its own history, adopting it and converting it into binding law.

For sure, this sounds rather pathetic, but in this special case, it is commensurate with the matter at hand. For it is the historically unique signature of the 21st century that a global civilization has currently arisen, not only on the levels of technical, economic, and communicative processes, but that a worldwide, normative agreement has also come forth which, in spite of all cultural and religious differences of humanity, is clear on this particular point: That every human being ought to have the right to develop as freely as possible, for no other reason than that he or she is a human being.

2. Of course, "as freely as possible" will not be understood in the same way everywhere, but that is no objection to the equally astonishing, as well as actually matter-of-course fact, that human rights (with their core of the

positive and negative autonomy of each individual) are no longer a mere utopia of some idealists, but an indisputable, world-societal reality bringing about multiple effects.

This is astonishing because the universality of this thought was still being challenged as a matter of principle in the 20th century: In the name of powerful racist, imperialist and totalitarian ideologies, enemy concepts and deadly oppositions ruled in many parts of the world, denying to the other in each case the equality of birth on principle. The other person was – as an "enemy of the people" or as an "Untermensch" (subhuman) – nothing but the rightless object of foreign superiority.

Of course, I do not claim that such matters of antihuman deprivation of rights are no longer happening. But the novelty and singularity of the present resides in the fact that the established human right to develop as freely as possible proscribes them as such and stigmatizes them immediately as injustice.

3.   And yet: Is it not a matter of course for us human beings to be able to "walk in the shoes of another person"? Is it not precisely this basic social act which allows for cooperation and civilizing progress? Is it not thus the elementary experience of primary similarity and equality of human beings – or, if you wish: The primary experience of the rightfulness of human-rights-claims – the ground on which human vitality was able to develop in the first place? If the question is formulated in this way, the reply is clear. All the more pressing is the discourse on its causes which could block, and keep blocking, a clear answer and its consequences.

4.   Human rights are an idea with de facto effects: A normative power opposing reigning circumstances in multiple aspects. This becomes most evident when it is all about realizing human rights, i. e. to turn general demands into concrete claims and commitments.

Every human being ought to be able to lead a self-determined life so far as possible. Each person should be able to exist in peace and security. Each person ought to be able to say what he or she means. She should learn what she is capable of doing. We ought to be allowed to join whomsoever we wish to; and so on. And therefore also: We should be allowed to be healthy – not victims of illnesses and circumstances, which can all too easily be decoded as the result of avoidable bad luck and unjust burdens.

The problem of realizing the idea of human rights – and in particular focusing on the right to health – enables us to perceive what immense tasks are tied to its assertion. But in working towards fulfilling these tasks we are equally able to experience where and how they are to be accomplished. We learn that realizing human rights is an objective that is far from having been accomplished but it need not be a poor utopia.

---

*   This chapter was originally written by the author
    in German and translated into English by Salomé
    Hangartner.

Introduction

Mary Robinson and Andrew Clapham

The run up to the 2008 election in the United States focused at one point on the nature of health care in America. During the second presidential debate, the candidates were asked the following question: "Is health care in America a privilege, a right, or a responsibility?" Senator Obama (as he then was) replied as follows:

> "Well, I think it should be a right for every American. In a country as wealthy as ours, for us to have people who are going bankrupt because they can't pay their medical bills – for my mother to die of cancer at the age of 53 and have to spend the last months of her life in the hospital room arguing with insurance companies because they're saying that this may be a pre-existing condition and they don't have to pay her treatment, there's something fundamentally wrong about that."[1]

Many of us have a similar sense that there is something wrong when individuals face life threatening diseases and are unable to receive the care they need. We all probably have felt the frustration of knowing that more could be done to ensure that an adequate health care system, accessible and affordable for all, was in place in every country. We may even have made the connection to rights and sometimes human rights. But we now have to go a little deeper and ask: "Even if we are convinced that everyone deserves to have access to the basic requirements of health – which includes not only health care but also the underlying determinants of health such as proper nutrition, adequate sanitation, safe drinking water and education – how does affirming a right to health change the realities in communities and nations around the world?"

We can start to answer by inquiring – what does it mean, precisely, to say that health is a human right? Despite the fact that the World Health Organization declared in 1946 that the "enjoyment of the highest attainable standard of health is one of the fundamental rights of every human being" and that over 70% of all nations have ratified the 1966 International Covenant on Economic, Social and Cultural Rights which makes the right to health an international legal obligation that must be progressively realized at the national level, the reality is that the right to health is still not universally recognized as a fundamental human right. Like other economic, social and cultural rights, it has been neglected and violated on a massive scale in too many parts of the world.

The chapters in this Swiss Human Rights Book explain the scope of the right to health enshrined in the Covenant. Of course, the Covenant actually speaks of the "the right of everyone to the highest attainable standard of physical and mental health", but we would suggest that the expression "right to health" has become the acceptable shorthand, and indeed later human rights instruments such as the 1988 San Salvador Protocol to the American Convention on Human Rights use the expression "the right to health".[2] Scholars in this field have concluded that the phrase "right to health" is "best, in line with the international treaty provisions that proclaim not only the right to health care services, but also the right to a number of underlying preconditions for health, such as safe drinking water, adequate sanitation, environmental health, and occupational health."[3]

But we have chosen to move beyond the treaties and look more generally at the international institutions, partnerships and civil society organizations that are tackling the right to health in new and exciting ways. Global health and human rights are both issues that define Geneva. The home of the UN Office of the High Commissioner for Human Rights, the Human Rights Council and the Committee on Economic, Social and Cultural Rights is also known as the headquarters of the World Health Organization, and now a growing number of health institutions and initiatives such as UNAIDS, the Global Fund to Fight AIDS, Tuberculosis and Malaria, the GAVI Alliance, the Medicines for Malaria Venture and the Drugs and Neglected Diseases Initiative. All these initiatives recognize that we need to broaden the range of actors traditionally associated with human rights. We need a

21st century approach that highlights the multiple actors involved in ensuring the right to health for all.

The essays in this book aim to contribute to that goal by exploring what it means to take a rights-based approach in the various fields where the authors have experience. The UN Special Rapporteur on the right to health and others have encouraged human rights and health advocates to think, not only about strictly legal strategies, but also about how the underlying principles of human rights and the right to health can help inform and shape policymaking and action concerning health interventions at all levels.

In understanding what human rights-based approaches add to existing efforts, consider, for example, the importance of health indicators. Concern for human rights focuses attention on the disadvantaged and requires the active and informed participation of individuals and communities. A clearer picture often emerges when indicator data is disaggregated on various grounds, such as sex, race and ethnicity. Disaggregated indicators can reveal whether or not some disadvantaged individuals and communities are suffering from de facto discrimination. Equally important, for the most part, existing health indicators are rarely designed to monitor issues like participation and accountability, although these are essential in ensuring better access to health care.

Policy interventions that are grounded in human rights with a strong gender dimension can help inform and support efforts to strengthen health systems and improve their performance. Human rights require not only that quality health systems are available, accessible and acceptable to all but that positive action is taken to address the economic, social and political inequalities behind mortality and ill-health. A human rights approach helps to ensure a holistic and integrated approach to health delivery, with a focus on prevention.

Understanding and addressing influences such as gender, poverty, culture and age is a crucial part of the process. These powerful determinants of health shape the distribution of diseases, access to and use of health services, and the course of health outcomes. Attention to the human rights principles of non-discrimination and equality can highlight differential treatment of distinct population groups, moving beyond averages to focus attention on the health needs of vulnerable or marginalized groups, and thus help to ensure that health systems meet the health needs of all segments of a population.

In the end, nothing could be more important to promoting greater enjoyment of the right to health than strengthening health systems around the world. A nation's health system is its life-force and a marker of the priority it gives to its most vulnerable and marginalized members of society. When the right to health is debated in national elections, we know this is an issue whose time has come. A country's health is fundamental not only to its wellness, but to its social cohesion, its prosperity and perhaps even to its political stability. The strength, therefore, of every country's health system and within every country, its local and community-based capacities – is of paramount importance.

1   Full transcript available at http://edition.cnn. com/2008/POLITICS/10/07/presidential.debate. transcript/.

2   See e.g. Article 10 Right to Health: (1) Everyone shall have the right to health, understood to mean the enjoyment of the highest level of physical, mental and social well-being.

3   Brigit Toebes, 'The Right to Health' in A. Eide, C. Krause and A. Rosas (eds.) *Economic, Social and Cultural Rights: A Textbook* (2nd edition, Dordrecht: Nijhoff, 2001) 169–190 at 170; see also Virginia A. Leary, 'The Right to Health in International Human Rights Law' 1(1) *Health and Human Rights* (1994) 24–56 at 26.

01

HEALTH: A HUMAN RIGHTS PERSPECTIVE

The Human Right to Health: Conceptual Foundations

Eibe Riedel

Introduction

Health is a fundamental human right, indispensable for the exercise of many other human rights, and necessary for living a life in dignity. The right to the highest attainable standard of health as a normative standard was first enunciated in 1946 in the Constitution of the World Health Organization (WHO), and has since been reiterated in a number of WHO declarations, foremost amongst them the 1978 Alma-Ata Declaration on Primary Health Care and the 1998 World Health Declaration. But of course there were precedents. Prior to the eighteenth century, responsibility in case of disease or illness predominantly fell into the hands of private entities, such as churches and charities. State institutions usually only intervened in cases of epidemic or pandemic diseases, mostly laying down forms of quarantines. At the centre of all these mostly communal health considerations were efforts to provide adequate sanitation, particularly in the larger cities.[1] In the 18th century, awareness of public health and its importance for society grew rapidly, yet the concept of modern public health only developed in the days of the industrial revolution, when unhealthy working and living conditions, caused to a large extent by mass production, led to epidemics and other grave health problems, epitomized in the novels by Charles Dickens.

The spread of epidemics beyond national borders soon elevated these questions to the international level, as they were considered as threats to international trade, and were therefore discussed at the first international conferences on sanitation. In 1903, one of these conferences set up the

Office International d'Hygiène Publique (OIHP) which was later associated to the League of Nations, and ultimately became the Health Organization of the League of Nations. The concept of primary health care for all was first discussed at a conference convened by this new organization and was later taken up by the United Nations.

Work-related issues of health were also taken up in the International Labour Organization (ILO), founded in 1919. During the Second World War, the ideas of social rights and, in particular, health as a human right, were further developed and institutionalized. A milestone in that respect was Franklin D. Roosevelt's Four Freedoms speech in 1941, in which he proclaimed the crucial importance of the freedom from want. At the United Nations (UN) Conference on International Organization in San Francisco in 1945, this issue was taken up, and was later reflected in Article 55 of the UN Charter, and elaborated in the World Health Organization as a specialized agency of the UN. The right to health has been subsequently firmly established in numerous instruments at the international, regional and national levels.

The UN Charter-based protection

Under the so-called UN Charter-based system of human rights protection, Article 55 of the UN Charter says that "... the United Nations shall promote: a. higher standards of living, ... b. solutions of international economic, social health, and related problems ..., and c. universal respect for, and observance of human rights and fundamental freedoms for all without distinction as to race, sex, language, or religion." Health is also referred to in Articles 57 and 62 of the UN Charter, as one of the fields of responsibility of the Economic and Social Council (ECOSOC). The most influential and basic document in this respect is, however, the Universal Declaration of Human Rights of 1948 (UDHR), which, when adopted by the UN General Assembly, was initially legally non-binding in nature, but has since assumed the status of customary international law for most of its provisions, affirming in Article 25(1) that "everyone has the right to a standard of living adequate for the health of himself and his family, including food, clothing, housing and medical care, and necessary social services".

The right to health set out in Article 25 of the UDHR has been the subject of work by the UN Human Rights Council, the former UN Commission on Human Rights, and the human rights special procedures. In particular, a Special Rapporteur on the right of everyone to the highest attainable standard of physical and mental health was appointed by the Commission on Human Rights in April 2002.[2] Since the creation of this mandate, the Special Rapporteur has submitted annual thematic reports and reports on country missions to the Human Rights Council (and the former Commission). The members of the Human Rights Council and its predecessor body have also adopted a number of resolutions on the right to health, for example resolutions on human rights and HIV/AIDS[3] (and endorsement of the International Guidelines on HIV/AIDS and Human Rights[4]), and on access to medication in the context of HIV/AIDS.[5]

The WHO, like most specialized agencies of the UN system, places great emphasis in its work on formulating policies, strategies and programmes of action, rather than laws. The primarily policy-oriented approach adopted by the WHO has nevertheless proved to be very successful. Member States of the WHO have followed the policies, programmes and recommendations elaborated since 1948, have contributed to the eradication or near-eradication of many diseases, and have helped to combat major pandemics and endemic diseases. The treaty approach has, by contrast, been utilized by the ILO in relation to workers' rights. The tripartite structure of that organization favoured such a legal approach. The organization's awareness of health problems is exemplified in Conventions No. 155 on Occupational Safety and Health (1981), No. 161 on Occupational Health Services (1985), and No. 169, the Indigenous and Tribal Peoples Convention (1989). The latter considers equal but culturally sensitive health care and protection an important factor with respect to indigenous peoples' labour rights.

Specifically, Article 3(d) of ILO Convention No. 182 against worst forms of child labour deems children's health as an essential criterion for the definition of the term "worst forms of child labour". It must be noted that the ILO Conventions are legally binding documents for those states that are parties to them, and in such cases apply immediately to states, labour unions and employer organizations.

Under the UN Charter-based system, various declarations have been elaborated, dealing with health matters, such as the Vienna Declaration and Programme of Action of 1993, alluding to the right to health in several of its paragraphs, acknowledging, in particular, the importance of health care and protection.

The UN Millennium Declaration of 8 December 2000, adopted by the UN General Assembly, also stresses the importance of health care and prevention of disease by committing states to the improvement of maternal and child health, and the combat against HIV/AIDS, malaria, and other major diseases. Of the eight UN Development Goals (MDGs), three have a direct healthcare dimension (goals 4, 5 and 6), while target 17 of MDG No. 8 calls for cooperation with pharmaceutical companies, in order to provide access to affordable essential drugs in developing countries. By way of example only, let us refer here to a number of texts that elaborate health issues: the Standard Minimum Rules for the Treatment of Prisoners (1977), as well as the Basic Principles for the Treatment of Prisoners (1990), include many references to health care and protection; or the UN Principles for Older Persons (1991) stress the importance of access to adequate health care facilities "to maintain or regain the optimum level of physical, mental and emotional well-being and to prevent or delay the onset of illness"; or the UN Principles for the protection of persons with mental illness and the improvement of mental health care (1991), and the UN Declaration of Commitment on HIV/AIDS (2001); indicating international awareness regarding this most perilous epidemic.

While all these instruments with relevance to health matters have either been adopted or approved by the UN General Assembly or the ECOSOC, strictly speaking they have no legally binding effect on states and governments. Still, the mere fact that these instruments have been followed by states, as if they were binding, has illustrated that they form an important component within the international movement to promote and protect the physical and mental health of all persons worldwide. Thus, a strategy fully applied voluntarily by states is as good as a treaty that has to undergo a cumbersome ratification and adoption process at the universal and national levels.

The treaty-based protection system

By contrast, the international treaty-based system works on the assumption that states will apply the international obligations for human rights protection in their own domestic law system as binding legal obligations. The international human rights system, as a consequence, has developed considerably over the last forty years. A large majority of states have by now ratified the key human rights treaties, such as the two Covenants, the International Covenant on Economic, Social and Cultural Rights (ICESCR) and the International Covenant on Civil and Political Rights (ICCPR) of 1966, in force since 1976, or the Convention on the Rights of the Child (CRC) of 1989, or the Convention on the Elimination of All Forms of Discrimination Against Women (CEDAW) of 1979. As a result, a solid blanket of human rights norms has been spread out, on which issues of human rights protection can be monitored at the international level.

In relation to the right to health, the ICESCR manifests the human right to health in its Article 12, stating that:

> "1. The States Parties to the present Covenant recognize the right of everyone to the enjoyment of the highest attainable standard of physical and mental health. 2. The steps to be taken by the States Parties to the present Covenant to achieve the full realization of this right shall include those necessary for: (a) The provision for the reduction of the stillbirth-rate and of infant mortality and for the healthy development of the child; (b) The improvement of all aspects of environmental and industrial hygiene; (c) The prevention, treatment and control of epidemic, endemic occupational and other diseases; (d) The creation of conditions which would assure to all medical service and medical attention in the event of sickness."

Other articles in the ICESCR address different aspects in the context of health, thus contributing to a comprehensive and integrated protection of the human right to health.

The ICCPR, as the parallel Covenant on civil and political rights, in its Article 6, stresses that States Parties are under an obligation to protect every human being's inherent right to life, and some States Parties have used this provision also in relation to the right to health, where no specific provision for that is to be found in constitutional or other legislative documents. In the area of international humanitarian law, the Geneva Conventions (1949) in their Common Article 3, as well as in both Additional Protocols of 1977 stress the eminent role for health care and protection in international and internal armed conflict situations.[6]

The network of international treaty law instruments with significance for the right to health is very elaborate.[7] A listing of all relevant health-related norms would exceed the scope of this overview. To single out a recent addition, having direct effect on the realization of the right to health, let us note the WHO Framework Convention on Tobacco Control of 2003, setting up a secretariat and annual meetings in conferences of States Parties, has opted for the avenue of a legally binding instrument rather than mere statements of policies and strategies to achieve its aims. The WHO thus is beginning to elaborate the possibilities of the legal approach alongside the well-tried policy approach.

The international treaties of recent years increasingly focus on vulnerable, disadvantaged or marginalized individuals and groups, and often highlight discrimination issues. The right to health is, however, also contained in regional international standards, such as the African Charter on Human and Peoples' Rights ("Banjul Charter"), Article 16; The African Charter on the Rights and Welfare of the Child, Article 14; the Revised European Social Charter, Articles 11 and 13; and the Additional Protocol to the American Convention on Human Rights in the Area of Economic, Social and Cultural Rights ("Protocol of San Salvador"), Article 10. Indirect protection of health is also afforded by the American Convention on Human Rights, the Inter-American Convention on the Prevention, Punishment and Eradication of Violence against Women, and the European Convention for the Protection of Human Rights and Fundamental Freedoms and its 14 Protocols.

The right to health is also recognized in numerous national constitutions,[8] either directly, as in South Africa, or indirectly, as in India. Such indirect protection can be effected by judicial pronouncements, incorporating the right to health aspects in other human rights, explicitly guaranteed at the national level.[9] In some countries, where the Constitution does not provide specifically for the right to health, elementary health care issues can be deduced from a more generic human rights provision, such as the human dignity provision read in conjunction with a "social state" or solidarity principle, as under the German Basic Law in Articles 1 and 20. These chapeau provisions serve as an umbrella of human rights protection, albeit restricted to guaranteeing the survival kit, the existential minimum, without which a life in dignity cannot be led.[10]

Right to health: Freedom and entitlements

If one looks at the complex nature of the right to health, several quite distinct dimensions have to be borne in mind: On the one hand, the right contains the freedom to make decisions about one's own health data; on the other hand, the right to health also embraces an entitlement to a system of health care protection. So the availability of health services, facilities and products of good quality represents a comprehensive dimension, while the actual individual rights guarantee represents another, equally important dimension.

In 2000 the Committee on Economic, Social and Cultural Rights (CE-SCR) adopted General Comment No. 14 which outlines in great detail the various dimensions of the right to health.[11] The freedom dimension of the right to health includes questions of sexual and reproductive health, the right to be free from interference, such as non-consensual medical treatment. The entitlement dimension addresses such issues as the right to emergency medical services, and to the underlying determinants of health, such as adequate sanitation, safe and potable water, adequate food and shelter, safe and healthy working conditions, and a healthy environment. If these underlying determinants of health are not met, the right itself cannot properly be protected.

A lot of discussion centred on the question of entitlement to emergency medical treatment, particularly as regards undocumented immigrants. From a human rights perspective, such people are particularly vulnerable and in greatest need of immediate protection. Most developed countries, as receiving countries, resist such arguments, however, fearing that they cannot cope with the health problems of potentially huge numbers of undocumented immigrants. While General Comment No. 14 takes a broad approach which covers primary, secondary (specialist) and tertiary (high cost intensive medical treatments) health care, in the Committee's practice such people seem to be entitled to emergency treatment only, until such time that status questions are resolved. From the beginning non-governmental organizations have taken a broader view. But it must be remembered that General Comments set out to state the human rights law, as it is conventionally agreed, not what might be considered to be desirable. The Committee, like all treaty bodies, has to draw a fine line between interpreting – which it is entitled to do – and legislating, which is up to the contracting states. In the monitoring practice of the state reporting procedure, this distinction is not always applied strictly. Committee members may ask questions on the treatment availability for undocumented aliens, hoping that the State Party engages in a constructive dialogue on the issue. This way, the Government concerned may get recommendations from the Committee on how to change the legal bases of alien treatment situations at home, and the Committee can then follow up these recommendations in the next dialogue with the State Party.

Right to health: Availability, accessibility, acceptability and quality

General Comment No. 14 starts out by saying that the expression "right to highest attainable standard of health" in Article 12 of ICESCR is very broadly phrased, perhaps too broadly. But it certainly cannot be understood as a right to be healthy.[12] Thus the right contains both freedoms and entitlements. The notion of the "highest attainable standard of health" in Article 12(1) of ICESCR takes into account both the individual's biological and socio-economic preconditions, and the state's available resources. A number of important aspects cannot, however, be addressed solely within the relationship between the state and individuals. In particular, good health cannot be ensured by a state, nor can states provide protection against every conceivable cause of human ill health. Thus, genetic factors, individual susceptibility to ill health or the adoption of unhealthy or risky lifestyles, albeit important, cannot be attributed to the state. General Comment No. 14, therefore, restricts the right to health to a right to the enjoyment of a variety of facilities, goods, services and conditions necessary for the realization of the right to health.[13] The right to health, as interpreted by the CESCR, contains four essential and inter-related elements: Availability, accessibility, acceptability and quality (the AAAQs).[14]

It is clear that health facilities, goods and services must be available in sufficient quantity within a given country. This includes, inter alia, hospitals, clinics, trained medical personnel, and availability of essential medicines according to the 20 or so essential drugs that the WHO Essential Drugs List contains. But it also comprises preventive public health strategies and promotional activities, such as awareness-raising campaigns against HIV/AIDS, or information as regards safe drinking water and adequate sanitation facilities. The issues connected with sanitation and water were only flagged in General Comment No. 14, but the right to water and sanitation was later elaborated in General Comment No. 15.[15] The right to water and sanitation has now been given additional prominence by the institution of an Independent Expert on that issue, established by the Human Rights Council in 2008. The availability of health personnel is crucial in rural areas in many countries.

The dimension of accessibility without discrimination is next addressed in General Comment No. 14: It comprises non-discrimination, particularly for the marginalized and disadvantaged sections of the population, in law and in fact.[16] It also addresses physical accessibility, i.e. within safe physical reach for all sections of the population, especially for the most vulnerable groups, such as ethnic minorities, indigenous peoples, women, children, adolescents, older persons, persons with disabilities, and particularly persons with HIV/AIDS. Thus, to take but one example, in many Saharan countries, girls have to walk a long way to collect water, and frequently are accosted by young men, so safe access to water is a clear priority for them. Most critical is the further aspect of economic accessibility (affordability); equity demands that poorer households should not be disproportionately burdened with health expenses as compared to richer households. If a health centre charges user fees and those in need cannot pay the fee, the centre is not economically accessible. Needless to say, the exact amounts to be assessed are up to democratically elected parliaments and other processes at the national level.

The right to health also requires that health facilities must be respectful of medical ethics, they must also be culturally appropriate and gender-sensitive. There should be acceptability. Thus health workers need to be aware of cultural sensitivities in the provision of health care. For example, when women are examined by male doctors, a female nurse should be in attendance. Lastly, the quality of health care is a decisive factor. Facilities must be scientifically and medically appropriate, and of good quality. Thus, for example, provision of an expensive mammography machine to a health centre may not be scientifically and medically appropriate where human and technical resources are scarce, as in many less developed countries, and where the main issue for women is cervical cancer.[17] Where health education is offered, it must be ensured that such education is of high quality.

The right to health, like all ESC-rights, is subject to progressive realization and resource availability. In the past, this has given rise to fundamental misunderstandings: This progressive nature was taken by some governments to mean that, unlike civil and political rights, economic, social and cultural rights merely represented programmatic goals or promotional obligations, non-self-executing norms, whereby it would be up to the State Parties concerned to decide, by way of discretion, if, and how, the right promised at the international level would be operationalized at the national level. As long as no implementation steps were taken at the domestic level, the right would only be subject to vague and general reporting and monitoring at the international level. It would amount only to very soft obligations. However, ever since its General Comment No. 3 in 1990, the Committee has consistently emphasized that this approach clearly contravenes the object and purpose of the Covenant. Progressive realization and resource availability, mentioned in Article 2(1) of the Covenant, simply mean that states have to show how they have progressed in the realization of rights protection between two reporting phases, i.e. how the situation has improved over the last four years. This is not merely a programmatic obligation, but a clear and immediate obligation of the State Party.[18] If no progress was made, or there was even regression, then the State Party is under a stringent legal obligation to explain why it could not fulfil the Covenant obligation. The question of resource availability, to which Article 2(1) also refers, is not a *carte blanche* for states to do as they please. While setting out a general standard, developed countries start from a higher level of rights realization than developing countries, which start from a much lower level of rights realization, on account of their economic situation. Nonetheless, even the developing country must take reasonable and deliberate targeted steps towards better realization of the right to health. Thus, for example, some obligations are not resource-dependent at all, but apply across the board, such as non-discrimination or equality issues. In addition, where developing countries are unable to meet even these minimal requirements, they are under an obligation to seek international cooperation and assistance. Developed countries as a corollary have an international obligation under Article 2(1) ICESCR to provide such cooperation and assistance, even though that obligation is not specified in any detail by way of concrete amounts. Many developed countries do indeed provide such assistance, but do so as a voluntary exercise, and consequently do not regard this assistance as part of their international legal obligations. The Committee, from the very beginning, has taken a different view, as recently outlined in its Statement on Resource Allocation,[19] which the Human Rights Council requested the Committee to outline in connection with the adoption of the Optional Protocol to the ICESCR at the end of 2008.

Levels of protection for the right to health

Article 12 of ICESCR imposes three levels of obligation for States Parties: The first type of obligation, the obligation to respect, requires states to refrain from interfering directly or indirectly with the enjoyment of the right to health.[20] The state, as a matter of principle, has to avoid any action or activity which would hamper the equal enjoyment of access to preventive, curative or palliative health services, e.g. access to contraceptives, health-related information or traditional preventive care, healing practices and medicines.

In General Comment No. 14, several examples are given to outline specific legal obligations resting on States Parties, such as preventing unequal access to health facilities, including for prisoners or detainees, asylum-seekers and undocumented immigrants, and the obligation to abstain from enforcing discriminatory health practices as a state policy, particularly vis-à-vis women, or the obligation to prevent the marketing of unsafe drugs and from applying coercive medical treatments, unless this is for the treatment of mental illness in exceptional and closely defined circumstances, or for the prevention and control of communicable diseases.

The State Party furthermore has obligations to protect which include, inter alia, the adoption of legislation, or the taking of other measures ensuring equal access to health care and health-related services provided by third or private parties. This means that the state, although not directly responsible for the administration of a particular health matter, still remains indirectly responsible, ensuring that the marketing of medical equipment, and of medicines provided by third parties, remain under the state's control. Thus, under this control function, the state has to ensure that medical practitioners, and other health professionals, meet appropriate standards of education, skills, and ethical codes of conduct. States also remain responsible for protecting their population from harmful traditional practices, interfering with access to pre and post-natal care and family planning, and to combat female genital mutilation where this still represents a widespread social practice.[21]

Under the obligation to fulfil, states are required, inter alia, to give sufficient recognition to the right to health in the national political and legal systems, and to adopt a national health policy containing detailed plans for realizing the right to health. States Parties must also provide adequate health care, including immunization programmes against the major infectious diseases. Public health infrastructures should also provide for sexual and reproductive health services, particularly in rural areas. Many other examples are given in General Comment No. 14, paragraph 36. States are also required to formulate, implement and review periodically a coherent national policy to minimize the risk of occupational accidents and diseases.[22]

While these obligations seem to require a lot from each State Party, the Committee in General Comment No. 14 has made it abundantly clear that despite the multifarious legal obligations in relation to the freedom aspects of the right to health and the entitlement components of that right, a relatively small but essential number of core obligations can be made out which all states, whether rich or poor, should be able to meet in all circumstances, because they are not resource-dependent, or only to a very limited degree, comparable to any civil or political rights situation. These core right to health obligations affect the "survival kit" or "existential minimum" which every person needs for survival and for leading a life in dignity. Furthermore, these core obligations reflect the actual practice of very many states at their domestic law level, and may be regarded as part of customary international law or even as general principles of law in the sense of Article 38(1) (c) of the Statute of the International Court of Justice (ICJ). Accordingly, states without exception are obliged:

"(a) To ensure the right of access to health facilities, goods and services on a non-discriminatory basis, especially for vulnerable or marginalized groups, (b) to ensure access to the minimum essential food which is nutritionally adequate and safe, to ensure freedom from hunger to everyone, (c) to ensure access to basic shelter, housing and sanitation, and an adequate supply of safe and potable water, (d) to provide essential drugs, as from time to time defined under the WHO Action Programme on Essential Drugs, (e) to ensure equitable distribution of all health facilities, goods and services, and (f) to adopt and implement a national public health strategy and plan of action, on the basis of epidemiological evidence, addressing the health concerns of the whole population ..."

These then are the minimum core obligations of the right to health which states must meet. Other obligations of comparable priority cover reproductive, maternal and child health care, and other duties outlined in the General Comment No. 14, paragraph 44.[23]

Accountability structures

Increasingly, international attention is focussing on mechanisms of accountability in realizing the right to health. While the State Party reporting to treaty bodies provides some form of international control, more effective implementation of international obligations at the national level is required. A number of accountability mechanisms are available for that purpose.[24] Accountability involves states being answerable for their acts or omissions regarding their right to health obligations. If no accountability mechanisms exist, the right to health will be largely meaningless or ineffective for right holders. Several different types of accountability mechanisms can be distinguished:

1. Judicial;
2. quasi-judicial;
3. administrative;
4. political; and
5. social.

Under judicial review of executive action or statutory or constitutional interpretation, at the national level, many examples can be given from various countries. To pick out but one, *Minister of Health v. Treatment Action Campaign,* the Constitutional Court of South Africa applied sections 27 and 28 of the South African Constitution when the question of access to essential drugs for HIV/AIDS patients was at issue, and drew on General Comments by the Committee to determine that health policy had to be reasonable in development and implementation. For a policy to be "reasonable", it had to be comprehensive, coordinated between the various levels of government, and focussed on those in greatest need.[25]

In many common law jurisdictions, quasi-judicial accountability mechanisms are a preferred option, such as dispute resolution by patients' rights commissions or tribunals, health care commissions, and complaints tribunals or procedures, to be found in many other countries as well. In the United Kingdom, for example, the Health Care Commission submitted a review of maternity services in January 2008,[26] which revealed that only one in four National Health Service maternity services could be described as "best performing". The Commission has indicated that it will conduct a follow-up review to check on progress on the recommendations made.

As far as administrative accountability mechanisms are concerned, there is an increasing use of the practice of requiring human rights impact assessments, borrowed from similar and well-tried practices in relation to environment protection measures.[27] That process seeks to reduce large scale potential negative impacts, and to enhance the potential positive impacts of a proposed action.

Another accountability mechanism centres on political processes, and obviously varies tremendously from one state to another. In this form of action, parliamentary committee review of budget allocations and the use of public funds is at stake, and is usually exercised through democratically elected, or appointed, health councils and health care commissions.

Last, but certainly not least, social accountability is effected by civil society involvement, ranging from independent or collaborative forms of monitoring healthcare issues, and conducting public hearings and social audits, and frequently involving and attracting media attention.

When the right to health is reviewed for the effects it is having at the national level, the accountability mechanisms are a key component for the solution of health problems, but often there are no specific remedies. The international treaty-based system of protection is relatively weak, lacking concrete implementation at the domestic level. For this reason, international attention increasingly focuses on effective remedies. Providing quasi-judicial international monitoring, such as the production of views under communication procedures under the Optional Protocol of the ICCPR and under the Optional Protocol to the ICESCR, does not provide the real answer. For the right to health to be really meaningful, it needs to be given teeth: There must be adequate legal or other remedies provided at national level, open to any rights-holder claiming that his or her right to health has been violated.[28] The remedies available can be variegated, ranging from restitution or rehabilitation, via compensation, satisfaction and guarantees of non-repetition. To illustrate this, the case of *Grootboom and others v. Government of the Republic of South Africa and others*[29] may be looked at.[30] A group of adults and children had moved onto private land from an informal settlement. They were subsequently forcibly evicted from the private land, and camped on a sports ground in the area. They could not erect sufficient shelter, as most of their belongings had been destroyed during the eviction measure. During the High Court proceedings, various levels of government (municipal, regional and national) made offers to ameliorate the immediate crisis situation for the group, which they accepted. When four months later it appeared that none of the government levels had fulfilled their promises, the Constitutional Court made an order which included the provision of a specified number of temporary toilets and taps pending the construction of permanent toilets and water taps on the sports ground. As a matter of the rule of law, many jurisdictions will not allow courts to replace policy decisions of parliament or of the executive by its own policy choice, unless – as in the *Grootboom* case – there is a discretion reduction to zero, where only one possible lawful answer remains. In that case only can a court adjudicate accordingly. And this obviously applied in the *Grootboom* case.

In state practice, courts on the whole will tread very cautiously when it comes to decisions involving allocation of large sums of money. Thus, in the case of *Soobramoney v. Minister of Health, Kwa-Zulu-Natal*[31] in view of a shortage of funds, a policy had been adopted in which automatic access to dialysis was limited to patients suffering from acute renal failure. For those suffering from chronic renal failure, access to dialysis was provided only if they were eligible for a kidney transplant. A medical ethics commission had assessed that more people could be kept alive through application of this policy than if untreatable patients were allowed to use the few available dialysis machines. The applicant did not belong to the class of beneficiaries on account of his chronic renal failure, having also had unsuccessful kidney transplants, and as he also suffered from multiple forms of cancer. His claim that his right of access to health care services under Article 27 of the South African Constitution had been violated was rejected by the Constitutional Court. Justice Sachs observed that "[w]hen rights by their very nature are shared and inter-dependent, striking appropriate balances between the equally valid entitlements or expectations of a multitude of claimants" is a matter of "defining the circumstances in which the rights may most fairly and effectively be enjoyed".[32] Hence the Court concluded that the circumstances in which dialysis treatment could most fairly and effectively be enjoyed were not those of the applicant. So no violation of the right to health was found.

Health indicators and benchmarks

Another difficulty that health rights activists have addressed in recent years is the fact that very often the country analysis does not lend itself to in-depth analysis, because neither the Committee as treaty body, nor the State Party, are fully aware what data should be utilized in measuring the performance of the state during the reporting period. For that reason, indicators have been elaborated which should facilitate that task. Numerous research projects have been carried out in recent years in this respect, but while everyone agrees that only a relatively small number of health indicators should be employed, manageable for the reporting state, as soon as one delves further into the matter by asking WHO specialists and other health officials for indicators, soon a huge number of such indicators are proposed. The ideal of having just a handful of key indicators for each human right has proved to be illusory. Utilization of benchmarks, which are self-set targets set by States Parties, can be of assistance here. But as the Indicators, Benchmarks, Scoping and Assessment Project of Mannheim University has shown (the IBSA process),[33] once agreed benchmarks have been applied, and then measured ("assessed") five years later, there may well be clearer notions of relevant indicators to be used for monitoring purposes. But so far, although several of the Committee's recent General Comments have reminded states of the benchmarking of indicators, no state has actually negotiated with the Committee as yet on the details of such focussed monitoring. Two developed countries have recently indicated that they are prepared to begin such new forms of focussed reporting.[34] In the reporting guidelines of the Committee, quite a few indicators are already to be found, and it now only needs a renewed conceptual effort in a spirit of cooperation between the State Party concerned and the Committee. While the CESCR probably has advanced most in this sphere so far, other treaty bodies, and the Office of the High Commissioner for Human Rights itself, are presently analysing this approach, across all major human rights treaties. Realizing the right to health will undoubtedly benefit from this approach and may become more effective at the normative international level, and particularly when it comes to implementing that right at the national level.

The way ahead

The right to health has by now been recognized as a fundamental human right, and case law from several countries underpins the international treaty obligations. In the years and decades to come, questions surrounding healthcare, health conditions and protection of everyone's right to health will continue to play a prominent role in international and national efforts to improve lives, especially of those who suffer under harsh living conditions and whose other human rights are utterly neglected. In particular, the right to health will increasingly be intertwined with the fight against extreme poverty and hunger, with further regimes regulating intellectual property (including patents), as well as connecting to decisions about scientific and genetic research, and with overarching issues of environment protection. For instance, it will be interesting to observe whether the right to health and the Agreement on Trade-Related Aspects of Intellectual Property Rights, Including Trade in Counterfeit Goods (TRIPS) can be harmonized, in order to make drugs, especially those which are essential for the battle against epidemics like HIV/AIDS, available to everyone in need. The exceptions to the General Agreement on Tariffs and Trade (GATT) might be read more with a human rights focus than purely from the perspective of a market economy.[35] Along with international intellectual property law, international trade law will have to, at least, integrate issues related to health care and protection into its relevant rules.

Another key aspect that will continue to be central to this debate, and which signals dangers for the universal realization of the right to health, is the concept of privatization, whether directly in the field of healthcare, or on the periphery (access to water, education, use of infrastructure). It will be incumbent on states and on the international community to strike the right balance between (private) economic interests and basic human needs. The Committee on Economic, Social and Cultural Rights, as the Covenant monitoring body, has regularly addressed these issues and emphasized that, while the policy choices involved are left to the discretion of states, nevertheless, the human rights effects of such actual policy choices will be closely monitored, in line with Article 12 of ICESCR. Most states now accept that the right to health is a fundamental human right, and are now beginning to take a rights-based approach in their national law implementation measures. But much still remains to be done to get the greatest possible attention to this human right at the domestic level, so that in particular, the marginalized and disadvantaged groups of society will be able to realize their elementary health needs, necessary for survival and for leading a dignified life.

1 The earliest known water supply and drainage systems were set up in ancient Egypt, India and Greece, and by the Inca society in America, see Eibe Riedel, 'The International Protection of the Right to Health', in Rüdiger Wolfrum et al. (eds.) *Encyclopedia of Public International Law* (Heidelberg: Max Planck, 2008); see also Brigit C.A. Toebes, *The Right to Health as a Human Right in International Law* (Antwerp: Intersentia, 1999), at 7 et seq.; Jonathan Mann, Laurence Gostin, Sofia Gruskin, Troyen Brennan, Zita Lazzarini, Harvey Fineberg, 'Health and Human Rights' in *Health and Human Rights* (New York/London: Routledge, 1999), at 9 et seq.

2 UN Commission on Human Rights, Resolution 2002/31, 22 April 2002; See also the Human Rights Council, Resolution 6/29, 14 December 2007.

3 See, e.g., Commission on Human Rights, 'The protection of human rights in the context of human immunodeficiency virus (HIV) and acquired immune deficiency syndrome (AIDS)', Resolution 1999/49, 27 April 1999.

4 Commission on Human Rights, 'International Guidelines on HIV/AIDS and Human Rights', UN Doc. E/CN.4/1997/150 (1997).

5 Commission on Human Rights, 'Access to medications in the context of pandemics such as HIV AIDS, tuberculosis and malaria', Resolution 2003/29, 22 April 2003.

6 For example, Article 11 of Additional Protocol I, which protects the "physical and mental health and integrity of persons", and Article 4 of Additional Protocol II prohibits "violence to the life, health and physical well-being of persons".

7 Eibe Riedel, 'New Bearings to the State Reporting Procedure: Practical Ways to Operationalize Economic, Social and Cultural Rights – the Example of the Right to Health', in S. von Schorlemer (ed.) *Praxishandbuch UNO* (Berlin: Springer, 2003), at 345–358.

8 Cf. E. Kinney and B. Clark, 'Provisions for Health and Health Care in the Constitutions of the Countries of the World', 37 *Cornell International Law Journal* 2004, at 285.

9 For a good case study, see H. Potts, 'Accountability and the Right to the Highest Attainable Standard of Health', Open Society Institute, Public Health Programme, University of Essex, Human Rights Centre, 2008, Appendix I, case studies 3 and 4 – India, at 33–35.

10 Eibe Riedel, 'International Law Shaping Constitutional Law', in Eibe Riedel (ed.), *Constitutionalism: Old Concepts, New Worlds* (Berlin: Berliner Wissenschafts-Verlag, 2005, p. 105–121, at 115.

11 Committee on Economic, Social and Cultural Rights (CESCR), *General Comment No. 14 on the right to the highest attainable standard of health*, 11 August 2000, UN Doc. E/C.12/2000/4.

12 Ibid., at para. 8.

13 Ibid., at para. 9, last sentence.

14 Ibid., at para. 12 a–d.

15 Committee on Economic, Social and Cultural Rights (CESCR), *General Comment No. 15 on the right to water*, 20 January 2003, UN Doc. E/C.12/2002/11.

16 The CESCR is presently preparing General Comment No. 20 on Article 2(2) of ICESCR, addressing non-discrimination.

17 Cf. Potts, *supra* note 9 , at 10.

18 General Comment No. 14, *supra* note 11, at para. 30.

19 Statement on Evaluation of the Obligation to Take Steps to the "Maximum of Available Resources" under an Optional Protocol to the Covenant, 10 May 2007, UN Doc. E/C12/2007/1; for details see Eibe Riedel, 'Zur Durchsetzung wirtschaftlicher, sozialer und kultureller Rechte im Völkerrecht', in Th. Giegerich, A. Zimmermann, U. Heinz (eds.) *Wirtschaftliche, soziale und kulturelle Rechte im globalen Zeitalter* (Berlin: Dunker and Humblot, 2008), 71–93, at 83–85.

20 General Comment No. 14, *supra* note 11, at para. 34.

21 Ibid., at para. 35.

22 Ibid., at para. 36.

23 Paragraph 44 of General Comment No. 14 states: "The Committee also confirms that the following are obligations of comparable priority: (a) To en-

sure reproductive, maternal (pre-natal as well as post-natal) and child health care; (b) To provide immunization against the major infectious diseases occurring in the community; (c) To take measures to prevent, treat and control epidemic and endemic diseases; (d) To provide education and access to information concerning the main health problems in the community, including methods of preventing and controlling them; (e) To provide appropriate training for health personnel, including education on health and human rights."

24 See Potts, *supra* note 9, at 13 et seq.

25 *Minister of Health v. Treatment Action Campaign* (TAC) (2002) 5 SA 721 (CC).

26 See United Kingdom Healthcare Commission, 'Key finding of the 2007 Maternity Service Review', 25 January 2008, available at http://www. healthcarecommission.org.uk/_db/_documents/ Maternity_FINAL_BRIEFING_NOTE.doc.

27 See Paul Hunt and Gillian MacNaughton, 'Impact Assessments, Poverty and Human Rights: A Case Study Using the Right to the Highest Attainable Standard of Health', available at http://www2. essex.ac.uk/human_rights_centre/rth/projects. shtm; Potts, *supra* note 9, at 20.

28 On the violations approach, see generally Audrey Chapman, 'The Right to Health', in Audrey Chapman and Sage Russell (eds.), *Core Obligations: Building a Framework for Economic, Social and Cultural Rights* (Antwerp: Intersentia, 2002) at 185–216.

29 *The Government of South Africa v. Grootboom,* Constitutional Court of South Africa, 2000 ICHRL 72, 21 September 2000.

30 Cf. Eibe Riedel, 'Measuring Human Rights Compliance: The IBSA Procedure as a Tool of Monitoring', in Andreas Auer, Alexandrew Flückiger, Michel Hottelier (eds.) *Études en l'honneur du Professeur Giorgio Malinverni : Les Droits de l'homme et la constitution* (Geneva, Schulthess, 2007), 251–272, at 256 et seq.; Riedel, *supra* note 7, at 117.

31 CCT 32/97, 27 November 1997; discussed in Susan Marks and Andrew Clapham, *International Human Rights Lexicon* (Oxford: Oxford University Press, 2005) 197–208, at 207.

32 *Soobramoney v. Minister of Health KwaZulu Natal* 1997 (12) BCLR 1696, at para. 54.

33 Riedel, *supra* note 7, at 256 et seq.; Eibe Riedel, 'Monitoring the 1966 International Covenant on Economic, Social and Cultural Rights', in International Labour Organization (ILO), *Protecting Labour Rights as Human Rights: Present and Future of International Supervision,* (Geneva: ILO, 2007) at 3–13, particularly at 8–9.

34 In 2008 France and Australia informally indicated that they are, in principle, prepared to engage in such a new type of reporting.

35 For an insightful and critical analysis in relation to the right to food as a corollary to the right to health, see H. M. Haugen, *The Right to Food and the TRIPS Agreement* (Leiden/Boston: Brill, 2007), particularly at 213–251.

Health Systems and the Right to the Highest Attainable Standard of Health

Paul Hunt and Gunilla Backman*

The right to the highest attainable standard of health depends upon the interventions and insights of medicine and public health. Equally, the classic, long-established objectives of medicine and public health can benefit from the newer, dynamic discipline of human rights. At an abstract level, a few far-sighted people understood this when the World Health Organization (WHO) Constitution was drafted in 1946, and the Declaration of Alma-Ata was adopted in 1978, which is why both instruments affirm the right to the highest attainable standard of health. The Ottawa Charter of Health Promotion of 1986 also reflects the connections between public health and human rights.

However, these connections were general and abstract. At the time, the right to the highest attainable standard of health was only dimly understood and attracted limited support from civil society. It was little more than a slogan. Others have surveyed the evolution of health and human rights since Alma-Ata and Ottawa, and we will not repeat this exercise here.[1] To the credit of everyone responsible, *The Health and Human Rights Journal* has played an indispensable role in this evolution.

One vital part of this evolutionary process has been a deepening understanding of the right to the highest attainable standard of health. Although neglected in much of the literature, this fundamental human right must surely be the cornerstone of any consideration of health and human rights. Through the endeavours of innumerable organizations and individuals, the content of the right to the highest attainable standard of health is now sufficiently well understood to be applied in an operational, systematic and sustained manner. Crucially, this understanding is new: It dates from within the last ten years or so. Of course, much more work is needed to grasp all the implications of the right to the highest attainable standard of health, but it can no longer be seen (or dismissed) as merely a rhetorical device. In these circumstances, it is timely to revisit Alma-Ata, and examine health systems, from the new, operational perspective of the right to the highest attainable standard of health.

In any society, an effective health system is a core institution, no less than a fair justice system or democratic political system.[2] In many countries, however, health systems are failing and collapsing,[3] giving rise to an extremely grave and widespread human rights problem. At the heart of the right to the highest attainable standard of health lies an effective and integrated health system, encompassing medical care and the underlying determinants of health, which is responsive to national and local priorities, and accessible to all. Without such a health system, the right to the highest attainable standard of health can never be realized. It is only through building and strengthening health systems that it will be possible to secure sustainable development, poverty reduction, economic prosperity, improved health for individuals and populations, as well as the right to the highest attainable standard of health.

There is an analogy between, on the one hand, court systems and the right to a fair trial and, on the other hand, health systems and the right to the highest attainable standard of health. The right to a fair trial is widely recognized to have strengthened many court systems. It has helped to identify the key features of a fair court system, such as independent judges, trials without undue delay, the opportunity to call witnesses and make legal argument, legal aid for impecunious defendants in serious cases, and so on. The right to a fair trial has exposed unfair judicial processes and led to welcome reforms. Significantly, many features arising from the right to a fair trial have major budgetary implications.

In much the same way, the right to the highest attainable standard of health can help to establish effective, integrated and accessible health systems. If this is to happen, however, greater clarity is needed about the key features of a health system that arise from the right to the highest attainable standard of health.

Importantly, the right to the highest attainable standard of health is recognized in the constitution of many states.[4] Also, it is enshrined in numerous binding international human rights treaties, such as the International

Covenant on Economic, Social and Cultural Rights (ICESCR) and the Convention on the Rights of the Child (CRC), which has been ratified by every state of the world, except for two (the United States of America (USA) and Somalia).

This chapter identifies some of the key right-to-health features of a health system. It considers health systems from the new, operational perspective of the right to the highest attainable standard of health. All of the features and measures identified here are already found in some health systems, recognized in some international health instruments (such as the Declaration of Alma-Ata), or advocated in the health literature. But they are not usually recognized as human rights issues. The chapter outlines how the right to the highest attainable standard of health underpins and reinforces an effective, integrated, accessible health system – and why this is important.[5]

A right-to-health approach to strengthening health systems

In the last decade, states, international organizations, international and national human rights mechanisms, courts, civil society organizations, academics and many others have begun to explore what the right to the highest attainable standard of health means and how it can be put into practice.[6] Health workers are making the most decisive contribution to this process.[7] Drawing upon this deepening experience, and informed by health good practices, this section briefly outlines the general approach of the right to the highest attainable standard of health towards the strengthening of health systems.

At the centre: The well being of individuals, communities and populations. A health system gives rise to numerous technical issues. Of course, experts have an indispensable role to play in addressing these technical matters. But there is a risk that health systems become impersonal, "top-down" and dominated by experts. Additionally, as a recent WHO publication observes, "health systems and services are mainly focused on disease rather than on the person as a whole, whose body and mind are linked and who needs to be treated with dignity and respect."[8] The publication concludes, "health care and health systems must embrace a more holistic, people-centred approach."[9] This is also the approach required by the right to the highest attainable standard of health. Because it places the well being of individuals, communities and populations at the centre of a health system, the right to health can help to ensure that a health system is neither technocratic nor removed from those it is meant to serve.

Not only outcomes, but also processes. The right to the highest attainable standard of health is concerned with both processes and outcomes. It is not only interested in what a health system does (e.g. providing access to essential medicines and safe drinking water), but also how it does it (e.g. transparently, in a participatory manner, and without discrimination).

Transparency. Access to health information is an essential feature of an effective health system, as well as the right to the highest attainable standard of health. Health information enables individuals and communities to promote their own health, participate effectively, claim quality services, monitor progressive realization, expose corruption, hold those responsible to account, and so on. The requirement of transparency applies to all those working in health-related sectors, including states, international organizations, public private partnerships, business enterprises and civil society organizations.

Participation. All individuals and communities are entitled to active and informed participation on issues bearing upon their health. In the context of health systems, this includes participation in identifying overall strategy, policy-making, implementation and accountability. The importance of community participation is one of the principal themes recurring throughout the Declaration of Alma-Ata. Crucially, states have a human rights responsibility to establish institutional arrangements for the active and informed participation of all relevant stakeholders, including disadvantaged communities.[10]

Equity, equality and non-discrimination. Equality and non-discrimination are among the most fundamental elements of international human rights, including the right to the highest attainable standard of health. A state has a legal obligation to ensure that a health system is accessible to all without discrimination, including those living in poverty, minorities, indigenous peoples, women, children, slum and rural dwellers, people with disabilities, and other disadvantaged individuals and communities. Also, the health system must be responsive to the particular health needs of women, children, adolescents, the elderly, and so on. The twin human rights principles of equality and non-discrimination mean that outreach (and other) programmes must be in place to ensure that disadvantaged individuals and communities enjoy, in practice, the same access as those who are more advantaged.

Equality and non-discrimination are akin to the critical health concept of equity. There is no universally accepted definition of equity, but one definition is "equal access to health-care according to need."[11] All three concepts have a social justice component. In some respects, equality and non-discrimination, being reinforced by law, are more powerful than equity. For example, if a state fails to take effective steps to tackle race discrimination in a health system, it can be held to account and required to take remedial measures. Also, if a health system is accessible to the wealthy but inaccessible to those living in poverty, the state can be held to account and required to take remedial action.

Respect for cultural difference. A health system must be respectful of cultural difference. Health workers, for example, should be sensitive to issues of ethnicity and culture. Also, a health system is required to take into account traditional preventive care, healing practices and medicines. Strategies should be in place to encourage and facilitate indigenous peoples, for example, to study medicine and public health. Moreover, training in some traditional medical practices should also be encouraged.[12] Of course, cultural respect is right as a matter of principle. But, additionally, it makes sense as a matter of practice. As Thoraya Obaid, Executive Director of the United Nations Population Fund (UNFPA), observes: "Cultural sensitivity ... leads to higher levels of programme acceptance and ownership by the community, and programme sustainability."[13]

Medical care and the underlying determinants of health. The health of individuals, communities and populations requires more than medical care. For this reason, international human rights law casts the right to the highest attainable standard of physical and mental health as an inclusive right not only extending to timely and appropriate medical care, but also to the underlying determinants of health, such as access to safe water and adequate sanitation, an adequate supply of safe food, nutrition and housing, healthy occupational and environmental conditions, access to health-related education and information, including on sexual and reproductive health, and freedom from discrimination.[14] The social determinants of health, such as gender, poverty and social exclusion, are major preoccupations of the right to the highest attainable standard of health. In his work, for example, the first United Nations Special Rapporteur on the right to health consistently looked at medical care and the underlying determinants of health, including the impact of poverty and discrimination on health. In short, the right to the highest attainable standard of health encompasses the traditional domains of both medical care and public health. This is the perspective that the right to the highest attainable standard of health brings to the strengthening of health systems.

Progressive realization and resource constraints. The right to the highest attainable standard of health is subject to progressive realization and resource availability. In other words, it does not make the absurd demand that a comprehensive, integrated health system be constructed overnight. Rather, for the most part, human rights require that states take effective measures to progressively work towards the construction of an effective health system that ensures access to all. The disciplines of medicine and public health take a similar position; the Declaration of Alma-Ata, for example, is directed to "progressive improvement."[15] Also, the right to health is realistic, it demands more of high-income than low-income states. That is to say, implementation of the right to health is subject to resource availability.

These two concepts – progressive realization and resource availability – have numerous implications for health systems, some of which are briefly explored later in this chapter. For example, because progressive realization does not occur spontaneously, a state must have a comprehensive, national plan, encompassing both the public and private sectors, for the development of its health system. The crucial importance of planning is recognized in the health literature, the Declaration of Alma-Ata, and General Comment No. 14 on the right to the highest attainable standard of health of the United Nations Committee on Economic, Social and Cultural Rights.[16]

Another implication of progressive realization is that an effective health system must include appropriate indicators and benchmarks, otherwise there is no way of knowing whether or not the state is improving its health system and progressively realizing the right to the highest attainable standard of health. Moreover, the indicators must be disaggregated on suitable grounds, such as sex, socio-economic status and age, so that the state knows whether or not its outreach programmes for disadvantaged individuals and communities are working. Indicators and benchmarks are already commonplace features of many health systems, but they rarely have all the elements that are important from a human rights perspective, such as disaggregation on appropriate grounds.[17]

A third implication arising from progressive realization is that at least the present level of enjoyment of the right to the highest attainable standard of health must be maintained. This is sometimes known as the principle of non-retrogression.[18] Although rebuttable in certain limited circumstances, there is a strong presumption that measures lowering the present enjoyment of the right to health are impermissible.

Finally, progressive realization does not mean that a state is free to choose whatever measures it wishes to take so long as they reflect some degree of progress. A state has a duty to adopt those measures that are most effective, while taking into account resource availability and other human rights considerations.

Duties of immediate effect: Core obligations. Although subject to progressive realization and resource availability, the right to the highest attainable standard of health gives rise to some core obligations of immediate effect. A state has "a core obligation to ensure the satisfaction of, at the very least, minimum essential levels" of the right to the highest attainable standard of health.[19] What, more precisely, are these core obligations? Some are discussed later in this chapter. Briefly, they include an obligation to:

—— Prepare a comprehensive, national plan for the development of the health system.

—— Ensure access to health-related services and facilities on a non-discriminatory basis, especially for disadvantaged individuals, communities and populations; this means, for example, that a state has a core obligation to establish effective outreach programmes for those living in poverty.

—— Ensure the equitable distribution of health-related services and facilities e.g. a fair balance between rural and urban areas.

—— Establish effective, transparent, accessible and independent mechanisms of accountability in relation to duties arising from the right to the highest attainable standard of health.

Also, a state has a core obligation to ensure a minimum "basket" of health-related services and facilities, including essential food, to ensure freedom from hunger, basic sanitation and adequate water, essential medicines, immunization against the community's major infectious diseases, and sexual and reproductive health services including information, family planning, pre-natal and post-natal services, and emergency obstetric care. Some states have already identified a minimum "basket" for those within their jurisdiction. Some international organizations have also tried to identify a minimum "basket" of health services. This is a difficult exercise, not least because health challenges vary widely from one state to another and therefore, in practice, the minimum "basket" may vary between countries. In some countries the challenge is undernutrition, elsewhere it is obesity.

Much more work has to be done to help states identify the minimum "basket" of health-related services and facilities required by the right to the highest attainable standard of health. However, that vital task is not the purpose of this chapter. The aim here is to identify a number of additional, and frequently neglected, features arising from the right to the highest attainable standard of health, and informed by health good practices, that are required of all health systems. These include, for example, access on the basis of equality and non-discrimination, an up-to-date health plan, effective accountability for the public and private health sector, and so on.

Quality. All health services and facilities must be of good quality. For example, a health system must be able to ensure access to good quality essential medicines. If rejected in the North because they are beyond their expiry date and unsafe, medicines must not be recycled to the South. Because medicines may be counterfeit or tampered with, a state must establish a regulatory system to check medicine safety and quality. The requirement of good quality also extends to the manner in which patients and others are treated. Health workers must treat patients and others politely and with respect.

A continuum of prevention and care with effective referrals. A health system should have an appropriate mix of primary (community-based), secondary (district-based) and tertiary (specialized) facilities and services, providing a continuum of prevention and care. The system also needs an effective process when a health worker assesses that their client may benefit from additional services, and the client is referred from one facility or department to another. Referrals are also needed, in both directions, between an alternative health system (e.g. traditional practitioners) and "mainstream" health system. The absence of an effective referral system is inconsistent with the right to the highest attainable standard of health.

Vertical or integrated? There is a longstanding debate about the merits of vertical (or selective) health interventions, which focus on one or more diseases or health conditions, and a comprehensive, integrated approach. By drawing off resources, vertical interventions can jeopardize progress towards the long-term goal of an effective health system. They have other potential disadvantages, such as duplication and fragmentation. However, in some circumstances, such as during a public health emergency, there may be a place for vertical intervention. When these circumstances arise, the intervention must be carefully designed, so far as possible, to strengthen and not undermine a comprehensive, integrated health system.

Coordination. A health system, as well as the right to the highest attainable standard of health, depends upon effective coordination across a range of public and private actors (including non-governmental organizations) at the national and international levels. The scope of the coordination will depend upon how the health system is defined. But, however it is defined, coordination is crucial. For example, a health system and the right to the highest attainable standard of health demand effective coordination between various sectors and departments, such as health, environment, water, sanitation, education, food, shelter, finance and transport. They also demand coordination within sectors and departments, such as the Ministry of Health. The need for coordination extends to policy-making and the actual delivery of services.

Health-related coordination in many states is very patchy and weak. Alone, the Cabinet is an insufficient coordination mechanism for health-related issues. Other coordination mechanisms are essential.

Health as a global public good: The importance of international cooperation.[20] Public goods are goods that benefit society as a whole. The concept of "national public goods", such as the maintenance of law and order, is well established. In an increasingly interdependent world, much more attention is being paid to "global public goods". They address issues in which the international community has a common interest. In the health context, global public goods include the control of infectious diseases, the dissemination of health research, and international regulatory initiatives, such as the WHO Framework Convention on Tobacco Control. Although it remains very imprecise, the concept of "global public goods" confirms that a health system has both national and international dimensions.

The international dimension of a health system is also reflected in states' human rights responsibilities of international assistance and co-operation. These responsibilities can be traced through the Charter of the United Nations, the Universal Declaration of Human Rights, and several more recent international human rights declarations and binding treaties.[21] They are also reflected in the outcome documents of several world confer-ences, such as the Millennium Declaration, as well as numerous other initi-atives, including the Paris Declaration on Aid Effectiveness (2005).

As a minimum, all states have a responsibility to cooperate on trans-boundary health issues and to "do no harm" to their neighbours. High-in-come states have an additional responsibility to provide appropriate inter-national assistance and cooperation in health for low-income countries. They should especially assist low-income countries to fulfil their core obli-gations arising from the right to the highest attainable standard of health. Equally, low-income states have a responsibility to seek appropriate inter-national assistance and cooperation to help them strengthen their health systems.The relationship between health "global public goods" and the hu-man rights responsibility of international assistance and cooperation in health demands further study.

Striking balances. Few human rights are absolute. Frequently, balances have to be struck between competing human rights. Freedom of informa-tion, for example, has to be balanced with the right to privacy. Moreover, there are often legitimate but competing claims arising from the same hu-man right, especially in relation to those numerous rights that are subject to resource availability. In the context of health systems, finite budgets give rise to tough policy choices. Should the government build a new teaching hospital, establish more primary health care clinics, strengthen community care for people with disabilities, improve sanitation in the capital's slum, improve access to anti-retrovirals, or subsidize an effective but expensive cancer drug? Human rights do not provide neat answers to such questions, anymore than do ethics or economics. But human rights require that the questions be decided by way of a fair, transparent, participatory process, taking into account explicit criteria, such as the well being of those living in poverty, and not just the claims of powerful interest groups.[22]

Because of the complexity, sensitivity and importance of many health policy issues, it is vitally important that effective, accessible and independent mechanisms of accountability are in place to ensure that reasonable balances are struck by way of fair processes that take into account all relevant considerations, including the interests of disadvantaged individuals, communities and populations.

Monitoring and accountability. Rights imply duties, and duties demand accountability. Accountability is one of the most important features of human rights – and also one of the least understood. Although human rights demand accountability, that does not mean that every health worker or specialized agency becomes a human rights enforcer. Accountability includes the monitoring of conduct, performance and outcomes. In the context of a health system, there must be accessible, transparent and effective mechanisms of accountability to understand how those with responsibilities towards the health system have discharged their duties. The crucial role of monitoring and accountability is explored later in this chapter.

Legal obligation. The right to the highest attainable standard of health gives rise to legally binding obligations. A state is legally obliged to ensure its health system includes a number of the features and measures signalled in the preceding paragraphs. The health system must have, for example, a comprehensive, national plan; outreach programmes for the disadvantaged; a minimum "basket" of health-related services and facilities; effective referral systems; arrangements to ensure the participation of those affected by health-decision making; respect for cultural difference; and so on. Of course, these requirements also correspond to health good practices. One of the distinctive contributions of the right to the highest attainable standard of health is that it reinforces such health good practices with legal obligation and accountability.

The "building blocks" of a health system

Informed by health good practices, the preceding section outlines the general approach of the right to the highest attainable standard of health towards the strengthening of health systems. This general approach has to be consistently and systematically applied across the numerous elements that together constitute a functioning health system. What are these functional elements of a health system? The health literature on this issue is very extensive. For its part, WHO identifies "six essential building blocks" which together make up a health system:[23]

___ Health services (medical and public health)
___ Health workforce
___ Health information system
___ Medical products, vaccines and technologies
___ Health financing
___ Leadership, governance, stewardship

Each "building block" has generated a huge literature over many years. For present purposes, three short points demand emphasis. First, these are not only "building blocks" for a health system; they are also "building blocks" for realizing the right to the highest attainable standard of health. Like a health system, the right to health requires health services, health workers, health information, medical products, financing and stewardship.

Second, in practice, the "building blocks" might not have all the features required by the right to the highest attainable standard of health. For example, a country might have a health information system, one of the WHO "building blocks". But the information system might not include appropriately disaggregated data, which is one of the requirements of the right to health. In short, an essential "building block" might be in place, but without all the features required by international human rights law.

Third, the crucial challenge is to apply – or integrate – the right to the highest attainable standard of health, as well as other human rights, across the six "building blocks". The general approach outlined in the preceding section has to be consistently and systematically applied to health services, health workers, health information, medical products, financing and stewardship – all the elements that together constitute a functioning health system.

The systematic application of the right to health to the six "building blocks" is likely to have a variety of results. In some cases, a focus on the right to health will reinforce existing features of the "building blocks" that routinely receive the attention they deserve. In other cases, the application of the right will identify existing features of the "building blocks" that tend to be overlooked in practice and that require much more attention, such as the disaggregation of data on appropriate grounds. It is also possible that the application of the right may identify features that, although important, are not usually regarded as forming any part of the six "building blocks".[24]

Applying the right-to-health approach to one of the "building blocks" of a health system

By way of illustration, this section begins to apply the right to the highest attainable standard of health to one of WHO's six "building blocks": Leadership, governance and stewardship. This is "arguably the most complex but critical building block of any health system."[25] It encompasses many elements, including planning, monitoring and accountability.

Planning

Planning is one of the weakest features of the development and strengthening of health systems. With a few honourable exceptions, the record of health planning is poor, while the history of health planning is surprisingly short. Many states do not have comprehensive, up-to-date health plans. Where they exist, plans "often fail to be implemented and remain grand designs on paper. Elsewhere plans may be implemented but fail to respond to the real needs of the population."[26]

However, from the perspective of the right to the highest attainable standard of health, effective planning is absolutely critical. Progressive realization and resource availability – two inescapable components of the international right to health – cannot be addressed without planning.[27]

Recognizing the critical role of effective planning, the United Nations Committee on Economic, Social and Cultural Rights designated the preparation of a health "strategy and plan of action" as a core obligation arising from the right to the highest attainable standard of health. The Committee also encouraged high-income states to provide international assistance "to enable developing countries to fulfil their core … obligations", including the preparation of a health plan.[28] According to the Declaration of Alma-Ata: "All governments should formulate national policies, strategies and plans of action to launch and sustain primary health care as part of a comprehensive national health system and in coordination with other sectors."[29]

Health planning is complex and many of its elements are important from the perspective of the right to the highest attainable standard of health, including the following.

The entire planning process must be as participatory and transparent as possible. It is very important that the health needs of disadvantaged individuals, communities and populations are given due attention. Also, effective measures must be taken to ensure their active and informed participation throughout the planning process. Both the process and plan must be sensitive to cultural difference. One example where the participatory approach was used was in the village of San Jose de Secce and the communities of Oqopeqa, Punkumarqiri, Sanuq and Laupay in the Ayacucho district, Peru, where high maternal mortality rates were registered. It was estimated that 94 per cent of the women gave birth at home, compared to 6 per cent in the health centres. This was due to various barriers, such as because the state health services did not take account of local cultural conceptions of health and sickness. In an attempt to reduce the maternal mortality, a culturally-adapted project was introduced which provided sexual and reproductive health services and promoted a participatory approach between health workers and the community, including the traditional birth attendants (TBA). As a result, the delivery room and care given during prenatal checkups, delivery and the postnatal period, were made culturally acceptable, for example, by providing a bed as well as sturdy rope, so that the women could give birth squatting and gripping the rope, as they were accustomed to. The protocol for care outlined, among others, that the person attending the birth should speak Quechua and preferably be female. Further, in line with the beliefs in the communities, the protocol included the requirement to deliver the placenta to the family member present so that it could be buried, and the opportunity for the user to remain in the health facility for up to eight days. An evaluation after the measures had been taken demonstrated a great increase in deliveries at health centres.[30]

Prior to the drafting of the plan, there must be a health situational analysis informed by suitably disaggregated data. The analysis should identify, for example, the characteristics of the population (e.g. birth, death and fertility rates), their health needs (e.g. incidence and prevalence by disease), and the public and private health-related services presently available (e.g. the capacity of different facilities).

The right to the highest attainable standard of health encompasses an obligation on the state to generate health research and development that addresses, for example, the health needs of disadvantaged individuals, communities and populations. Health research and development includes classical medical research into drugs, vaccines and diagnostics, as well as operational or implementation research into the social, economic, cultural, political and policy issues that determine access to medical care and the effectiveness of public health interventions. Implementation research, which has an important role to play with a view to dismantling societal obstacles to health interventions and technologies, should be taken into account when drafting the national health plan.

The plan must include certain features such as clear objectives and how they are to be achieved, time-frames, indicators and benchmarks to measure achievement, effective coordination mechanisms, reporting procedures, a detailed budget that is attached to the plan, financing arrangements (national and international), evaluation arrangements, and one or more accountability devices. In order to complete the plan, there will have to be a process for prioritizing competing health needs.

Before their finalization, key elements of the draft plan must be subject to an impact assessment to ensure that they are likely to be consistent with the state's national and international legal obligations, including those relating to the right to the highest attainable standard of health. For example, if the draft plan proposes the introduction of user fees for health services, it is vital that an impact assessment is undertaken to anticipate the likely impact of user fees on access to health services for those living in poverty. If the assessment confirms that user fees are likely to hinder access, the draft plan must be revised before adoption, otherwise it is likely to be inconsistent with the state's obligations arising from the right to the highest attainable standard of health.[31]

Of course, planning is only the means to an end: An effective, integrated health system that is accessible to all. The main task is implementation. Evaluation, monitoring and accountability can help to ensure that all those responsible for implementation discharge their duties as planned, and that any unintended consequences are swiftly identified and addressed.

Monitoring and accountability

As already discussed, monitoring and accountability have a crucial role to play in relation to human rights and health systems. Monitoring is a precondition of accountability. Accountability provides individuals and communities with an opportunity to understand how those with responsibilities have discharged their duties. Equally, it provides those with responsibilities the opportunity to explain what they have done and why. Where mistakes have been made, accountability requires redress. But accountability is not a matter of blame and punishment. It is a process that helps to identify what works, so it can be repeated, and what does not, so it can be revised. It is a way of checking that reasonable balances are fairly struck.

In the context of health systems, there are many different types of accountability mechanisms, including health commissioners, democratically elected local health councils, public hearings, patients' committees, impact assessments, maternal death audits, judicial proceedings, and so on. An institution as complex and important as a health system requires a range of effective, transparent, accessible, independent accountability mechanisms. The media and civil society organizations have a crucial role to play as well.

Accountability in respect of health systems is often extremely weak. Sometimes the same body provides health services, regulates and holds to account. In some cases, accountability is little more than a device to check that health funds were spent as they should have been. Of course, that is important. But human rights accountability is much broader. It is also concerned with ensuring that health systems are improving and the right to the highest attainable standard of health is being progressively realized, for all, including disadvantaged individuals, communities and populations.

In some states, the private health sector, while playing a very important role, is largely unregulated. Crucially, the requirement of human rights accountability extends to both the public and private health sectors. Additionally, it is not confined to national bodies; it also extends to international actors working on health-related issues.

Accountability mechanisms are urgently needed for all those – public, private, national and international – working on health-related issues. The design of appropriate, independent accountability mechanisms demands creativity and imagination. Often associated with accountability, lawyers must be willing to understand the distinctive characteristics and challenges of health systems, and learn from the rich experience of medicine and public health.

The issue of accountability gives rise to two related points. First, the right to the highest attainable standard of health should be recognized in national law. This is very important because such recognition gives rise to legal accountability for those with responsibilities for health systems. As is well known, the right is recognized in WHO's Constitution, as well as the Declaration of Alma-Ata. It is also recognized in numerous binding international human rights treaties. The right to the highest attainable standard of health is also protected by numerous national constitutions. It should be recognized in the national law of all states.

Second, although important, legal recognition of the right to the highest attainable standard of health is usually confined to a very general formulation that does not set out in any detail what is required of those with responsibilities for health. For this reason, a state must not only recognize the right to health in national law, but also ensure that there are more detailed provisions clarifying what society expects by way of health-related services and facilities. For example, there will have to be provisions relating to water quality and quantity, blood safety, essential medicines, the quality of medical care, and numerous other issues encompassed by the right to the highest attainable standard of health. Such clarification may be provided by laws, regulations, protocols, guidelines, codes of conduct and so on. WHO has published important standards on a range of health issues. Obviously, clarification is important for providers, so they know what is expected of them. It is also important for those for whom the service or facility is intended, so they know what they can legitimately expect. Once the standards are reasonably clear, it is easier (and fairer) to hold accountable those with responsibilities for their achievement.

In summary, there is a legal obligation arising from the right to the highest attainable standard of health to ensure that health planning is participatory and transparent; addresses the health needs of disadvantaged individuals, communities and populations; and includes a situational analysis. Before finalization, key elements of the draft plan must be subject to an impact assessment, and the final plan must include certain crucial features. These (and there are others) are not just a matter of health good practice, sound management, justice, equity or humanitarianism. They are a matter of international legal obligation. Whether or not the obligations are properly discharged should be subject to review by an appropriate monitoring and accountability mechanism.

Conclusion

Like other human rights, the right to the highest attainable standard of health is a site of struggle.[32] It is not, and never will be, a substitute for struggle. In recent years, the contours and content of the right to the highest attainable standard of health have become clearer, making it possible to tease through its practical implications for health policies, programmes and projects. The right brings a set of analytical, policy and programmatic tools. As always, the right retains its powerful rhetorical, campaigning qualities. The right to the highest attainable standard of health should be seen as one important element in a multidimensional strategy for progressive social change.

Whether the right to the highest attainable standard of health can successfully shape health systems depends upon multiple variables. Progressive governments must be persuaded to integrate the right across their policy-making processes, in accordance with their legal obligations. WHO and other international organizations must be prevailed upon to champion the right to the highest attainable standard of health. Civil society organizations have to campaign around health and human rights. Judges and lawyers have to be willing to learn from health workers and find innovative ways to vindicate the right to the highest attainable standard of health. Health workers must grasp the potential of the right to the highest attainable standard of health to help them achieve their professional objectives. Human rights mechanisms must take this fundamental human right seriously and its meaning must be further clarified. More right to health tools must be fashioned. Disadvantaged individuals, communities and populations must apprehend that the right to the highest attainable standard of health empowers them by granting entitlements which place legal and moral obligations on others.

Today, there are numerous health movements and approaches, including health equity, primary health care, health promotion, social determinants, health security, continuum of care, biomedical, macroeconomics, and so on. All are very important. It is misconceived, however, to regard human rights as yet another approach with the same status as the others. Like ethics, the right to the highest attainable standard of health is not optional – and, like ethics, it recurs throughout all other approaches. The right to the highest attainable standard of health is the only perspective that is both underpinned by universally recognized moral values and reinforced by legal obligations. Properly understood, the right to the highest attainable standard of health has a profound contribution to make towards building healthy societies and equitable health systems.

* This article is a shortened and revised version of the report of the UN Special Rapporteur on the right of everyone to the enjoyment of the highest attainable standard of physical and mental health, A/HRC/7/11, 31 January 2008. Also see Hunt and Backman, "Health Systems and the Right to the Highest Attainable Standard of Health", *Health and Human Rights: An International Journal,* Vol. 10, No. 1 (2008); and Backman and others, "Health Systems and the Right to Health: an Assessment of 194 Countries", *Lancet,* Vol. 372, No. 9655 (2008), at 2047–2085. In this article "the right to the highest attainable standard of health" or "the right to health" are used as short hand for thew full formulation of the right.

1 See for example J. Mann, S. Gruskin, M. Grodin and G. Annas (eds), *Health and Human Rights: A Reader* (New York and London: Routledge, 1999); S. Gruskin, M. Grodin, G. Annas and S. Marks (eds.), *Perspectives on Health and Human Rights* (New York and London: Routledge, 2005); A. Yamin, 'Journeys towards the Splendid City', 26 *Human Rights Quarterly* (2004), at 519; the report of the UN Special Rapporteur on the right to the highest attainable standard of health, A/HRC/4/28, 17 January 2007; and P. Hunt, 'The Health and Human Rights Movement: Progress and Obstacles', 16(1) *Journal of Law and Medicine* (2008) 15 JLM 714–724.

2 L. Freedman, 'Achieving the MDGs: Health Systems as core social institutions', 48 *Development* (2005), at 1.

3 World Health Organization, *Everybody's Business: Strengthening Health Systems to Improve Health Outcomes* (Geneva: WHO, 2007), at 1.

4 E. Kinney and B. Clark, 'Provisions for Health and Health Care in the Constitutions of the Countries of the World' 37 *Cornell International Law Journal* (2004) 285–355.

5 The literature reveals many definitions of a health system, each with carefully nuanced differences. In 2007, for example, WHO defined a health system as "all organizations, people and actions whose *primary intent* is to promote, restore or maintain health." Ibid. at 2 (italics in the original). For present purposes, there is no need to favour one definition over another because all the features and measures identified in this chapter should be part of any health system, however defined.

6 For surveys of the key international instruments and a selection of the case law, see the reports of the UN Special Rapporteur on the right of everyone to the enjoyment of the highest attainable standard of physical and mental health, E/CN.4/2003/58, 13 February 2003, and A/HRC/4/28, 17 January 2007.

7 Health workers include all those developing, managing, delivering, monitoring and evaluating preventive, curative and rehabilitative health in the private and public health sectors, including traditional healers.

8 WHO, *People at the Centre of Health Care* (Geneva: WHO, 2007), at V.

9 Ibid., at VII.

10 See H. Potts, *Human Rights in Public Health: Rhetoric, Reality and Reconciliation,* unpublished PhD thesis, Monash University, Melbourne, Australia, 2006. Also, participation in the context of the right to health has been explored in several reports of the UN Special Rapporteur on the right of everyone to the enjoyment of the highest attainable standard of physical and mental health, including E/CN.4/2006/48/Add.2 (on Uganda) and E/CN.4/2005/51 (on mental disability).

11 A. Green, *An Introduction to Health Planning for Developing Health Systems* (Oxford: Oxford University Press, 2007) at 64.

12 For more on indigenous peoples and the right to the highest attainable standard of health see, for example, the reports of the UN Special Rapporteur on the right of everyone to the enjoyment of the highest attainable standard of physical and mental health, A/59/422 and E/CN.4/2005/51/Add.3.

13 UNFPA, *Culture Matters* (Geneva : UNFPA, 2000), at V.

14 See, for example, Article 24 of the Convention on the Rights of the Child. Medical care includes dental care.

15 Paragraph VII(6).

16 For more on planning, see page 52.

17 For a human rights-based approach to health indicators, see the report of the UN Special Rapporteur on the right of everyone to the enjoyment of the highest attainable standard of physical and mental health, E/CN.4/2006/48, 3 March 2006.

18 Committee on Economic, Social and Cultural Rights (CESCR), *General Comment No. 14 on the right to the highest attainable standard of health*, 11 August 2000, UN Doc. E/C.12/2000/4, at para. 32.

19 Ibid., paras. 43–45.

20 This section draws extensively from United Kingdom Department of Health, *Health is Global: Proposals for a UK Government-Wide Strategy*, (London: Department of Health, 2007) especially at 46.

21 See S. Skogly, *Beyond National Borders: States' Human Rights Obligations in International Cooperation*, (Antwerp: Intersentia, 2006).

22 On prioritization, see the report of the UN Special Rapporteur on the right of everyone to the enjoyment of the highest attainable standard of physical and mental health, A/62/2/214, 8 August 2007.

23 WHO, *supra* note 3, at 3.

24 Such as ex-ante impact assessments (see paragraphs below on planning).

25 WHO, *supra* note 3, at 23.

26 Green, *supra* note 11, at 18.

27 See previous section on progressive realization and resource constraints.

28 General Comment No. 14, *supra* note 18, paras. 43–45.

29 Para. VIII.

30 P. Hunt and J. Bueno de Mesquita, *Reducing Maternal Mortality: The Contribution of the Right to the Highest Attainable Standard of Health* (2007), available at http://www2.essex.ac.uk/human_rights_centre/rth/docs/ReducingMaternalMortality.pdf.

31 See P. Hunt and G. MacNaughton, *Impact Assessments, Poverty and Human Rights: A Case Study Using the Right to the Highest Attainable Standard of Health*, 2006, available at http://www2.essex.ac.uk/human_rights_centre/rth/projects.shtm.

32 P. Hunt, *Reclaiming Social Rights: International and Comparative Perspectives*, (Aldershot, UK: Dartmouth, 1996) at 186 and Yamin, *supra* note 1, at 528.

Social Determinants of Health from a Rights-Based Approach

Barbara Wilson*

Introduction

The right to the highest attainable standard of health is a fundamental human right. It is indispensable to the exercise of other human rights and especially to the right to life. It is closely related to, and dependent upon, the realization of the rights to food, housing, work, education, non-discrimination, equality and the prohibition of ill-treatment, and respect of human dignity. It is also linked to the rights to privacy and family life, access to information and the freedoms of association, assembly and movement.[1]

A multitude of factors, either intrinsic or extrinsic, may hinder or even prevent the full enjoyment of the right to health, as guaranteed by Article 12, paragraph 1, of the International Covenant on Economic, Social and Cultural Rights.[2] Ill health is caused by, and the result of, poor living conditions. It is a direct consequence of an unhealthy and polluted environment, unsafe drinking water, and undernourishment. Dangerous working conditions also contribute to poor health.

Certain categories of the population are more at risk than others: prisoners and detainees, ethnic minorities and indigenous populations, disabled persons, older persons, asylum-seekers, refugees and migrant workers are all in danger of suffering from ill health. Due to gender inequality, inadequate access to health services and goods affects, in particular, women and girls.

Lack of enjoyment of the right to health also results from insufficient financial resources, either of individuals or of the state, but most frequently of both. The right to health will suffer from the general economic climate and the degree of economic development of a state. It will also be affected by disparities between different regions within a state, in particular, between urban and rural areas. The level of health enjoyed will vary according to the national origin and social status of different categories of the population, the most vulnerable generally being the worst hit by insufficient public spending on health care.

The right to health may also be affected by natural or man-made disasters. In addition, trade or financial agreements may adversely impact upon the right to health. In this respect, not only states but also third parties have a responsibility to eliminate factors and obstacles which may impede or block the full enjoyment of the right to health. The "brain drain" of qualified medical personnel to the private sector, or to foreign countries, can reduce the effectiveness of public health care systems particularly in developing countries.

Even though many factors of a national and international nature may interfere with the right of everyone to enjoy the best possible level of health, the greatest hindrance to the full enjoyment of this right is poverty. More than 2.8 billion people in the world are living in conditions of abject poverty, with little or no hope of accessing adequate health facilities, goods and services.[3] Poverty erodes or nullifies economic and social rights, such as the right to health, adequate housing, clothing, food and safe water. It also promotes unhealthy lifestyles, such as prostitution, drug addiction, alcoholism and begging.

Poverty is not a phenomenon confined to developing countries. It is a global condition and is experienced by all states in varying degrees. Many developed states have categories of the population who experience poverty: people belonging to ethnic minorities, indigenous populations and migrant workers often live in appalling conditions, such as slums and temporary settlements without proper infrastructure. Women are more likely to live in poverty than men, and frequently have the sole responsibility for the care of children.[4] Furthermore, children who grow up in poverty are severely, and often permanently, disadvantaged.[5]

The aim of this chapter is to pinpoint and analyse, as far as possible, the principal social factors or determinants which may impair or prevent the

full enjoyment, without discrimination, of the right to the highest standard of health possible.[6]

Discrimination

Health facilities, goods and services must be accessible to everyone without discrimination.[7] The various prohibited grounds of discrimination are
laid down in many international human rights instruments and, notably,
in Article 2, paragraph 2, of the Covenant on Economic, Social and Cultural
Rights. Despite this legally binding guarantee which is immediately applicable,[8] access to health facilities, goods and services is, in practice, not always
guaranteed to everyone on an equal footing. Vulnerable and marginalized
groups, such as ethnic or religious minorities, women and children, older
persons and the disabled, are often victims of limited or even lack of access
to health care and the underlying determinants of health. This is largely due
to the disproportionately high cost of health services and goods in relation
to the financial means of these people.

Income and property

Everyone should have access to hospitals, clinics and other health care facilities, as well as to trained medical personnel and essential drugs[9] without discrimination.[10] Equally, health facilities, services and goods must be
affordable for all. Payment for such goods and services must therefore be
based on the principle of equity.[11] Whatever measures have been taken to
ensure social security benefits,[12] and whether health care insurance be provided by a public, private or mixed system, the state is obliged to ensure
that adequate health care is economically accessible to everyone, including
socially disadvantaged groups.[13]

Inevitably, the health of the poorest and most vulnerable persons in society will suffer if the cost of health care is prohibitive. In this respect, the
right to health is directly linked to the right to social security,[14] as well as
the right of everyone to work, and to earn a decent living for themselves
and their families, as guaranteed by Articles 6 and 7 of the Covenant on
Economic, Social and Cultural Rights.[15]

Lack of universal coverage of health care schemes, privatization of medical facilities and services and the departure of trained medical personnel
to the private sector all constitute significant obstacles to the right of every-

one to receive adequate health care without discrimination. Large-scale privatization in a number of countries has been shown to affect not only the cost but also the quality and availability of health services and goods. This impacts, in particular, on the poorest categories of the population.[16]

Racial or ethnic origin

Persons belonging to racial or ethnic minorities must have safe physical and economic access to health facilities, services and goods without discrimination.[17] Unfortunately, due to their ethnicity or the colour of their skin, these persons are often victims of de facto and even multiple discrimination in relation to health care. In some cases, for example, Roma are reportedly denied access to health services, including emergency aid services; they are segregated in hospitals, and discriminated against by medical practitioners, who allegedly provide medical services of lower quality to them, or extort from them unjustified amounts of money.[18]

Indigenous peoples

In indigenous communities, the health of the individual is closely linked to the society as a whole[19] and the organization of health care takes on an autonomous aspect. Indigenous communities often develop and practise their own traditional health care system, using their own particular healing techniques and medicines. In this context, indigenous peoples should benefit from "specific measures" which enable them to have access to appropriate health services and goods that are culturally acceptable. If they are deprived of the necessary resources, or even access to their ancestral lands, which allow them to carry out traditional preventive care, healing practices and cultivate vital medicinal plants, their health may be seriously impaired. The means to provide the medicinal plants, animals and minerals necessary to the health of these peoples depends largely on freedom of access to their lands. Moreover, any break with the "symbiotic relationship" which they have with their traditional territories may have an adverse effect on their physical and mental health.[20] In addition, indigenous peoples are often victims of discrimination in access to public health services.[21]

Gender and sexual orientation

Despite the economic growth achieved by a state, lack of expenditure on health care sometimes means that significant proportions of the population, in particular, women and girls, have limited or no access to basic health care services and goods. This situation results, in some cases, in high rates of maternal and infant mortality, as well as a high incidence of tuberculosis and other communicable diseases.[22]

Even in states where comprehensive legislation on equality between men and women may have been adopted, widespread gender inequalities and cultural stereotypes often continue to prevail, negatively affecting the equal enjoyment of economic, social and cultural rights for women and especially for those belonging to disadvantaged and marginalized groups.[23] Single mothers, in particular, experience multiple forms of discrimination and often encounter difficulties in access to health facilities, services and goods.[24] They also are at risk from a lack of adequate reproductive health services,[25] especially in rural areas.[26]

Discrimination on the basis of sexual orientation is still widespread in certain states and affects the enjoyment of economic, social and cultural rights by many people. Homosexuals experience discrimination in access to employment, housing and, in particular, health services. In some cases, the lack of access to essential health care and goods can seriously affect the health of these persons, especially those suffering from HIV/AIDS.[27]

National or social origin

This prohibited ground of discrimination overlaps to a large extent with ethnicity. It does however encompass a wider segment of the population to include refugees, asylum-seekers, migrant workers and all other non-nationals under the state's jurisdiction. It also protects persons considered as belonging to "socially inferior" groups.

In spite of constitutional and legislative provisions prohibiting caste-based discrimination, de facto discrimination persists with impunity in some states.[28] Persons belonging to these groups are often victims of discrimination in relation to many of the rights guaranteed by the Covenant and, in particular, with regard to coverage from universal healthcare schemes.[29] Refugees, asylum-seekers, migrant workers and other non-nationals may also be victims of discrimination in access to basic health care[30] and, as a result, are more likely to suffer from poor health than the rest of the population.

The Committee on Economic, Social and Cultural Rights is particularly concerned about the wide disparities in the quality of health care between rural and urban areas.[31] Persons living in rural or remote areas, especially refugees and indigenous peoples, may also experience discrimination in access to primary health care,[32] increased susceptibility to disease and reduced life expectancy.[33]

Food and nutrition

Food, along with water, is essential not only to good health but also to life. In spite of the fact that there is enough food in the world today to feed everyone sufficiently, at least 854 million people are currently suffering from food insecurity and two billion people are suffering from malnutrition.[34] The consequences of this chronic crisis on the state of health of those affected is self-evident: vitamin deficiency leads to increased susceptibility to all kinds of diseases, malformation of babies and growing children, blindness, brain damage and mental retardation. Even death will result from severe undernourishment. The enjoyment of the right to adequate food and the right to be free from hunger, as guaranteed by Article 11 of the Covenant on Economic, Social and Cultural Rights, is therefore of paramount importance.

The right to adequate food is not only essential to health but it is "indivisibly linked to the inherent dignity of the human person" and is "indispensable for the fulfilment of other human rights enshrined in the International Bill of Human Rights."[35] Furthermore, the right to food which is nutritionally adequate and safe, and the right to be free from hunger, are considered to be part of the core obligations of state parties.[36]

There are many causes of lack of adequate food and nutrition: climate change, the use of agrofuels, imbalances of power in the food production and distribution chain, speculation on the agricultural commodity markets, and soaring food prices are but a few.[37] Poverty – not only of the individual but also of the state – is however the principal cause of the lack of enjoyment of the right to adequate food. In theory, all categories of the population may be affected but, in practice, it is the most vulnerable groups who are the worst hit by lack of food, malnutrition and hunger.[38] Access to food may be hampered by inefficiency, corruption and discrimination in the distribution of food. Once again, it is the disadvantaged and marginalized groups of society who are excluded.[39]

In all circumstances, states have a core obligation to take the necessary action in order to ensure the availability and the accessibility of sufficient food, in ways which do not interfere with the enjoyment of the right to health.[40]

Housing and living conditions

Safe physical and economic access to health care and goods implies that medical services and the underlying determinants to health, such as safe and potable water and adequate sanitation facilities, are accessible to all categories of the population, including those who reside in rural areas.[41]

A large number of individuals and families on low incomes live in sub-standard housing and thus in unsafe, unhygienic and unhealthy conditions.[42] Persons belonging to racial, ethnic and national minorities, especially migrant workers and persons of foreign origin, are especially affected.[43] In addition, they also have inadequate access to health care facilities.[44] For example, many Roma live in informal settlements or slums which lack basic infrastructure and services, such as safe water, electricity, gas, heating and adequate sewage and garbage disposal.[45] They are frequently denied access to social housing and are increasingly victims of forced evictions, often without any provision of adequate alternative housing.[46] Women and, in particular, migrant women or those belonging to ethnic minorities, older persons, and persons with disabilities are subject to lack of security of tenure and forced evictions.[47] Indigenous peoples are often deprived of access to their ancestral lands.[48] All these negative living conditions will take their toll on the health of the people concerned.

In many states, prisoners and detainees live in appalling circumstances. Overcrowded and unhygienic conditions in prisons, as well as lack of appropriate health care, have all given rise to a high rate of tuberculosis and other serious health problems, such as HIV/AIDS, among the prison population.[49]

Homelessness affects more than 100 million people in the world. It is the cause of much ill-health,[50] affects marginalized and vulnerable groups[51] and may even lead to suicide.[52] Although there is no sole and easily identifiable cause of homelessness, a certain number of risk factors have been pinpointed by states: lack of affordable housing, speculation in housing and land for investment purposes, urban migration, unemployment, poverty, domestic violence, drug addiction and mental illness are but a few reasons which make people vulnerable to homelessness.[53]

Forced displacement

Persons may be displaced within the territory of a state for various reasons: internal armed conflict often makes people flee their homes, seeking refuge in safer regions. Violence, armed conflict and natural disasters have one tragic common denominator: they all lead to the forced displacement of large numbers of people which, in turn, can cause serious damage to mental and physical health.[54]

Urban development projects, real estate speculation, or the preparation for mega-events, such as the Olympic Games, lead to forced evictions of city dwellers.[55] Equally, land acquisition by private and state actors, for the purposes of constructing dams and mines, may result in the displacement of indigenous peoples, against their will, from their traditional territories and environment, thus depriving them of their essential sources of nutrition and the means for preparing their own traditional medicines.[56]

Lack of employment sometimes forces the rural population to move to urban areas in search of work.[57] Many of these immigrants end up living in squalid and unsafe settlements, deprived of the most basic services such as clean water, sufficient space and health care.[58]

Displacement is also caused by natural disasters, such as earthquakes, tsunamis and cyclones. Those persons affected not only become vulnerable to serious communicable diseases requiring urgent medical attention, they also find themselves cut off from their regular sources of health care and goods. Even when special, emergency measures have been taken to alleviate suffering, delays and inadequacies in the distribution of health care and vital medicines may occur leading to an increased risk to health.[59]

Natural disasters and armed conflict

Natural disasters always leave a trail of devastation in terms of human life and sickness. States have a joint and individual responsibility to provide disaster relief and humanitarian assistance in times of emergency. Priority should be given to supplying medical aid, food and water to the victims and to ensuring that any financial assistance given, actually reaches the most vulnerable or marginalized groups of the population.[60] Psychiatric help is frequently required by victims and especially by those who not only are displaced, but have also lost members of their families.[61]

Whether it be internal or international, armed conflict always causes violence, hardship, suffering and disease. At a time when urgent medical help is vital to health and even to life, access to the usual health services and goods may break down irreparably. It is then important that humanitarian aid be brought to victims of the conflict.[62]

Persons belonging to vulnerable categories of the population, such as women, children, ethnic minorities, older persons, handicapped persons and non-nationals of a state, always suffer most from the disastrous consequences of armed conflict. Their health, although fragile in peace-time, will often deteriorate even further and require emergency aid. All too often, the most needy will not receive the urgent medical help they so desperately require.

As in the case of natural disasters, states have immediate obligations to allow humanitarian aid to reach the victims of armed conflict and to do all in their power to facilitate this type of assistance.[63] In the aftermath of armed conflict, severely damaged infrastructures may hinder the mobility of persons and access to goods and essential public services, namely health care facilities.[64] In such cases, the Committee on Economic, Social and Cultural Rights urges state parties to provide adequate and immediate assistance, in order to alleviate the adverse impact of the conflict on all members of the population.[65] In particular, persons belonging to vulnerable and marginalized groups should benefit from special temporary measures.[66]

Harmful lifestyles and physical and mental violence

It should be underlined that good health cannot be ensured by the state, nor can a state provide protection against all causes of ill-health.[67] Nevertheless, preventive measures, such as awareness campaigns and public information schemes, should be introduced in order to alert the population to the potential risks engendered by unhealthy living. In this respect, the Committee on Economic, Social and Cultural Rights encourages state parties to adopt measures aimed at informing the public of the dangers linked to drug or alcohol abuse,[68] both active and passive smoking[69] and unsafe sex.[70] Furthermore, the Committee recommends that state parties analyse the motives for committing suicide, "with a view to developing effective

measures aimed at the prevention of suicide among vulnerable groups",
such as young people, homosexuals, persons addicted to drugs and/or alcohol, detainees and older persons.[71] The promotion of a healthy lifestyle, especially amongst young people, is paramount.[72]

Harmful traditional medical or cultural practices which are discriminatory towards women and girls, such as female genital mutilation, child marriages, witch-hunting, honour killings, and the preferential nourishment
and care of male children are strictly condemned as being serious violations
of the right to health and physical integrity.[73]

Physical or mental violence takes many different forms and concerns a
wide spectrum of victims. However, women and children belonging to disadvantaged or marginalized groups are usually the most affected. Domestic violence is unfortunately widespread in many states and frequently goes
unreported and therefore unpunished.[74] It is not only confined to developing states but is often prevalent in economically developed states.[75] Spousal
rape and sexual abuse of children have tragically become common-place.[76]
In many cases, domestic violence will have disastrous effects on physical
and mental health and can even lead to death.[77] The Committee has reiterated on many occasions the necessity to criminalize such acts and to provide shelter and medical assistance to the victims.[78]

In a broader context, women and children are vulnerable to exploitation, whether it be economic,[79] or sexual,[80] or both.[81] In particular, trafficking in persons remains a serious problem in many states causing considerable physical and mental suffering.[82] The victims of such practices require
specific protection and medical attention which are all too often sadly lacking.[83] Children are often victims of forced labour or hazardous working conditions.[84] This type of exploitation is in direct contradiction with Articles
6 and 7 of the Covenant and the International Labour Organization's Convention No. 182 on the Worst Forms of Child Labour.[85] It is also contrary to
the right of every child to receive a basic education.[86] In addition, millions
of children live in the streets and are amongst the most vulnerable to sexual
exploitation and forced labour,[87] as well as to health risks, such as alcohol or
drug addiction and HIV/AIDS.[88]

There is also a strong prevalence of HIV/AIDS among high-risk groups
such as sex workers, drug users and incarcerated persons. These people
are also frequently victims of discrimination by health care institutions.[89]
Trade in human organs, particularly in kidneys, is prevalent in some states
and is on the increase.[90] Such practices are an affront to human dignity and

constitute a serious violation of the right to physical integrity. They affect primarily the poorest and most vulnerable categories of the population.

Safe and healthy working conditions and a healthy environment

As guaranteed by Article 7(b) of the Covenant on Economic, Social and Cultural Rights, state parties must recognize the right of everyone to the enjoyment of just and favourable conditions of work, which include safe and healthy working conditions.[91]

Despite the obligation to ensure industrial safety and hygiene, occupational accidents and diseases are on the increase,[92] affecting greatly the enjoyment of the right to health of the active population.

Occupational accidents and illnesses often have irreparable consequences. Unsafe or unhygienic working conditions can lead to serious accidents and industrial diseases, such as lead poisoning and asbestos-related illnesses. Article 12(2)(b) of the Covenant urges state parties to take preventive measures and to minimize, as far as is reasonably practicable, the causes of health hazards inherent in the working environment.[93]

Despite legal guarantees, many serious accidents occur in coalmining,[94] in the construction sector[95] and in the transportation industry.[96] It must be pointed out that not only state authorities, but also non-state actors, such as private employers, have the responsibility to create a healthy and safe working environment.[97]

In addition, generally poor conditions of work, such as excessive working hours, lack of sufficient rest breaks and lack of periodic holidays with pay, are not only contrary to Article 7(d) of the Covenant, they are also dangerous to health.[98]

More generally, environmental degradation has a strong negative impact on the health of the whole population.[99] Exposure to a dangerous, or polluted environment, can have serious consequences on the enjoyment of the right to health:[100] Pollution of water, air and soil, radiation and exposure to harmful chemicals or heavy metals can all seriously impair the health of an entire community. For instance, survivors of the 1984 gas leak in a pesticide plant in Bhopal are continuing to suffer serious long-term effects on health from exposure to gas.[101] Reported incidents and lack of security in nuclear plants, as well as an absence of information about the risks to the health of those persons living in close proximity to nuclear installations are constant reminders that transparency is all important.[102] In such cases, state parties are strongly advised to adopt measures for preventing nuclear accidents and for ensuring rapid intervention should a serious incident occur.[103] In this context, states have a general obligation to inform the population of any dangers to the environment which could harm the health or life of the community.[104]

Access to information, education and effective remedies

Access to health-related education and information, including information on sexual and reproductive health, is an important determinant of the right to health.[105] This means that the right to seek, receive and to communicate health issues must be respected.[106] In addition, the population should be associated with, and participate in, all health-related decision-making in the community at local, national and international levels.[107] However, access to health information does not mean that personal health data, which should be treated with confidentiality, may be divulged.[108]

The prevention, treatment and control of epidemic, endemic and occupational and other diseases require states to draw up and adopt prevention and education programmes.[109] Information on health should also be made available throughout the state territory, including remote rural or mountainous areas.[110]

More generally, lack of education and illiteracy present serious obstacles to the full enjoyment of the right to health. The phenomenon of early marriages, the high rate of maternal mortality, and the rapid spread of HIV/AIDS and other sexually transmitted diseases, can largely be attributed to the lack of sex and reproductive education which is still viewed by some states as taboo.[111] Children and girls in particular are often deprived of access to education, thus barring them from obtaining basic schooling and hence valuable knowledge on health issues. Equally, adults who have never had the possibility to receive a basic education are severely handicapped when accessing health goods and services. Due to their lack of understanding of the written word, at best they are likely to experience difficulties and bureaucratic problems when dealing with health personnel and, at worst, they may be victims of discrimination and lack of access to health care,[112] without any hope of redress.

Access to effective judicial or other remedies without discrimination constitutes an essential determinant of the right to health.[113] Without the possibility to claim health entitlements within the legal order of a state, the most vulnerable and needy may find themselves deprived of the means to exercise their right to receive basic health care.

The Committee on Economic, Social and Cultural Rights recommends that state parties ensure redress for victims of violations of the right to equal access to health care services, facilities and goods.[114] States should also provide information on the number and nature of cases brought before the courts in relation to violations of the right to health and physical integrity.[115]

National and international trade and financial agreements

Trade and financial agreements may have negative effects on the cost of health services and especially that of essential drugs.[116] They may even have an impact on access to health care, social security and the intellectual property regimes protecting, inter alia, access to generic medicines, biodiversity, water and the right of indigenous communities to these resources.[117]

The Committee on Economic, Social and Cultural Rights strongly recommends that state parties assess ex ante the potential adverse impact of trade or financial agreements and development policies on the right to health of their populations and, in particular, on the health of the most vulnerable groups.[118] In order to ensure that the rights to health, adequate food and a decent standard of living are not adversely affected, states should also eliminate dependency of small-scale farmers on multinational corporations.[119]

The failure of a state to respect its legal obligations regarding the right to health when entering into bilateral or multilateral agreements with other states, international organizations and multinational corporations constitutes a violation of the standards laid down in Article 12 of the Covenant,[120] which can result in serious damage to physical and mental health.

Concluding remarks

Although many factors in society today may lead to ill-health, there are two main root causes: poverty and hunger.

Despite rapid economic development in recent years, poverty persists in many states, disproportionately affecting persons belonging to marginalized and vulnerable groups, such as ethnic minorities, immigrants, indigenous peoples, women and the rural population. Disparities in income, and in the enjoyment of an adequate standard of living, continue to widen between the rich and the poor.[121] In some states, the number of people living in extreme poverty has even increased.[122] The absence of a poverty line which would enable states to define the extent of poverty and to monitor and evaluate progress in alleviating poverty, is deeply regrettable.[123] Poverty is also one of the main social determinants of health.

In addition to being poor, 100 million people will go to bed hungry tonight. Although the causes of the current food crisis are numerous and hotly debated in the international community, one hard fact stands out: food prices are too high for the poorest nations and peoples in the world to afford adequate nourishment. As a result, food insecurity and hunger are on the increase, leading inevitably to ill-health and, in many cases, to death.

Unless these two important obstacles to health and well-being can be tackled and overcome with success in the short, medium, and long-term, the health of millions of people will suffer irreparably. This is an intolerable situation, because it is a preventable one.[124]

The realization of the right to health, like other human rights, requires states to pursue international cooperation in order to identify and eliminate the obstacles to the full enjoyment of this right by everyone.[125] This obligation implies that states must protect effectively the right to health by regulating and monitoring the activities, not only of national authorities, but also of private actors in order to ensure that the right to health is respected and promoted.

Although the health of all sectors of the population is affected by poor living conditions, an unhealthy and unsafe environment, together with increasing violence, the most vulnerable and marginalized groups will always suffer the most from poverty and hunger. As a matter of priority, states must address the root causes which undermine the enjoyment of the right to health in order to promote the well-being and safety of the entire population.

* This article reflects the personal opinions of the author in her capacity as Professor of Human Rights Law and not as member of the Committee on Economic, Social and Cultural Rights.

1 See Committee on Economic, Social and Cultural Rights (CESCR), General Comment No. 14 on the right to the highest attainable standard of health, 11 August 2000, UN Doc. E/C.12/2000/4, at para. 1 and para. 3; unless otherwise stated, all General Comments referred to are those of the Committee on Economic, Social and Cultural Rights.

2 Hereinafter referred to as the 'Covenant' or the 'Covenant on Economic, Social and Cultural Rights'.

3 General Comment No. 14, *supra* note 1, para. 5; see also, Statement on Poverty and the International Covenant on Economic, Social and Cultural Rights, adopted by the Committee on Economic, Social and Cultural Rights, 4 May 2001, E/C.12/2001/10, para. 4.

4 General Comment No. 19 (2007) on the right to social security (art. 9), para. 32.

5 Statement on Poverty, *supra* note 3, para. 5.

6 In August 2008, a report on the topic of social determinants of the right to health was published by the Commission on the Social Determinants of Health at the World Health Organization. This chapter does not address this report and was written before this report was issued. However, for those interested in this topic, it is recommended that readers consult the Commission on Social Determinants of Health, *Closing the Gap in a Generation: Health Equity Through Action on the Social Determinants of Health* (Geneva: WHO, 2008), available at http://www.who.int/social_determinants/final_report/en/index.html.

7 General Comment No. 14, *supra* note 1, para. 12(b) and para. 18.

8 General Comment No. 3 (1990) on the nature of states parties' obligations (art. 2 para. 1), para. 1.

9 For a list of essential drugs, see, WHO Model List of Essential Medicines, revised in March 2007 (for adults); WHO Model List of Essential Medicines for Children, revised in October 2007.

10 General Comment No. 14, *supra* note 1, para. 12(a) and (b).

11 Ibid., para. 12(b)(III); see also, Concluding Observations on the second periodic report of Ireland, E/C.12/1/Add.77, para. 22.

12 General Comment No. 19, *supra* note 4, para. 4(a) and (b): the schemes instituted may be contributory or insurance-based (such as social insurance) or non-contributory (such as universal schemes) or targeted social assistance (for those in need) or other forms of social security (such as self-help, community-based or mutual schemes).

13 Ibid., para. 2 and para. 23; General Comment No. 14, *supra* note 1, para. 36; Concluding Observations on the initial report of Switzerland E/C.12/1/Add.30, para. 24 and para. 36.

14 General Comment No. 19, *supra* note 4, para. 12(a) and (b), para. 22 and para. 23.

15 See also, General Comment No. 18 (2005) on the right to work (art. 6), para. 1, para. 2 and para. 7.

16 Concluding Observations on the second to fifth periodic report of India, E/C.12/IND/CO/5, para. 38.

17 General Comment No. 14, *supra* note 1, para. 12(b) (II).

18 Concluding Observations on the third periodic report of Hungary, E/C.12/HUN/CO/3, para. 25.

19 General Comment No. 14, *supra* note 1, para. 27.

20 Ibid., para. 27; see also, Concluding Observations on the second periodic report of Bolivia, E/C.12/BOL/CO/2, para. 24.

21 Concluding Observations on the second periodic report of Bolivia, *supra* note 20, para. 15.

22 Concluding Observations on the second to fifth periodic report of India, *supra* note 16, para. 33; Concluding Observations on the second periodic report of Algeria, E/C.12/1/Add.71, para. 21.

23 Concluding Observations on the second to fifth periodic report of India, *supra* note 16, para. 16 and para. 33; Concluding Observations on the initial report of Zambia, E/C.12/1/Add.106, para. 30.

24 Concluding Observations on the third periodic report of France, E/C.12/FRA/CO/3, para. 13.

25 Concluding Observations on the second periodic report of Nepal, E/C.12/NPL/CO/2, para. 26.

26 Concluding Observations on the second periodic report of Benin, E/C.12/BEN/CO/2, para. 25.

27 Concluding Observations on the second to fifth periodic report of India, *supra* note 16, para. 13, para. 52 and para. 73.

28 Concluding Observations on the second periodic report of Nepal, *supra* note 25, para. 13; Concluding Observations on the second to fifth periodic report of India, *supra* note 16, para. 13 and para. 14.

29 Concluding Observations on the second to fifth periodic report of India, *supra* note 16, para. 38.

30 Concluding Observations on the second periodic report of Senegal, E/C.12/1/Add.62, para. 33; Concluding Observations on the third periodic report of France, *supra* note 24, para. 26 and para. 46; Concluding Observations on the third periodic report of Belgium, E/C.12/BEL/CO/3, para. 21 and para. 35; see also, Committee on the Elimination of Racial Discrimination, General Recommendation XXX on discrimination against non-citizens (2005), para. 3, para. 29 and para. 36.

31 Concluding Observations on the fifth periodic report of Ukraine, E/C.12/UKR/CO/5, para. 27.

32 Concluding Observations on the initial report of Serbia and Montenegro, E/C.12/1/Add.108, para. 33.

33 Concluding Observations on the fourth periodic report of the Russian Federation, E/C.12/1/Add. 94, para. 31 and para. 33.

34 Statement on the World Food Crisis of the Committee on Economic, Social and Cultural Rights, 19 May 2008, E/C.12/2008/1, para. 2; see also, Olivier de Schutter, Background Note: Analysis of the World Food Crisis by the Special Rapporteur to the United Nations on the Right to Food, 2 May 2008, para. 2, available at www2.ohchr.org/english /issues/food/docs/SRRTFnotefoodcrisis.pdf.

35 Statement on the World Food Crisis, *supra* note 34, para. 6; General Comment No. 12 (1999) on the right to food, para. 4; see also, Human Rights Council, 7th Special Session, Resolution S-7/1: the negative impact of the worsening of the world food crisis on the realization of the right to food for all, adopted by consensus, 22 May 2008.

36 General Comment No. 14, *supra* note 1, para. 43(b).

37 Address by the UN Special Rapporteur on the Right to Food, Olivier de Schutter, at the High-Level Conference on World Food Security: The Challenges of Climate Change and Bioenergy, Rome, 3–5 June 2008.

38 Concluding Observations of the second periodic report of Benin, *supra* note 26, para. 22: 43% of the population suffer from chronic malnutrition; ibid., para. 23: prisoners and detainees suffer from severe undernourishment; Concluding Observations on the second periodic report of Nepal, *supra* note 25, para. 22: almost a quarter of the population is undernourished, rural communities and persons belonging to the lower castes are particularly vulnerable to food insecurity; Concluding Observations on the initial report of Uzbekistan, E/C.12/UZB/CO/1, para. 27 and para. 31: 28% of the population (approx. 6.7 million people, two thirds of whom reside in rural areas) live below the poverty line and do not have enough food for their basic needs. Consequently, there is a high incidence of malnutrition in the state party.

39 Concluding Observations on the second to fifth periodic report of India, *supra* note 16, para. 28.

40 General Comment No. 12, *supra* note 35, para. 8.

41 General Comment No. 14, *supra* note 1, para. 12(b) (II).

42 Concluding Observations on the third periodic report of France, *supra* note 24, para. 22 and para. 23.

43 Concluding Observations on the third periodic report of Belgium, *supra* note 30, para. 14.

44 Ibid., para. 21; Concluding Observations on the third periodic report of France, *supra* note 24, para. 21.

45 Concluding Observations on the fifth periodic report of Ukraine, *supra* note 31, para. 25; Concluding Observations on the third periodic report of Hungary, *supra* note 18, para. 22; Concluding Observations on the initial report of Greece, E/C.12/1/Add.97, para. 22.

46 Concluding Observations on the third periodic report of Hungary, *supra* note 18, para. 22.

47 Miloon Kothari, Statement by the Special Rapporteur on Adequate Housing on World Habitat Day, 1 October 2007, available at http://www.un hchr.ch/huricane/huricane.nsf/view01/E23B1F14 F3D942FBC125736700705408?opendocument.

48 Concluding Observations on the second periodic report of Bolivia, *supra* note 20, para. 23: whilst indigenous peoples make up 62% of the population, almost 70% of the land is controlled by only 7% of the population.

49 Concluding Observations on the fifth periodic report of Ukraine, *supra* note 31, para. 29; Concluding Observations on the second to fifth periodic report of India, *supra* note 16, para. 35; Concluding Observations on the initial report of Uzbekistan, *supra* note 38, para. 34. See also, Paul Hunt, Report of the Special Rapporteur on the right of everyone to the enjoyment of the highest attainable standard of physical and mental health: Summary of communications sent to and replies received from Governments and other sectors, 4 March 2008, A/HRC/7/11/Add.1.

50 Concluding Observations on the fourth periodic reports of the United Kingdom of Great Britain and Northern Ireland, the Crown Dependencies and the Overseas Dependent Territories, E/C.12/1/Add.79, para. 19: the homeless often suffer from alcoholism or mental illness.

51 Concluding Observations on the fifth periodic report of Ukraine, *supra* note 31, para. 22 and para. 45: children leaving state-run school orphanages are particularly vulnerable to becoming homeless.

52 Concluding Observations on the third periodic report of France, *supra* note 24, para. 25 and para. 27.

53 See, for example, Third periodic report of France, E/C.12/FRA/3, para. 193–199; Miloon Kothari, Report of the Special Rapporteur on adequate housing as a component of the right to an adequate standard of living, E/CN.4/2005/48.

54 Concluding Observations on the implementation of the Covenant in the Republic of the Congo (in the absence of a written report), E/C.12/1/Add.45, para. 22: as a result of the violence and the ensuing massive displacements, epidemics of diseases and diarrhoea occurred.

55 Concluding Observations on the initial report of China E/C.12/1/Add.107, para. 31; Concluding Observations on the initial report of Greece, *supra* note 45, para. 21.

56 General Comment No. 14, *supra* note 1, para. 27; Concluding Observations on the second to fifth periodic report of India, *supra* note 16, para. 31.

57 Concluding Observations on the combined second, third and fourth periodic report of Costa Rica, E/C.12/CRI/CO/4, para. 19.

58 Miloon Kothari, Statement by the Special Rapporteur on Adequate Housing, *supra* note 47.

59 Concluding Observations on the second to fifth periodic report of India, *supra* note 16, para. 32.

60 General Comment No. 14, *supra* note 1, para. 40; see also, Concluding Observations on the second to fifth periodic report of India, *supra* note 16, para. 32 and para. 72.

61 Concluding Observations on the second periodic report of Japan, E/C.12/1/Add.67, para. 27.

62 General Comment No. 14, *supra* note 1, para. 10.

63 Ibid., para. 16; see, also: Concluding Observations on the implementation of the Covenant by the Republic of the Congo, *supra* note 54, para. 22 and para. 28.

64 Concluding Observations on the second periodic report of Nepal, *supra* note 25, para. 10; Concluding Observations on the fourth periodic report of the Russian Federation, *supra* note 33, para. 10 and para. 38.

65 Concluding Observations on the initial report of Bosnia and Herzegovina, E/C.12/BIH/CO/1, para. 39.

66 Concluding Observations on the second periodic report of Nepal, *supra* note 25, para. 36.

67 General Comment No. 14, *supra* note 1, para. 9.

68 Concluding Observations on the third periodic report of Austria, E/C.12/AUT/CO/3, para. 16; Concluding Observations on the fourth periodic report of Spain, E/C.12/1/Add.99, para. 23.

69 The Committee commends states which have enacted legislation banning smoking in public places: Concluding Observations of the third periodic report of France, *supra* note 24, para. 9; public awareness campaigns should be conducted to reduce tobacco use and alcohol consumption: Concluding Observations on the initial report of Latvia, E/C.12/LVA/CO/1, para. 52.

70 Concluding Observations on the initial report of China, *supra* note 55, para. 60.

71 Concluding Observations on the third periodic report of France, *supra* note 24, para. 47.

72 Concluding Observations on the fifth periodic report of Finland, E/C.12/CO/FIN/5, para. 27.

73 General Comment No. 14, *supra* note 1, para. 21, 37 and 51: See for example: Concluding Observations on the second to fifth periodic report of India, *supra* note 16, para. 25; Concluding Observations on the second periodic report of Benin, *supra* note 26, para. 19 and para. 26.

74 Concluding Observations on the intial report of Latvia, *supra* note 69, para. 21.

75 See, for example: Concluding Observations on the fourth periodic report of Norway, E/C.12/1/Add.109, para. 15; Concluding Observations on the third periodic report of France, *supra* note 24, para. 19.

76 See, for example: Concluding Observations on the initial report of Greece, *supra* note 45, para. 16 and para. 17; Concluding Observations on the second periodic report of Benin, *supra* note 24, para. 17; Concluding Observations on the second to fifth periodic report of India, *supra* note 16, para. 26.

77 Concluding Observations on the fourth periodic report of Spain, *supra* note 68, para. 17.

78 See, for example: Concluding Observations on the third periodic report of France, *supra* note 22, para. 39; Concluding Observations on the third periodic report of Belgium, *supra* note 30, para. 32; Concluding Observations on the fifth periodic report of Ukraine, *supra* note 31, para. 42.

79 Concluding Observations on the second periodic report of Benin, *supra* note 26, para. 20; Concluding Observations on the fourth periodic report of Mexico, E/C.12/MEX/CO/4, para. 22.

80 Concluding Observations on the second periodic report of Benin, *supra* note 26, para. 18.

81 Concluding Observations on the second and third periodic reports of Paraguay, E/C.12/PRY/CO/3, para. 12(h).

82 Concluding Observations on the initial report of Greece, *supra* note 45, para. 18.

83 Concluding Observations on the second to fifth periodic report of India, *supra* note 16, para. 27; Concluding Observations on the fifth periodic report of Ukraine, *supra* note 31, para. 20 and para. 43.

84 Concluding Observations on the initial report of China, *supra* note 55, para. 23: hazardous occupations include mining; Concluding Observations on the second periodic report of Nepal, *supra* note 25, para. 19: some children continue to work in conditions of bonded labour; Concluding Observations on the second periodic report of Bolivia, *supra* note 20, para. 14(d): indigenous children, in particular, are exploited and frequently victims of the harmful practice of 'criaditos' which constitutes forced domestic labour of children.

85 On the need to protect children from all forms of work which are likely to interfere with their development or physical or mental health, see, General Comment No. 18, *supra* note 15, para. 15.

86 As guaranteed by art. 13 of the Covenant; see also, General Comment No. 13 (1999) on the right to education (art. 13), para. 1.

87 Concluding Observations on the second periodic report of Georgia, E/C.12/1/Add.83, para. 20.

88 Concluding Observations on the fifth periodic report of Ukraine, *supra* note 31, para. 22; Concluding Observations on the initial report of Latvia, *supra* note 69, para. 23; Concluding Observations on the initial report of the Former Yugoslav Republic of Macedonia, E/C.12/MKD/CO/1, para. 21: hundreds of children in cities, primarily Roma, live on the streets and do not attend school or benefit from adequate health care.

89 Concluding Observations on the fifth periodic report of Ukraine, *supra* note 31, para. 28.

90 Concluding Observations on the second to fifth periodic report of India, *supra* note 16, para. 39.

91 See also, General Comment No. 18, *supra* note 15, para. 2.

92 Concluding Observations on the fourth periodic report of Spain, *supra* note 68, para. 14; Concluding Observations on the initial report of Latvia, *supra* note 69, para. 18.

93 See also, General Comment No. 14, *supra* note 1, para. 15; ILO Convention No. 155, Occupational Safety and Health Convention (1981), art. 4 para. 2.

94 Concluding Observations on the fifth periodic report of Ukraine, *supra* note 31, para. 16; Concluding Observations on the initial report of China, *supra* note 55, para. 24.

95 Concluding Observations on the fourth periodic report of Spain, *supra* note 68, para. 14.

96 Concluding Observations on the third periodic report of Hungary, *supra* note 18, para. 15.

97 Concluding Observations on the fourth periodic report of the Russian Federation, *supra* note 33, para. 47; Concluding Observations on the initial report of Latvia, *supra* note 69, para. 42: the Committee urges state parties to sanction employers who fail to observe safety regulations in the work-place; see, also: General Comment No. 14, *supra* note 1, para. 35; Andrew Clapham, *Human Rights Obligations of Non-State Actors* (Oxford: Oxford University Press, 2006) 326.

98 Concluding Observations on the initial report on China, *supra* note 55, para. 24 and para. 53; Concluding Observations on the second periodic report of Japan, *supra* note 61, para. 19; Concluding Observations on the combined second, third and fourth periodic report of Costa Rica, *supra* note 57, para. 18.

99 Concluding Observations on the initial report of Uzbekistan, *supra* note 38, para. 28.

100 General Comment No. 14, *supra* note 1, para. 15; Concluding Observations on the second and third periodic reports of Paraguay, *supra* note 81, para. 16: the expansion of soybean cultivation has fostered the indiscriminate use of toxic agro-chemicals, leading to illness and even death among children and adults, contamination of the water supply and the disappearance of ecosystems.

101 Concluding Observations on the second to fifth periodic report of India, *supra* note 16, para. 36 and para. 76.

102 Concluding Observations on the second periodic report of Japan, *supra* note 61, para. 22.

103 Ibid., para. 49.

104 See, at a regional level: European Court of Human Rights, *Guerra v. Italy,* judgment of the Grand Chamber of 19 February 1998, Reports of Judgments and Decisions 1998-I, para. 60; *Oneryildiz v. Turkey,* judgment of the Grand Chamber of 30 November 2004, Reports of Judgments and Decisions 2004-XII, para. 90.

105 General Comment No. 14, *supra* note 1, para. 11.

106 See, in this context, art. 19(2) of the International Covenant on Civil and Political Rights.

107 General Comment No. 14, *supra* note 1, para. 11; see also, Statement on Poverty, *supra* note 3, para. 12.

108 General Comment No. 14, *supra* note 1, para. 12(b) (IV).

109 Ibid., para. 16.

110 Ibid., para. 36; see, for example: Concluding Observations on the second to fifth periodic report of India, *supra* note 16, para. 77; Concluding Observations on the second periodic report of Benin, *supra* note 26, para. 46.

111 Concluding Observations on the second to fifth periodic report of India, *supra* note 16, para. 37.

112 Concluding Observations on the second periodic report of Bolivia, *supra* note 20, para. 14(g) and para. 15; Concluding Observations on the second to fifth periodic report of India, *supra* note 16, para. 42: adult illiteracy rates continue to remain high, especially amongst women and disadvantaged and marginalized groups.

113 General Comment No. 3, *supra* note 8, para. 5.

114 Concluding Observations on the second to fifth periodic report of India, *supra* note 16, para. 52; see, also: Concluding Observations on the fourth periodic report of the Russian Federation, *supra* note 33, para. 32 and para. 60: legislation on the rights of patients concerning, inter alia, professional ethics and redress for medical errors is necessary.

115 Concluding Observations on the second periodic report of Benin, *supra* note 26, para. 47: on cases related to female genital mutilation; Concluding Observations on the third periodic report of Hungary, *supra* note 18, para. 42: concerning victims of domestic violence.

116 Concluding Observations on the third periodic report of Morocco, E/C.12/MAR/CO/2, para. 29.

117 Concluding Observations on the combined second, third and fourth periodic report of Costa Rica, *supra* note 57, para. 27.

118 Concluding Observations on the third periodic report of Morocco, *supra* note 116, para. 56; Concluding Observations on the combined second, third and fourth periodic report of Costa Rica, *supra* note 57, para. 48; see, also: Statement on the World Food Crisis, *supra* note 34, para. 13.

119 Concluding Observations on the second to fifth periodic report of India, *supra* note 16, para. 69.

120 General Comment No. 14, *supra* note 1, para. 50.

121 Concluding Observations on the fourth periodic report of Mexico, *supra* note 79, para. 23.

122 Concluding Observations on the second and third periodic reports of Paraguay, *supra* note 81, para. 12 a).

123 Concluding Observations on the fifth periodic report of Finland, *supra* note 72, para. 17; Concluding Observations on the initial report of China, *supra* note 55, para. 30; see also, Concluding Observations on the second to fifth periodic report of India, *supra* note 16, para. 28: in its pursuit of economic growth, the state party defined the poverty threshold exclusively in terms of consumption. In addition, economic, social and cultural rights have yet to be fully integrated into poverty-reduction strategies.

124 Olivier de Schutter, Background Note: Analysis of the World Food Crisis, *supra* note 34, para. 2.

125 See, UN Charter, art. 56; Covenant on Economic, Social and Cultural Rights, art. 2, para. 1, and art. 23; Vienna Declaration and Programme of Action, adopted at the Vienna World Conference on Human Rights, 14–25 June 1993, A/CONF.157/23, 12 July 1993.

Access to Essential Medicines as a Component of the Right to Health

Stephen P. Marks

Introduction

In *Human Rights Obligations of Non-State Actors,* Andrew Clapham wrote, "Perhaps the most obvious threat to human rights has come from the inability of people to achieve access to expensive medicine, particularly in the context of HIV and AIDS."[1] He was referring to threats to human rights from intellectual property agreements under the World Trade Organization, which are often seen as obeying a different – and many would say utterly incompatible – logic than human rights. The right to health, in the interpretation of the Committee on Economic Social and Cultural Rights, means that "States Parties ... have a duty to prevent unreasonably high costs for access to essential medicines."[2]

This chapter will explain the significance and place of the human right to essential medicines as a derivative right within the broader right to the highest attainable standard of physical and mental health. As a component of the right to health, the right to essential medicines depends not only on the production, distribution, and pricing of medicines, but also on the incentives for research and development of drugs needed to treat diseases in developing countries, on functioning health systems, so that drugs are part of a rational system of quality treatment and care, as well as on infrastructure, so that they can be delivered to all areas where they are needed. Considering that these broader issues are examined in other chapters, this chapter will focus more on the impediment to the realization of the right to essential medicines caused by the protection of intellectual property. This chapter begins with an overview of some of the basic data about the health impact of the current level of access to medicines, especially in developing countries. Then the essential features of the international trade regime that affect access to medicines are discussed, including how that regime functions in constant tension with the international human rights regime. The recent trend in legislation, litigation, and advocacy to favour access to essential medicines over protection of patent-holders will then be examined before analysing the most salient formulations of the right to access to essential medicines. Finally, several of the proposals currently under consideration to overcome the economic obstacles to realizing the right to essential medicines are presented.

Access to medicines in the global burden of disease

The trend in access to medicines, particularly in poor countries, provides the evidence for policies in global heath to increase access at all stages of the process from setting research priorities for the development of new drugs, to manufacturing, pricing, marketing, and distribution. "Essential medicines", according to the World Health Organization (WHO), are those that "satisfy the priority health care needs of the population" and "are intended to be available within the context of functioning health systems at all times in adequate amounts, in the appropriate dosage forms, with assured quality, and at a price the individual and the community can afford."[3] The United Nations Development Group defines "access" in this context as "having medicines continuously available and affordable at public or private health facilities or medicine outlets that are within one hour's walk from the homes of the population."[4]

In 1975, half of the world's population was without access to life-saving and other essential medicines.[5] While the proportion has decreased to about one-third of the world's population, the absolute number has remained constant at approximately two billion people.[6] According to the WHO, expanding access to existing interventions, including medicines, for infectious diseases, maternal and child health, and noncommunicable diseases would save more than 10.5 million lives a year by 2015.[7]

Significantly, the MDG Gap Task Force addressed the relation between the MDG issue of access to medicines and the right to health by noting that:

> "... the national constitutions define the fundamental political principles
> of a country and usually guarantee certain rights to their people. Health
> is a fundamental human right recognized in at least 135 national consti-
> tutions. Access to health care, including access to essential medicines, is
> a prerequisite for realizing that right. However, only five countries specif-
> ically recognize access to essential medicines and technologies as part of
> the fulfilment of the right to health."[8]

The MDG Gap Task Force also notes "Most national constitutions do not specifically recognize access to essential medicines or technologies as part of the fulfilment of the right to health."

The Working Group on Access to Essential Medicines of the United Na-
tions Millennium Project approached the problem from the human rights perspective. It opened its report by stating: "The lack of access to life-sav-
ing and health-supporting medicines for an estimated 2 billion poor people stands as a direct contradiction to the fundamental principle of health as a human right."[9] The Group gave priority consideration to improving ac-
cess to medicines in resource-poor settings and promoting research on new medicines for diseases of poverty. It identified six barriers to access the medicines: Inadequate national commitment, inadequate human resources, failure of the international community to keep its promises to developing countries, lack of coordination of international aid, obstacles created by the Trade-Related Aspects of Intellectual Property Rights (TRIPS) agreement, and the current incentive structure for research and development of medicines and vaccines to address priority health needs of developing countries.[10] In examining the solutions to the problem, the UN Working Group underscored the "consensus that human rights should incorporate the ability of individuals to maintain and restore good health through access to at least a basic level of primary care, including essential medicines"[11] and listed among the general principles underpinning issues of increasing access to medicines the human right to health, as well as women's inequality and gender disparities.[12]

Among the Working Group's recommendations to improve availability of medicines is improving the rate and relevance of innovation and developing more reliable procurement and supply systems at the national and

international levels.[13] The Group also recommended specific steps for promoting the safety, affordability, and appropriate use of medicines.[14] Finally, it devoted attention to the barrier created by the system of intellectual property protection, specifically citing the conclusion of the UN Millennium Project Task Force on Trade that the TRIPS agreement, and "TRIPS Plus" provisions of free-trade agreements, will over time probably have a negative impact on access to drugs in developing countries.[15] This trend clearly creates tension with the obligations of states to realize the right to health under the international human rights regime.

The tension between the international trade regime and the international human rights regime

In dissenting from the Working Group report just discussed, the representative of the pharmaceutical industry explained,

> "We do not believe that the main problem in barring medicines to the poor is patent protection, nor do we accept that individual company pricing practices are fundamental to explaining why one-third of the world's poor lack access to basic, low-cost essential medicines. An inaccurate and subjective link is forged between rights, 'monopoly' pricing, and global inequities in access to medicines ... We also believe that our private sector research model is worthy of preserving rather than abandoning on the risky premise that more public investment will by itself yield miracle cures against the complex scientific challenge of fighting resistant strains of infectious disease ... In short, the report fails to provide the balanced and accurate perspective necessary to stimulate fresh policy approaches that could make a real difference in the lives of the poor."[16]

From the perspective of the primary legal regime governing trade in products invented and manufactured by business entities, essentially transnational corporations, the issues of access to medicines is a clear-cut matter of the patenting of a new chemical product and the process for its use, as well as the protection of the patents involved in the markets where the producers intend to sell them. The patents, which protect the inventor from anyone copying the product without license, and allow the inventor to set the price, are protected internationally under the WTO Agreement on Trade-Related Aspects of Intellectual Property Rights (TRIPS). TRIPS requires WTO members to protect patents of pharmaceuticals for 20 years, thus giving drug companies exclusive rights to prevent unauthorized use, subject to domestic and international enforcement. Countries that fail to protect patents may be brought before the dispute settlement body of the WTO. As a result in part of the outcry over drug pricing in countries confronted by the HIV/AIDS pandemic, the least-developed countries, who were originally supposed to comply by 2006, now have until 1 January 2016 to implement TRIPS. However, all other WTO Members are bound, and even the poorest countries will be bound in less than a decade.

In addition to the delayed compliance until 2016, developing countries may avail themselves of "flexibilities" to avoid patent protections through parallel importing (importing cheaper versions of drugs from countries where pharmaceuticals are not patented or where their term of protection has expired) and compulsory licensing (manufacturing generic versions of patented medicines without the patent holder's authorization under certain conditions).[17] Most agree that the patent system is necessary and beneficial to promote innovation in the pharmaceutical industry, but there are various barriers to developing countries taking full advantage of the flexibilities, and hundreds of free trade agreements impose greater restrictions than TRIPS ("TRIPS-plus" provisions).

Access to patented medicines – as the pharmaceutical dissent to the Working Group report quoted above stresses – is not the sole or even the principal obstacle to adequate provision of health products and medical devices to the poor population of developing countries. In fact, one study by Amir Attaran claims that, of the 319 products on the WHO Model List of Essential Medicines, only seventeen are patentable. Furthermore, many of those are not actually patented, bringing the patent incidence down to 1.4%.[18] The author not only challenges the assumptions among activists that patents cause lack of access to affordable medicines in poor countries and within the pharmaceutical industry,[19] and that IPRs are necessary to protect to assure future research and development, but also expresses doubt that compulsory licensing can be made practicable, considering that "zero generic medicines have been manufactured this way in the past decade, treating zero patients in any country worldwide."[20] In response to Attaran's study, the Director of Medicines Policy and Standards at WHO wrote that "a statement on the percentage of patented medicines on the Model List is therefore not possible without specifying the geographical area and the specific time" and "a few patented medicines can greatly affect health

expenditure", noting that "the economic value and public health importance of the market of ARVs and future essential medicines for neglected
disease are buried in the statistics" of the quoted study.[21] Be that as it may,
the point for the purposes of a putative human right to essential medicines
is that challenging IPRs and urging use of TRIPS flexibilities do not constitute the only path toward realizing that right.

Numerous factors contribute to making essential medicines available
in poor countries, including affordable prices; government commitment
through a well conceived and implemented national medicines policy (NMP);
adequate, sustainable and equitable public sector financing; generic substitution; transparent and widely disseminated consumer information; efficient distribution; control of taxes, duties and other markups; and careful
selection and monitoring.[22]

As thoroughly demonstrated by Lisa Forman, corporate innovation for
diseases affecting poor countries does not occur for commercial reasons but
in response to "growing public pressure over corporate failures to address
developing country needs".[23] Drawing on the experience of the 1997 to 2001
litigation and trade pressure by the US Government and 40 pharmaceutical companies to resist South African's law aimed at gaining access to affordable medicine, which she considers the "tipping point" of the struggle,
Forman demonstrates how the Treatment Action Campaign case "brought
human rights arguments drawn from international and domestic law, arguing that the right to health provided constitutional authority for the legislation itself, and was a legal interest that should be prioritized over corporate property rights."[24] She concludes that this experience "can be seen to
provide a strategic roadmap for advancing the completion of the process of
normative diffusion, so that access to medicines as a human right starts to
assume a 'taken for granted' quality in politics, law, and public opinion."[25]

The "normative diffusion" is reflected by the Intergovernmental Working Group on Public Health, Innovation and Intellectual Property (IGWG),
whose Global Strategy and Plan of Action was adopted by the World Health
Assembly on 24 May 2008.[26] This group was set up in 2006 as a follow-up
to the Commission on Intellectual Property Rights, Innovation and Public Health with the aim of "securing an enhanced and sustainable basis for
needs-driven, essential health research and development relevant to diseases that disproportionately affect developing countries".[27] The IGWG considered inputs not only from governments but also from academia, public-
private partnerships, product-development partnerships and industry.[28] In

its Global Strategy, the IGWG both acknowledges that intellectual property rights are "an important incentive for the development of new health-care products" and quotes the provisions of the Universal Declaration of Human Rights on sharing in scientific advances and its benefits and protection of moral and material interest resulting from scientific production.[29]

Thus, for the IGWG, the "context" of its global strategy includes intellectual property rights, human rights and the importance of flexibilities in intellectual property agreements to facilitate "increased access to pharmaceutical products by developing countries".[30] Given the diversity of stakeholders involved, it is significant that the importance of all three was acknowledged. In enumerating the "principles" of the strategy, the IGWG inserted the following: "The enjoyment of the highest attainable standard of health is one of the fundamental rights of every human being without distinction of race, religion, political belief, economic or social condition."[31] It is clear from this effort, which will continue through the further elaboration and implementation of the elements and plan of action, that the claim of a human right to essential medicines has been a difficult case to make. But over the past decade, the tide appears to have shifted in favour of the human right to essential medicines and perhaps even more broadly to health products and medical devices.

Affirmation of the human right to essential medicines

As mentioned above, the human right to essential medicines is much broader than a claim against the negative impact of IPRs. Nevertheless, the withdrawal of the challenge by 40 pharmaceutical companies to South Africa's access to drugs law, the Doha Declaration, the deliberations of IGWG and similar events have used the tension with the international trade regime as a motivation for the affirmation of this right.

The TRIPS flexibilities provide a legal basis for poor countries to avoid the consequences of the patent system with regard to their capacity to make essential medicines available to their populations. The international trade regime is based on the logic of the global market and globalization. It has adjusted to the political imperative of promoting development and strategies defined by the international financial institutions in the poverty reduction programmes and the UN system in the Millennium Development Goals. It has not, so far, been receptive to the claim that a human right to health, including access to essential medicines, prevails over TRIPS. With the exception of the approach taken by the Working Group on Access to Essential Medicines of the UN Millennium Project (discussed above), these development approaches rarely articulate the human right to essential medicines. The affirmation of this right from the human rights perspective can be made, however, on the basis of core human rights instruments. These instruments have been applied to the problem of access to medicines by UN bodies including: the Office of the High Commissioner for Human Rights, the Commission on Human Rights and its Sub-Commission, the Committee on Economic, Social and Cultural Rights, and the Special Rapporteur on the right of everyone to the enjoyment of the highest attainable standard of physical and mental health, as well as by a number of non-governmental and academic initiatives.

The right to essential medicines in the core human rights instruments

Access to essential medicines can be affirmed as a human right on the basis, not only of the right to health (Article 12 of the International Covenant on Economic, Social and Cultural Rights (ICESCR)) but also on two other rights set out in the ICESCR, namely, the rights "to the protection of the moral and material interests resulting from any scientific, literary or artistic production" (Article 15(1)(c)) and "to share in scientific advancement and its benefits" (Article 15(1)(b)). The former is the human rights basis for intellectual property protection, according to which creative ideas and expressions of the human mind that possess commercial value receive the legal protection of property rights called "intellectual property rights" (IPRs). The major legal mechanisms for protecting IPRs are copyrights, patents, and trademarks. IPRs enable owners to select who may access and use their property, and to protect it from unauthorized use.

There is an apparent contradiction between these two rights when applied to access to medicines: Article 15(1)(c) seems to protect the "right" of pharmaceutical companies to earn a profit from the drugs they develop, by setting prices that render medicines inaccessible to the destitute sick, while Article 15(1)(b) seems to protect the "right" of those destitute sick to benefit from the development of new drugs. The way out of this dilemma is to distinguish intellectual property rights from human rights and consider them a temporary monopoly established for the valid social purpose of encouraging scientific invention and artistic creation. In other words, an IPR is a legally protected interest of a lower order than a human right, which implies a superior moral and legal claim. This distinction should not be interpreted to imply that IPRs do not have social value for, indeed, they have a very high value, justifying limiting Article 15 rights reasonably to promote innovation and creativity.

Human rights organs have progressively addressed this dilemma, articulating in different stages the human right to essential medicines. The Commission on Human Rights adopted a resolution in 2001, in which it recognized "that access to medication in the context of pandemics such as HIV/AIDS is one fundamental element for achieving progressively the full realization of the right of everyone to the enjoyment of the highest attainable standard of physical and mental health."[32] Among a list of measures, it called on states, "to refrain from taking measures which would deny or limit equal access for all persons to preventive, curative or palliative pharmaceuticals or medical technologies used to treat pandemics such as HIV/AIDS or the most common opportunistic infections that accompany them"[33] and, clearly with TRIPS in mind, "to ensure that their actions as members of international organizations take due account of the right of everyone to the enjoyment of the highest attainable standard of physical and mental health and that the application of international agreements is supportive of public health policies which promote broad access to safe, effective and affordable preventive, curative or palliative pharmaceuticals and medical technologies."[34] The United States was the only government to abstain from this resolution, which was adopted on 23 April 2001 by 52 votes with no votes against.

The Office of the High Commissioner prepared a report in 2001 on the impact of the TRIPS Agreement on human rights;[35] and the Sub-Commission on the Promotion and Protection of Human Rights took this up in its resolution the same year on "Intellectual Property Rights and Human Rights."[36] The resolution, adopted by consensus, referred to the "actual or potential conflict ... between the implementation of the TRIPS Agreement and the realization of economic, social and cultural rights."[37] In the context of the upcoming Doha Ministerial meeting of the WTO, the Sub-Commission alluded to the "need to clarify the scope and meaning of several provisions of the TRIPS Agreement, in particular of Articles 7 and 8 on the objectives and principles underlying the Agreement in order to ensure that states' obligations under the Agreement do not contradict their binding human rights obligations."[38] It reminded "all governments of the primacy of human rights obligations under international law over economic policies and agreements, and request[ed] them, in national, regional and international economic policy forums, to take international human rights obligations and principles fully into account in international economic policy formulation."[39] Significantly, it urged "all governments to ensure that the implementation of the TRIPS Agreement does not negatively impact on the enjoyment of human rights as provided for in international human rights instruments by which they are bound."[40]

One of the most significant events, legally and politically, for the right to essential medicines was indeed the Doha Ministerial meeting of the WTO, which adopted the Doha Declaration on the TRIPS Agreement and Public Health. In an unusually direct statement emanating from the WTO, better known for highly technical and legally complex sentences, the meeting declared: "The TRIPS agreement does not and should not prevent members from taking measures to protect public health ... in particular to promote access to medicines for all."[41] To be perfectly clear, the Declaration added, "In this connection, we reaffirm the right of WTO members to use, to the full, the provisions in the TRIPS Agreement, which provide flexibility for this purpose," meaning parallel importing and compulsory licensing. The text acknowledges that "[e]ach member has the right to grant compulsory licences and the freedom to determine the grounds upon which such licences are granted ... [and] the right to determine what constitutes a national emergency or other circumstances of extreme urgency, it being understood that public health crises, including those relating to HIV/AIDS, tuberculosis, malaria and other epidemics, can represent a national emergency or other circumstances of extreme urgency."[42] The next paragraph instructed the Council for TRIPS to find an expeditious solution to the problem of compulsory licensing for countries "with insufficient or no manufacturing capacities in the pharmaceutical sector,"[43] which was done in August, 2003. The Doha Declaration also extended the deadline to 1 January 2016 for the least-developed countries to apply provisions on pharmaceutical patents.

Position of the Committee on Economic, Social and Cultural Rights
The Committee threw down the gauntlet at the time of the Seattle Third Ministerial meeting of the WTO in 1999 when it "urged WTO members to ensure that their international human rights obligations are considered as a matter of priority in their negotiations which will be an important test-

ing ground for the commitment of States to the full range of their international obligations."[44] Two years later, on 26 November 2001, the Committee held a "day of general discussion" on Article 15(1)(c), following which it issued a "Statement on Human Rights and Intellectual Property", in which it considered that "intellectual property rights must be balanced with the right ... to enjoy the benefits of scientific progress and its applications."[45] It made explicit reference to the development of new medicines in the context of the Doha Declaration on the TRIPS Agreement and Public Health as an example of the need to strike a balance between the right to enjoy the benefits of scientific progress and its applications under Article 15(1)(b) and the right to benefit from the protection of the moral and material interests under Article 15(1)(c).[46] The Committee concluded by calling for "a mechanism for a human rights review of intellectual property systems."[47]

The Committee clarified further the human right to essential medicines in two of its General Comments, an earlier one on the right to health, and one based on the 2001 Statement. Indeed, in 2000, the Committee, in its General Comment No. 14, had interpreted the obligation under Covenant Article 12(2)(d) of the Covenant ("The creation of conditions which would assure to all medical service and medical attention in the event of sickness") to include "the provision of essential drugs."[48] In clarifying the obligations of states parties, the Committee included among the facilities, goods and services which must be available in sufficient quantity within the state "essential drugs, as defined by the WHO Action Programme on Essential Drugs".[49] As part of their obligation to protect, states parties have a duty "to control the marketing of medical equipment and medicines by third parties,"[50] which strongly suggests that the states should intervene where marketing of drugs by pharmaceutical companies is detrimental to the right to health.

But it was in General Comment No. 17, adopted in 2006, that the Committee challenged head-on the assumption of the international trade regime that the rights of companies holding patents over essential drugs were of the same order as the rights of those who need the drugs, by treating the former as a temporary, revocable monopoly, and the latter as human rights. Indeed, the Committee affirmed,

> "In contrast with human rights, intellectual property rights are generally of
> a temporary nature, and can be revoked, licensed or assigned to someone
> else. While under most intellectual property systems, intellectual property

rights, with the exception of moral rights, may be allocated, limited in time and scope, traded, amended and even forfeited, human rights are timeless expressions of fundamental entitlements of the human person ..."[51]

"States Parties should," the Committee continued,

"... ensure that their intellectual property regimes constitute no impediment of their ability to comply with their core obligations in relation to the right to health ... States thus have a duty to prevent that unreasonably high license fees or royalties for access to essential medicines ... undermine the right ... of large segments of the population to health ..."[52]

Non-governmental and academic promotion of the right to access essential medicines

Several non-governmental organizations (NGOs) have taken up the issue of access to medicines from a human rights perspective, principal among them are Médecins Sans Frontières (MSF) and Oxfam. In 1999, MSF launched the Campaign for Access to Essential Medicines and became the leader of the advocacy campaign aimed at improving access to existing medicines, diagnostics, and vaccines and at promoting the development of urgently needed better medical tools for people in poor countries.[53] In 2000 Oxfam also launched a major access to medicines campaign. This advocacy included focusing on a series of lawsuits from the pharmaceutical industry, including a frequently cited case against the South African government.[54]

Parallel to the advocacy work of NGOs are the vital private research initiatives, such as Management Sciences for Health (MSH), a private non-profit consultancy organization, which is headed by the former director of the WHO's essential medicines department. MSH has a strong focus on technical support and capacity building, and has expertise in supply chain management and delivery of medicines. One of its key programmes, "Strategies for Enhancing Access to Medicines", is funded by the Gates Foundation. The Gates Foundation is a major player in enhancing access to medicines, as is the Clinton Foundation, which has negotiated reduced prices for antiretrovirals by guaranteeing purchases and continuous demand. Other innovative financing mechanisms include UNITAID (which uses the proceeds of a solidarity tax on airline tickets to purchase drugs and diagnostics for HIV/AIDS, malaria and tuberculosis); Advance Market Commitments for vaccines (AMC) (which uses donor commitments to provide incentives to vaccine makers to produce vaccines for developing countries); The Global Fund to Fight AIDS, Tuberculosis and Malaria; and the United States President's Emergency Plan for AIDS Relief (PEPFAR). These efforts, however, rarely make reference to access to essential medicines as a human right.

Several academic initiatives have utilized an explicit human rights approach, including international officials and academics writing in scholarly journals.[55] A leading scholar, Thomas Pogge, has found the patent system "morally problematic" because patents on biological organisms and pharmaceutical products "directly or indirectly, impede the global poor's access to basic foodstuffs and essential medicines".[56] He proposes a "full-pull plan" (as opposed to a "push" plan, which funds a particular innovator) according to which all potential innovators, such as pharmaceutical companies, would have an equal chance for a substantial reward from public funds during the life of the patent, in proportion to the extent to which the new drug or other product reduces the global burden of disease (GBD).[57]

The University of Montréal hosted a workshop of scholars (including Pogge), national and international officials and NGO activists from 30 September to 2 October 2005, on "Human Rights and Access to Essential Medicines: The Way Forward". The meeting considered the burden of disease due to lack of access to medicines and adopted the Montréal Statement on the Human Right to Essential Medicines.[58]

After finding the current lack of access to medicines to be "contrary to ethical and legal duties, including human-rights obligations," the authors of the statement posit the obligation to make policies, rules, and institutions conducive to the realization of the right to essential medicines at the national and global levels.[59] Echoing the position taken in General Comment No. 14, the Montréal Statement, drawing on the WHO definition cited at the beginning of this chapter, defines essential medicines as "those that satisfy the priority health care needs of the population, in light of their public health relevance, proven quality, efficacy and safety, and comparative cost-effectiveness." The right to these medicines is part of the "core" obligations of parties to the ICESCR, requiring "immediate and effective measures and is not subject to progressive implementation."[60] The statement further calls on national governments in developing countries to allocate resources to making essential medicines available, and to update national lists of essential medicines, as well as to use trade flexibilities and safeguards, such as compulsory licensing and parallel importing. It calls on affluent countries to ensure fairer trade relations, alleviate crippling debt and increase assistance to facilitate this right.[61] Finally, the statement takes issue with the present system of incentives for innovation, which is based on "return on investment rather than priority health needs and outcomes", and advocates "alternative innovation systems that ensure that research and development are sufficient to meet priority health needs."[62]

Building on the Montréal Statement, a group of institutions, from Québec and Brazil, organized a workshop at the Université de Quebec on 20 November 2007, evaluating, from the right to development perspective, Target 17 of the Millennium Development Goals.[63] Other academic initiatives include Universities Allied for Essential Medicines (UAEM), which adopted the Philadelphia Consensus Statement at their annual conference held in Philadelphia at the beginning of October 2006, stating: "We believe that access to medical care and treatment is a basic human right."[64]

Draft Guidelines by the Special Rapporteur

As part of his mandate as UN Special Rapporteur on the right of everyone to the enjoyment of the highest attainable standard of physical and mental health, Paul Hunt submitted a report to the General Assembly in 2006 summarizing the responsibilities of states and of pharmaceutical companies with respect to access to medicines,[65] and circulated on 19 September 2007, a "Draft for Consultation" of a set of "Human Rights Guidelines for Pharmaceutical Companies in relation to Access to Medicines".[66]

Following consultation with states, NGOs, academics, pharmaceutical companies, UN agencies, national human rights institutions and other stakeholders, Hunt presented the Guidelines to the General Assembly in 2008, explaining that "the central objective of the Guidelines is to provide practical, constructive and specific guidance to pharmaceutical companies and other interested parties, including those who wish to monitor companies and hold them to account."[67] These forty-seven Guidelines deal with general policy; the disadvantaged; transparency; management, monitoring and accountability; corruption; public policy influence, advocacy and lobbying; quality; clinical trials; neglected diseases; patents and licensing; pricing, discounting and donations; ethical promotion and marketing; public-private partnerships; and associations of pharmaceutical companies. They call upon companies to recognize the importance of human rights in their corporate mission and provide board-level responsibility and accountability for its access to medicines strategy, with a public commitment to contribute to research and development for neglected diseases, and respect the right of countries to use TRIPS flexibilities. The Guidelines then address questions of management, including "an effective, transparent, accessible and independent monitoring and accountability mechanism", both internal and external, as well as participation from a human rights perspective. Other Guidelines would have companies comply with various international standards on corruption, good manufacturing practice, human subject research, and other areas. Special provisions relate to promoting research and development on neglected diseases. Regarding patents and licensing, the Guidelines call on drug companies to "respect the right of countries to use, to the full, the provisions ... TRIPS ..., which allow flexibility for the purpose of promoting access to medicines, including the provisions relating to compulsory licensing and parallel imports" and "respect the letter and spirit of the Doha Declaration ..."

Conclusion

The human right to essential medicines is a derivative right from the rights to health and to life. When the main human rights instruments were drafted, the idea that lack of access to medicines was contrary to human rights was not considered, except that access to medicines was one of a number of reasonable measures constituting healthcare. Subsequently, and particularly as a result of the AIDS pandemic, the vital need for treatment of HIV positive individuals contributed to the progressive acknowledgement that access to essential medicines, including antiretroviral treatments (ARTs), was an internationally recognized human right. This argument has been extended from HIV/AIDS to the full range of diseases that account for the disproportionate levels of mortality and morbidity in developing countries.

It may be useful to draw a parallel with the emergence of an implied derivative human right to water, formally acknowledged by the Committee on Economic, Social and Cultural Rights in 2002 in its General Comment No. 15 on the Right to Water.[68] The analogy with the right to water is reinforced by drawing on three main arguments used by the Committee, one based on evidence, one on logic, and the third on legal construction.

First, knowledge of the problem of water, created by the failure to guarantee access to it, was uncontested and acknowledged as requiring urgent action. The Committee noted that "[o]ver one billion persons lack access to a basic water supply, while several billion do not have access to adequate sanitation, which is the primary cause of water contamination and diseases linked to water."[69] Nearly two billion people do not have access to essential medicines and an estimated four million people could be saved annually in Africa and Southeast Asia if diagnosis and treatment with appropriate medicines were available. The criteria of magnitude and urgency of the problem are therefore met.

The second argument is based on a logical construction, according to which water as a human right is a necessary consequence of the nature of this commodity. The Committee argues as follows: "Water is a limited natural resource and a public good fundamental for life and health. The human right to water is indispensable for leading a life in human dignity. It is a prerequisite for the realization of other human rights."[70] Appropriate medicines are similarly indispensable to the health of people everywhere and the most basic drugs are a public good.[71]

The third basis for positing the right to water as a human right was the legal interpretation of existing human rights norms. The title of General Comment No. 15 mentions Articles 11 and 12 of the International Covenant on Economic, Social and Cultural Rights and the Committee explains how these two rights (adequate standard of living and health) are "inextricably related" to the right to water. The Committee relates the right to water to other human rights, including inter alia the right to life, the right to adequate food, the right to gain a living by work, the right to take part in cultural life. The right to essential medicines is similarly inseparable from the rights to an adequate standard of living, education, food, and housing.

Following the pattern of other general comments, the Committee then addresses the normative content of the right to water in terms of availability, quality, accessibility, and information, and devotes special attention to issues of discrimination and vulnerable groups. The Working Group on Access to Medicines organized its analysis and recommendations into three main categories: Availability, affordability, and appropriateness,[72] and then deals with quality[73] as well as crosscutting issues of human resources and gender.[74] In other words, the full range of essential and interrelated elements of the rights that treaty bodies cover in their general comments are applicable to the human right to essential medicines.

The developments described in this chapter are signs that the human right to essential medicines has advanced in terms of its normative content and its legal recognition, although it remains a daunting challenge to find accommodation with the international trade regime, bridge the gaps in political will, find incentives for innovation and affordable pricing, and create the availability of adequate human and financial resources to ensure distribution networks. All this needs to be achieved in order for this right to be of practical value for the two billion who currently lack access to essential medicines.

1 Andrew Clapham, *Human Rights Obligation of Non-State Actors* (Oxford: Oxford University Press, 2006), at 175.

2 Committee on Economic, Social and Cultural Rights, *General Comment No. 17 on the right of everyone to benefit from the protection of the moral and material interests resulting from any scientific, literary or artistic production of which he or she is the author*, UN doc. E/C.12/GC/17, 12 January, 2006, para. 35.

3 World Health Organization, 'Essential Medicines: Definition', available at http://www.who.int/medicines/services/essmedicines_def/en/. See also MDG Gap Task Force, *Millennium Development Goal 8: Delivering on the Global Partnership for Achieving the Millennium Development Goals: MDG Gap Task Force Report 2008* (New York: United Nations, 2008) at 36.

4 MDG Gap Task Force, *supra* note 3, at 35.

5 UN Millennium Project, *Prescription for Healthy Development: Increasing Access to Medicines, Report of Task Force on HIV/AIDS, Malaria, TB and Access to Essential Medicines*, Working Group on Access to Essential Medicines, 2005, at 4.

6 World Health Organization, *WHO Medicines Strategy 2000–2003: Framework for Action in Essential Drugs and Medicines Policy 2000–2003* (Geneva: WHO, 2000), available at www.who.int/medicines/strategy/strategy2000=2003.shtml.

7 The WHO Medicines Strategy 2004–2007, (Geneva: WHO, 2004), WHO/EDM/2004.5, p. 3.

8 MDG Gap Task Force, *supra* note 3, at 42.

9 Ibid., at 1.

10 Ibid., at 29–31.

11 Ibid., at 35.

12 Ibid., at 106.

13 Ibid., at 106–110.

14 Ibid., at 110–118.

15 Ibid., at 72–73.

16 Ibid., at 136.

17 TRIPS Art. 31 provides for the use of a patented product without the authorization of the right holder, under the following condition: "(f) Any such use shall be authorized predominantly for the supply of the domestic market of the Member authorizing such use;" and "(h) The right holder shall be paid adequate remuneration in the circumstances of each case, taking into account the

economic value of the authorization." Thus, compulsory licensing is not available to many countries without a significant pharmaceutical sector.

18 Amir Attaran, 'How Do Patents And Economic Policies Affect Access To Essential Medicines In Developing Countries?' 23(3) *Health Affairs* (2004), 155–156, at 157.

19 Ibid., at 159.

20 Ibid., at 161.

21 E-DRUG, 'WHO Model List of Essential Medicines and Patents', posting on essentialdrugs.org by Hans Hogerzeil on 23 March 2005, available at http://www.essentialdrugs.org/edrug/archive/200503/msg00071.php.

22 The WHO essential medicines strategy has the following seven components: (1) National policies on medicines; (2) National policies on traditional medicine and complementary and alternative medicine; (3) Sustainable financing mechanisms for medicines; (4) Supplying medicines; (5) Norms and standards for pharmaceuticals; (6) Regulation and quality assurance of medicines; (7) Using medicines rationally: World Health Organization, *WHO Medicines Strategy 2004–2007: Countries at the Core*, WHO publication No. WHO/EDM/2004.5, 2004, at 25–129.

23 Lisa Forman, "'Rights' and Wrongs: What Utility for the Right to Health in Reforming Trade Rules on Medicines?" 10(2) *Health and Human Rights: An International Journal* (2008).

24 Ibid.

25 Ibid.

26 WHO Resolution 61.21 adopted by the Sixty-first World Health Assembly on 24 May 2008. It is significant for the purpose of the present examination of the tensions between international trade and human rights to note the shift in the title of the Commission to that of the IGWG with respect both to the order of the terms and the deletion of "rights" attached to "intellectual property".

27 WHO Resolution 59.24 adopted by the Fifty-ninth World Health Assembly on 27 May 2006, para. 3.

28 World Health Organization, *Public Health, Innovation, and Intellectual Property: Progress Made by the Intergovernmental Working Group*, Report by

the Secretariat, 5 April 2007, WHO publication number A60/27, para. 4.

29 World Health Organization, *Global Strategy and Plan of Action on Public Health, Innovation, and Intellectual Property*, 24 May 2008, WHO publication number WHA61.21, annex, paras. 7 and 10.

30 Ibid., para. 12.

31 This language, taken form the WHO constitution, was retained after an additional provision on human rights was deleted following a divisive debate.

32 Commission on Human Rights resolution 2001/33, Access to medication in the context of pandemics such as HIV/AIDS, UN Doc. E/CN.4/RES/2001/33, 20 April 2001, para. 1.

33 Ibid., para. 3(a).

34 Ibid., para. 4(b).

35 UN Doc. E/CN.4/Sub.2/2001/13, 27 June 2001.

36 The Sub-Commission on the Promotion and Protection of Human Rights, Intellectual Property Rights and Human Rights, resolution 2001/21, UN Doc. E/CN.4/SUB.2/RES/2001/21, 16 August 2001.

37 Ibid., preamble.

38 Ibid.

39 Ibid., para. 3.

40 Ibid., para. 5.

41 World Trade Organization, Ministerial Conference, Fourth Session, Doha, 9–14 November 2001, Declaration on the TRIPS agreement and public health, adopted on 14 November 2001, Doc. WT/MIN(01)/DEC/2, 20 November 2001, para. 4, available at http://www.wto.org/English/thewto_e/minist_e/min01_e/mindecl_trips_e.htm.

42 Ibid., para. 5.

43 Ibid., para. 6.

44 *Statement of the United Nations Committee on Economic, Social and Cultural Rights to the Third Ministerial Conference of the World Trade Organization* (Seattle, 30 November to 3 December 1999), UN Doc. E/C.12/1999/9, 26 November 1999, para. 8.

45 *Human Rights and Intellectual Property: Statement by the Committee on Economic Social and Cultural Rights*, UN Doc. E/C.12/2001/15, 14 December 2001, para. 4.

46 Ibid., para. 17.

47 Ibid., para. 18.

48 Committee on Economic, Social and Cultural Rights (CESCR), *General Comment No. 14 on the right to the highest attainable standard of health*, 11 August 2000, UN Doc. E/C.12/2000/4, at para. 17.

49 Ibid., para. 12 (a).

50 Ibid., para. 35.

51 CESCR, *supra* note 2, at para. 2.

52 Ibid., para. 35.

53 MSF's Campaign is described at http://www.accessmed-msf.org/.

54 At the national level, major advances in the right to essential medicines were made by such NGOs as Treatment Action Campaign (TAC) in South Africa, which sued the South African government for not providing to pregnant women a drug known to reduce mother-to-child-transmission (MTCT) of HIV and won this case on the basis of the South African constitutional guarantee of the right to health: *Treatment Action Campaign (TAC) v Minister of Health*, Constitutional Court (2002) 5 SA 721 (CC). For other examples of judicial recognition of the right to essential medicines as part of the right to health, see Hans V. Hogerzeil et al. 'Is access to essential medicines as part of the fulfillment of the right to health enforceable through the courts?' 368 *The Lancet* (2006) 305–311; Mary Ann Torres 'The Human Right to Health, National Courts, and Access to HIV/AIDS Treatment: A Case Study from Venezuela,' 3(1) *Chicago Journal of International Law* (2002) 105–114.

55 See for example, Phillippe Cullet, 'Human Rights and Intellectual Property Protection in the TRIPS Era' 29(2) *Human Rights Quarterly* (2007) 403–430; Carlos María Correa, 'Implications of Bilateral Free Trade Agreements on Access to Medicines' 84(5) *Bulletin of the World Health Organization* (2006) 399–404; Michael A. Santoro, 'Human Rights and Human Needs, Diverse Moral Principles Justifying Third World Access to Affordable IV/AIDS Drugs' 31(4) *North Carolina Journal of International Law and Commercial Regulation* (2006) 923–942; Lisa Forman, 'Trade Rules, Intellectual Property, and the Right to Health', 21(3) *Ethics & International Affairs*, Volume (Fall 2007), 337–357. Hans V. Hogerzeil, 'Essential Medicines and Human Rights: What Can They Learn from Each Other?' 84(5) *Bulletin of the World Health Organization* (2006) 371–375, at 371; Hans Hogerzeil, 'Access to Essential Medicines as a Human Right' 33 *Essential Drugs Monitor* (2000) 25–26; Thomas Pogge, *World Poverty and Human Rights: Cosmopolitan Responsibilities and Reforms*, Second expanded edition (UK and Malden MA: Polity Press 2008), chapter 9 entitled 'Pharmaceutical Innovation: Must We Exclude the Poor?', 222–261.

56 Pogge, *supra* note 55, at 233.

57 Ibid., at 244–261. Under certain conditions, Norman Daniels considers that Pogge's incentive schemes could be "a way of moving some countries closer to satisfying a right to health, connecting the effort to human rights goals as he does.": Norman Daniels, *Just Health: Meeting Health Needs Fairly* (New York: Cambridge University Press, 2008), at 353.

58 The text is available in Thomas Pogge, 'Montréal Statement on the Human Right to Essential Medicines' 16(1) *Cambridge Quarterly of Healthcare Ethics* (2007), at 104–108.

59 Ibid., para. 3.

60 Ibid., paras. 4–5.

61 Ibid., paras. 6–11.

62 Ibid., paras. 14–15.

63 The participating institutions were l'Association pour la santé publique du Québec, Initiative luso-francophone sur l'accès au medicament et la protection du citoyen, Program on Human Rights in Development of the Harvard School of Public Health, Canadian Institutes of Health Research, le Réseau de recherche en santé des populations du Québec, and le Groupe d'étude sur l'interdisciplinarité et les représentations sociales de l'UQAM. Target 17 of the MDGs has been renumbered Target 8E.

64 See www.essentialmedicine.org.

65 Paul Hunt, *Report of the Special Rapporteur on the right to health*, 13 September 2006, UN Doc. A/61/338.

66 The online version of the Guidelines was made available at http://www2.essex.ac.uk/human_rights_centre/rth/.

67 Paul Hunt, *Report of the Special Rapporteur on the right to health,* 11 August 2008, UN Doc. A/63/263, at para. 46. Quotations from the Guidelines are from the version in the annex to that document.

68 CESCR, *General Comment No. 15 on the right to water,* 20 January 2003, UN Doc. E/C.12/2002/11 (2002).

69 The Committee cited WHO data for this claim. See, ibid., para. 1, note 1.

70 Ibid.

71 The full implications and related strategy for treating access to essential medicines as a public good are presented by Thomas Pogge in 'Human Rights and Global Health: A Research Program' which first appeared in Christian Barry and Thomas Pogge (eds.), 'Global Institutions and Responsibilities: Achieving Global Justice', special issue of *Metaphilosophy,* 36(1–2), January 2005, and currently available as 'Chapter 9: Pharmaceutical Innovation: Must We Exclude the Poor?', Pogge, *supra* note 55. The claim that essential medicines are a public good means that the innovation (formula for a new drug, device, etc.) is non-rivalrous, i.e., use of the formula for a drug to benefit one population will not compete with a similar use for another population, which is clearly the case if pharmaceutical knowledge is freely available. It must also be non-excludable, i.e., no one can be effectively excluded from access, which requires that the prices be brought down to the long-term marginal cost of production (as Pogge points out, *supra* note 55, at 240–244 and 264). As long as there is a temporary monopoly provided by the patent regime, essential medicines cannot be a public good.

72 *Supra* note 5, 58–82.

73 Ibid., 82–85.

74 Ibid., 21–22.

Advancing a Human Rights Approach on the Global Health Agenda

Lisa Oldring and Scott Jerbi*

Introduction

Increased attention to global health presents opportunities for governments to advance other shared objectives, including promotion of the broad international human rights agenda.

While some countries have pledged to integrate the promotion of human rights across all areas of foreign policy, in general terms policy approaches have concentrated primarily on civil and political rights issues such as the promotion of democratic governance and the rule of law. Relatively little emphasis has been placed on using the human rights framework concerning economic, social and cultural rights, including the right to the highest attainable standard of health, to advance international development or humanitarian objectives.

Recent foreign policy proposals in some countries and within inter-governmental fora suggest this may be changing. This chapter explores opportunities for integrating human rights into global health policy agendas, international development and aid effectiveness initiatives, and policies and partnerships to address specific global health challenges.

Global health and human rights on the international agenda

National health policies and strategies increasingly include a global health dimension, and governments in some countries are striving to improve coherence across domestic and foreign policies to address global health.[1] The increased attention to global health on foreign policy agendas has been motivated by a range of factors, such as national security interests, as well as by humanitarian concern and recognition of greater interdependence between nations brought about by the forces of globalization. This trend has created an important opportunity to improve health outcomes around the world.

Increased attention to global health also presents opportunities for governments to advance other shared objectives including promotion of the broad international human rights agenda, which includes the human right to the highest attainable standard of health. However, rarely has health been discussed as a matter of human rights in foreign policy settings at national, regional or global levels.

Since the adoption of the Universal Declaration of Human Rights in 1948, all states have endorsed the principle that human rights and freedoms are inalienable and inherent to all people. The principles of the Universal Declaration are now well-enshrined in international law, and civil, cultural, economic, political and social rights are reflected in a comprehensive framework of international and regional treaties, as well as in domestic constitutions and laws. At the same time, it must be acknowledged that traditional conceptions of norms concerning state sovereignty and non-intervention have, and in some cases continue to, come into conflict with global consensus around human rights and efforts by some governments to prioritize human rights in their foreign policies.

The Vienna Declaration and Programme of Action, adopted at the 1993 World Conference on Human Rights, asserted the promotion and protection of all human rights as both "a legitimate concern of the international community" and a "priority objective" of the United Nations (UN), and reaffirmed the universal and indivisible character of human rights. The establishment of ad hoc international criminal tribunals in the 1990's, and the subsequent creation of a permanent International Criminal Court, further signalled the commitment of the international community to ensure accountability for human rights abuses. The 2000 UN Millennium Summit reaffirmed global commitment to the Universal Declaration and to the broad international human rights framework, while legal developments in many countries have demonstrated the way in which human rights are given practical meaning at national and local levels.

More recently, at the 2005 World Summit, all UN Member States affirmed their primary responsibility to prevent crimes against humanity, war crimes, genocide and ethnic cleansing through "appropriate and necessary means".[2] They agreed that if they fail to do so, the international community, through the United Nations, must use "appropriate diplomatic, humanitarian and other peaceful means, in accordance with Chapters VI and VIII of the Charter", to help protect populations from such crimes. While the practical implications have yet to be explored, by committing to the "responsibility to protect" the international community has acknowledged that serious human rights violations, in and of themselves, require an international response.

Although the implicit tension between state sovereignty and the protection of individuals under international human rights law persists, today the notion that human rights are a legitimate concern of the international community is beyond challenge, and the indivisible and inter-dependent nature of human rights is now widely recognized. Economic, social and cultural rights have increasingly figured prominently on international human rights agendas, alongside issues of civil and political rights.[3]

While the contours and content of economic, social and cultural rights are yet to be fully explored and articulated, there is now a deeper appreciation of their importance to human dignity and well-being. There is also greater clarity around the principle of progressive realization, which guides the way in which these rights are to be implemented.[4] This principle recognizes that, particularly in resource-poor countries, economic, social and cultural rights may only be achieved over time. Nonetheless, states have an immediate obligation to ensure respect for these rights without discrimination, and to undertake all appropriate means towards their implementation, within the maximum extent of their available resources – including through international cooperation and assistance.

Health and human rights

Today there is growing recognition of the links between health and a wide range of human rights, as well as a growing appreciation of the right to the highest attainable standard of health itself. There is broad agreement that health policies, programmes and practices can have a direct bearing on the enjoyment of human rights, while a lack of respect for human rights can have serious health consequences.[5] Protecting human rights is recognized as key to protecting public health.

Policy interventions that are grounded in human rights with a strong gender dimension can help inform and strengthen public health responses.

Attention to the human rights principles of non-discrimination and equality can highlight differential treatment of distinct population groups, moving beyond averages to focus attention on the health needs of vulnerable or marginalized groups, and thus help to ensure that health systems meet the health needs of all segments of a population. Engaging individuals and communities actively in decisions bearing upon their health, including the development and implementation of health policies, strategies and programmes, helps ensure, for example, that disease-specific programmes do not skew the delivery of health interventions. By placing individuals at the centre of a health system, human rights provide a powerful standard by which to ensure that the health needs of all members of society are being met.

International human rights mechanisms regularly monitor health-related human rights issues within the scope of their mandates. The Committee on Economic, Social and Cultural Rights and other treaty monitoring bodies have clarified the normative content of the right to health, and regularly analyse foreign and domestic policies relevant to health through their consideration of country reports.[6]

In addition to various resolutions on the right to the highest attainable standard of health, the United Nations Human Rights Council and its predecessor, the Commission on Human Rights, have emphasized the need for intensified efforts to promote human rights in order to reduce vulnerability to HIV/AIDS, prevent HIV-related discrimination and stigmatization, and improve access to treatment.[7] The Human Rights Council now addresses health issues through its universal periodic review of the fulfilment by each state of its human rights obligations and commitments,[8] as well as through the work of the UN human rights special procedures. The UN Special Rapporteur on the right to health has examined states' domestic and foreign policies and practices through various country missions[9] and visits to international organizations, including the World Trade Organization, the International Monetary Fund and the World Bank.[10] Most recently, at the Human Rights Council, an optional protocol to the International Covenant on Economic, Social and Cultural Rights was adopted, which will make it possible for individuals, groups, or organizations acting on their behalf to seek justice at the international level for violations of the right to health and other economic, social and cultural rights.[11] These developments have helped to secure health prominently on the international human rights agenda.

Health and human rights in foreign policy: Recent examples

While a number of countries have incorporated human rights as a pillar of their foreign policy, few make explicit reference to the fulfilment of health-related human rights in this context. Recent foreign policy proposals in some countries suggest this may be changing. Some states have adopted a limited approach to human rights in their foreign policy through a commitment to respect, or "do no harm", in relation to health-related human rights, while others pursue a more robust foreign policy agenda which mirrors their domestic human rights commitments, including respect, protection and fulfilment of health-related human rights.

The Commission on the Future of Health Care in Canada underscored the promotion of human rights, including the right to health, as a fundamental principle of Canadian foreign policy and suggested that access to health care must become both a domestic policy priority and a key foreign policy objective.[12] A proposal for a government-wide global health strategy in the United Kingdom (UK) has set out a more limited objective of ensuring that the UK's domestic and foreign policies "do not prevent others from the progressive benefit"[13] of health-related human rights. The proposal notes that the UK global health strategy will have to ensure "that UK foreign and domestic policies – for example on trade, aid and debt relief – fully support and do not diminish countries' abilities to promote and protect the right to the highest attainable standard of health and the underlying determinants of health."[14]

While human rights have yet to become a mainstream part of foreign policy-making in the context of global health, governments have increasingly pursued health-related human rights objectives through policies adopted under the auspices of multilateral organizations. The 11th World Health Organization (WHO) General Programme of Work (GPW), adopted by the World Health Assembly in May 2006, outlines the promotion of health-related human rights, universal coverage, and gender equality as priority areas for all stakeholders to pursue as part of a global health agenda through 2015.[15] The GPW recalls the obligations of governments to work for the progressive realization of health-related human rights, and sets out the elements required to improve access to essential health services for the poor and other marginalized groups, including through health systems characterized by adequate and equitable financing and distribution of reliable health care; expanding access to sexual and reproductive health care for all; and ensuring the right of all groups in society to participate in the design,

implementation and monitoring of health policies, programmes and legislation. Human rights considerations also underpin the public health security provisions reflected in the revised International Health Regulations
(IHR), which entered into force on 15 June 2007.[16] For the first time, the
IHR provide explicitly for the protection of the human rights of travellers,
including respect for gender, socio-cultural, ethnic or religious considerations, and must be implemented "with full respect for the dignity, human
rights and fundamental freedoms of persons".

Human rights also have figured centrally in negotiations towards a
global strategy on health research and development. In its final report to
the World Health Assembly in 2006, the WHO Commission on Intellectual Property Rights, Innovation and Public Health underscored the human
rights imperative, both moral and legal, behind the need for solutions to
improve health outcomes in developing countries through the health innovation cycle.[17]

Building on the recommendations of the Commission, the World Health
Assembly tasked the WHO Inter-governmental Working Group on Public
Health, Innovation and Intellectual Property with developing a global strategy for identifying needs and promoting the discovery, development, and
delivery of medicines, with particular attention to neglected diseases that
primarily affect poor countries. In its final report to the World Health Assembly, the Working Group took forward many of the Commission's recommendations, although it was unable to achieve consensus at its final session
on a number of provisions, including language related to the implementation of states' health-related human rights obligations.[18] The Plan of Action
adopted by the WHA at its 61st session recognizes the right of everyone to
the enjoyment of the highest attainable standard of health, and aims to
promote new thinking on innovation and access to medicines and to provide a framework for essential health research and development.

Looking ahead: Opportunities for advancing human rights through health and foreign policy

Many factors tend to influence the place of human rights on a state's foreign policy agenda. Some countries have pledged to integrate human
rights across all areas of foreign policy, including through regional and global organizations.[19] Advancing the right to health in particular can help
to strengthen the coherence of states' human rights agendas, as well as

support the furthering of traditional human rights concerns such as democracy and rule of law. The effective implementation of health programmes at the national level requires, for example, transparency of information, accountability mechanisms and effective participation of affected communities. In short, the health agenda can serve as a platform, or entry point, for advancing a range of other human rights through foreign policy. By pursuing the integration of global health issues as matters of human rights, foreign ministries cannot only protect vital national interests, but also help advance their commitment to promoting human rights around the world.

Looking to the future, it seems likely that the links between health and human rights will become more prominent on government foreign policy agendas. A growing number of global initiatives point to the need for common frameworks and tools both to address the ethical and legal dimensions of global health policies, and to ensure greater accountability to affected individuals and communities. These include initiatives aimed at strengthening failing and inadequate health systems, increasing financing for health, addressing the global shortage of health workers and the migration of health professionals from the global south, and efforts to promote women's health, among others.

What steps should be taken to ensure that these global health policy initiatives are grounded in human rights and gender equality? What more could be done to advance human rights and gender equality through the work of global health partnerships, such as the GAVI Alliance and the Global Fund to Fight AIDS, Tuberculosis and Malaria? Equally important, what steps can be taken to ensure that human rights and gender equality are harnessed, for example, through development of relevant indicators and assessments, to advance the implementation of the Paris Declaration on Aid Effectiveness and achievement of the health-related Millennium Development Goals (MDGs)?

As a first step, urging governments to promote greater integration of health-related human rights into global health policy initiatives is a clear advocacy objective. WHO governing bodies have a critical role to play in fostering greater policy coherence with the UN human rights system around health-related human rights and the global health agenda. At the same time, the UN Human Rights Council should ensure that its thematic activities contribute to the promotion of human rights on global health agendas. Similarly, global health partnerships should strive towards greater coherence between their policies and programmes, and Member States' human rights commitments. The recent adoption by the GAVI Alliance of a gender policy, which aims to "promote increased coverage, effectiveness and efficiency of immunization and related health services by ensuring that all girls and boys, women and men, receive equal access to these services,"[20] is one example. Through this new policy the Alliance commits to "exercise leadership, and promote coordinated international efforts towards, the realization of existing international commitments to gender equality and health equity."

Making the case that it is not only in the national interest of governments to take such steps, but that such steps also contribute to better health outcomes for all, remains a challenge. Greater efforts should be made to highlight good practice examples which reveal the practical benefits of a human rights approach to health. By integrating human rights and global health as part of a coherent domestic and foreign policy, governments can contribute to improving global health outcomes while advancing shared commitments to human rights and the rule of law.

* This chapter is based on a background paper entitled 'Priority Areas for Action: Human Rights' prepared by Realizing Rights: The Ethical Globalization Initiative for the WHO Symposium on Foreign Policy and Global Health, May 2008.

1 See, for example, *Agreement on Foreign Health Policy Objectives,* adopted by the Swiss Federal Department of Foreign Affairs and the Swiss Federal Department of Home Affairs, 9 October 2006, available at www.bag.admin.ch/internatinal; R. Romanow, *Building on Values: The Future of Health Care in Canada* (Ottawa: Commission on the Future of Health Care in Canada; 2002), available at http://www.hc-sc.gc.ca/english/care/romanow/; *Council Conclusions on Health in All Policies* (HiAP), 2767th Employment, Social Policy, Health and Consumer Affairs Council meeting, Brussels, 30

November and 1 December 2006, available at www.eu2006.fi/news_and_documents/conclusions/vko48/en_GB1164897086637; United Kingdom Department of Health, *Health is Global: Proposals for a UK Government-Wide Strategy* (London: Department of Health Publications, 2007), available at http://www.dh.gov.uk/en/Publicationsandstatistics/Publications/PublicationsPolicyAndGuidance/DH_072697.

2 General Assembly resolution A/RES/60/1, 24 October 2005, paras. 138–139.

3 See UN Office of the High Commissioner for Human Rights, *Economic, Social and Cultural Rights: Information and Resources,* available at http://www2.ohchr.org/english/issues/escr/escr-general-info.htm#OHCHRpublic.

4 Economic and Social Council, *Report of the Unit-*

ed Nations High Commissioner for Human Rights, 25 June 2007, UN Doc. E/2007/82; Paul Hunt, *Report of the Special Rapporteur on the right to health to the General Assembly,* August 2007, UN Doc. A/62/214, 8; Paul Hunt, *Report of the Special Rapporteur on the right to health to the Commission on Human Rights,* 3 March 2006, UN Doc. E/CN.4/2006/48.

5 See WHO, *25 Questions & Answers on Health and Human Rights,* WHO Health and Human Rights Publication Series, Issue No. 1, July 2002, available at http://www.who.int/hhr/information/25%20 Questions%20and%20Answers%20on%20Health %20and%20Human%20Rights.pdf. See also Jonathan Mann et al. (eds.), *Health and Human Rights: A Reader* (New York: Routledge, 1999); and Sophia Gruskin et al. (eds.), *Perspectives on Health and Human Rights* (New York: Routledge, 2005).

6 See for example, ibid.; CEDAW, *General Recommendation No. 24 on women and health,* 20th session, 1999, UN Doc. A/54/38; Committee on the Rights of the Child (CRC), *General Comment No. 3 on HIV/AIDS and the rights of the child,* 17 March 2003, UN Doc. CRC/GC/2003/3; and CRC, *General Comment No. 4 on adolescent health,* 1 July 2003, UN Doc. CRC/GC/2003/4.

7 See, for example, Commission on Human Rights resolution 2005/84; *Report of the Secretary General on the protection of human rights in the context of HIV/AIDS,* 2 February 2007, UN Doc. A/HRC/4/110,; Human Rights Council decision 2/107, 'Access to medication in the context of pandemics such as HIV/AIDS, tuberculosis and malaria', 27 December 2006.

8 Human Rights Council resolution 5/1, 18 June 2007.

9 See, for example, Paul Hunt, *Report of the Special Rapporteur on the right to health: Mission to Sweden,* 28 February 2007, UN Doc. A/HRC/4/28/Add.2.

10 See the reports of the Special Rapporteur: Paul Hunt, *Report of the Special Rapporteur on the right to health: Mission to the World Bank, IMF and Uganda,* 5 March 2008, A/HRC/7/11/Add.2; and Paul Hunt, *Report of the Special Rapporteur on the Right to Health: Mission to the World Trade Organization,* 1 March 2004, E/CN.4/2004/49/Add.1.

11 See Human Rights Council resolution A/HRC/8/2 of 18 June 2008, and annex containing the Optional Protocol to the International Covenant on Economic, Social and Cultural Rights.

12 Romanow, *supra* note 1, at 240.

13 UK Department of Health, *supra* note 1, at 47.

14 Ibid., at 47.

15 *Engaging for Health, supra* note 6.

16 The International Health Regulations establish a legal framework "to prevent, protect against, control and provide a public health response to the international spread of disease in ways that are commensurate with and restricted to public health risks, and which avoid unnecessary interference with international traffic and trade": *Revision of the International Health Regulations,* 58th World Health Assembly, WHA58.3, Agenda item 13.1 (23 May 2005), available at www.who.int/csr/ihr/en/.

17 *Report of the WHO Commission on Intellectual Property Rights, Innovation and Public Health,* CIPIH/2006/1.

18 *Report of the Inter-Governmental Working Group on Public Health, Innovation and Intellectual Property,* A61/9, 19 May 2008, available at www.who.int/gb/ebwha/pdf_files/A61/A61_9-en.pdf.

19 See, for example, *Human Rights in Swedish Foreign Policy,* Government Communications 1997/98:89 and 2003/04:20.

20 *The GAVI Alliance Gender Policy,* GAVI Alliance and Fund Board Meeting 25–26 June 2008, Doc No. AF.2, available at www.gavialliance.org/resour ces/2_The_GAVI_Alliance_Gender_Policy.pdf.

02

PRIORITIZING WOMEN'S HEALTH

On the "Rights" Track: The Importance of a Rights-Based Approach to Reducing Maternal Deaths

Helen de Pinho

The Millennium Development Goals (MDGs), in particular MDG 5, have sharpened the world's focus on the critical need to reduce maternal mortality. Commitments have been made. One hundred and eighty nine countries signed on to the MDGs, committing their governments to achieving a 75% reduction in maternal mortality (based on the the 1990 figure) by the year 2015. International development partners have committed significant resources towards decreasing the number of women and newborns dying as a result of obstetric complications. NGOs have committed to advocating for action globally and locally to reduce maternal deaths. And at national levels in most developing countries there exists a strategic plan, a Road Map, a programme of work, even a budget – all geared towards reducing maternal mortality. But there has been little action. There is a huge gap between the plans and the actions, the rhetoric and the reality. It is generally recognized that of all the MDGs, progress towards meeting MDG 5 is deemed to have stalled.[1]

And yet the causes of maternal deaths are known, the interventions have been clearly articulated and the WHO estimates that 88–98% of maternal deaths are preventable.[2] Direct obstetric causes, which make up about 80% of all maternal deaths, are due to haemorrhage, pregnancy related hypertension and eclampsia, sepsis, complications secondary to unsafe abortions and obstructed labour. Increasingly in some countries, women are also dying of causes related to HIV or malaria.

There is general consensus that a three-pronged strategy is necessary to re-duce these maternal deaths: All women must have access to contraception to avoid unintended pregnancies; all pregnant women must have access to skilled care at the time of birth; and all women who experience complica-tions in pregnancy and childbirth must have timely access to quality emer-gency obstetric care.[3] This in turn requires a functioning and sustainable health system that engages communities and facilities[4] and that makes sure that health services are accessible to all women where the notion of accessi-bility encompasses principles of affordability, acceptability and availability.

The task is enormous. In many developing countries, the capacity of health systems to respond to the quiet tsunami of maternal deaths is ques-tionable. In these countries, health systems have deteriorated over the past three decades, some as a result of conflict, others because of a systematic undermining of government health systems and, in a handful of countries, as a result of inadequate governance.

Strengthening health systems will take more than simply tinkering around the edges. It will require a fundamental reframing of how govern-ments perceive health systems, the health care they deliver, and specifically how they take action to reduce maternal deaths. As Lynn Freedman indi-cates in her chapter in this book, it is no longer about "business as usual".

Why the need to reframe the way in which governments and develop-ment partners think about health systems? In short – history matters.

In 1985, at the end of the UN Decade for Women, the World Health Organization (WHO) reported that over 500 000 women per year were dy-ing as a result of obstetric complications. In the same year, Allan Rosen-field and Deborah Maine published their seminal article, "Maternal Mor-tality – A Neglected Tragedy: Where is the M in MCH [Maternal and Child Health]?",[5] challenging public health specialists to explain why most of the interventions traditionally bundled into maternal health care packages benefited the child and failed to address the key causes of maternal deaths. These two critical events galvanized the international community to focus on this previously disregarded and hidden crisis and led to the 1987 Safe Motherhood Conference in Kenya.[6]

The Nairobi Safe Motherhood Conference launched the Safe Mother-hood Initiative which, in turn, saw the formation of the Safe Motherhood Inter-Agency Group and a series of regional and national conferences that sought to entrench safe motherhood as an "accepted and understood term in the public-health realm" and core component of reproductive health.[7] In her paper, "Safe Motherhood Initiative: 20 Years and Counting",[8] Starrs describes how public health specialists and women's health advocates worked together to develop a comprehensive approach to reducing maternal deaths. This broad approach required action within the health systems – expanding the core elements of maternal health including antenatal care, clean, safe delivery, essential obstetric care and postnatal care from within the community through to the referral levels, as well as action to increase women's status, provide good nutrition to young girls, educate communities and provide family planning.

And yet, more than twenty years later, the WHO continues to report that over 500 000 women per year die as a result of obstetric complications.[9] The overall picture has barely changed. WHO reports that 99% of these deaths occur in developing countries, 13 countries account for 67% of the deaths.[10] Further analysis of these numbers reveals huge inequities in the maternal mortality ratios (MMRs) between developed and developing countries, and similar orders of difference within countries – urban to rural. Whereas women in the developed world face MMRs of less than 20 deaths per 100 000 live births, translating into a lifetime risk of death of less than 1 in 7300, this risk of dying increases exponentially to higher than 1 in 22, with MMRs soaring over 1000 maternal deaths per 100 000 live births for women in many developing countries, especially parts of Africa and Asia.[11] Where there has been a small decrease in the maternal mortality ratio over the past 10 years – an average of 1% decline per year, this decline is amongst countries that already have relatively low levels of maternal deaths.[12]

What went wrong?

Maine and Rosenfield argue that the Safe Motherhood Initiative lacked strategic focus,[13] especially if compared to the successful Child Survival Initiative. The Child Survival Initiative provided government and international agencies with a compact set of interventions that stopped children from dying, interventions captured under the acronym GOBI – growth monitoring, oral rehydration, breast-feeding and immunization – all of which could be delivered, if necessary, in the community and outside of a health facility. In comparison, the Safe Motherhood initiative was much broader, each action "clearly worthy and important goals, (but) only one, essential obstetric care, includes actions that can substantially reduce maternal deaths."[14]

Without a strategic focus, the Safe Motherhood Initiative was carved up into a menu of separate interventions from which donors, international agencies and governments could select, usually according to their resource levels, political expedience and, perceived cost-efficient "quick wins" and short cuts. Often excluded from the menu selection were the more "controversial" interventions, including access to family planning and provision of safe abortion care. Anti-abortionists came to regard safe motherhood as the Trojan horse for the introduction of legal abortion, and donors and international agencies became wary of providing support to the Safe Motherhood Initiatives.[15]

Selected Safe Motherhood interventions were generally implemented vertically through programmes outside of the national health system, with a lot of duplication and with little cohesion between them. Moreover, they were seldom evaluated with regard to their impact on reducing maternal deaths and the interventions were often fuelled by misconceptions.

Two key misconceptions resulted in widespread adoption of interventions that forced efforts to reduce maternal deaths down the wrong track. The first was that complications in pregnancy or childbirth in women most at risk could be prevented or predicted. Adopting a risk approach would identify some "high risk" women and could indeed reduce deaths amongst these women. But, such a focus on high-risk prediction would also create a false sense of security, generating the belief that it is possible to identify all women who will develop complications and require emergency care. This is not actually possible. In absolute numbers, more "low risk" women develop complications unexpectedly. Unfortunately, amongst these "low risk" women complications tend to be recognized late, there are inadequate systems to ensure timely referral to emergency care, and upon reaching these health services, appropriate care may not be available.

The second misconception was that training scores of traditional birth attendants (TBAs) in developing countries to assist women delivering at home would reduce maternal deaths. As a result, governments and international agencies invested lots of energy and millions of dollars in training TBAs to work in the community – regarded as a high coverage, cost-efficient approach.[16] Unfortunately, while TBAs may improve the routine delivery care that mothers and newborns receive, and have some impact on reducing newborn deaths, research has shown that they have proved ineffective in significantly reducing the maternal mortality ratio.[17] The TBAs are seldom supported by health services, many are unable or unwilling to refer a woman requiring emergency care, and they lack the infrastructure and life-saving skills necessary to manage complications effectively.

It is not by chance that Safe Motherhood programmes initiated in the 1990s favoured low cost interventions that could be delivered outside of a health system, nor was it accidental that these programmes were characterized by selective interventions and vertical programmes oftentimes associated with user fees. The failure to reduce maternal deaths over the past thirty years, or to reverse significant inequity in access to lifesaving health care, cannot be divorced from a political context shaped by a broader set of neo-liberal macro-economic policies that framed the associated health sector reforms underfoot in the 1990s. These reforms argued for: Decreased government spending on social services including health services; a shrinking role for government as service provider while at the same time expanding the role for the private sector and markets; changes in priority-setting mechanisms, with a focus on cost-efficiency analyses; the introduction of user fees masked as community participation; and the development of "essential packages of care".[18] In essence, these policies represented a technical response that embraced the commodification of health care as a product to be bought and sold, benefiting those "consumers" with resources.[19]

An approach which suggests "more of the same" is just not acceptable. If we are serious about making sure that even the most vulnerable woman in the most rural part of a country has access to family planning, skilled attendance at birth and, access to emergency obstetric care without delays, then we need to do more than deliver a set of technical interventions.

How would a rights-based approach reduce maternal mortality?

The fundamental right to the highest attainable standard of health is enshrined in the International Covenant on Economic, Social and Cultural Rights,[20] as well as other international human rights treaties including the Convention on the Elimination of All Forms of Discrimination Against Women.[21] As a consequence of these treaties, every woman's life is given equal value, and thus every woman has the right to a safe pregnancy, delivery and post-natal outcome, and access to emergency obstetric care should she develop complications.

Securing the right to health is a necessary step towards maternal mortality reduction, but is not sufficient to ensure action. We know that rights embedded in treaties do not automatically translate into services on the ground,[22] but a rights-based approach does shape how governments respond to the crisis of maternal deaths in a manner that is fundamentally different to the efficiency driven neo-liberal approach experienced over the past four decades. This is important.

A rights-based approach demands that states reject the notion of health and the delivery of health care as a commodity to be bought and sold in an open market. A rights-based approach requires that states understand the dynamics of power at work in structuring health outcomes, in this instance maternal death, and make visible the connections between poverty, discrimination, inequality and health.[23] A rights-based approach is ultimately about how communities, governments, development partners and other key stakeholders identify these workings of power and then employ a set of practices to demand, implement, and ensure the rearrangements of power necessary for change,[24] offering a counter to the decades of systematic undermining of health services.

The strength of using a rights-based approach to improve maternal health and reduce maternal mortality is that it provides both the formal mechanisms to hold governments accountable and expose rights violations, as well as defining a developmental approach based on a set of principles and values that guide the progressive realization of these rights. These principles of equity, transparency, accountability, participation and non-discrimination,[25] provide a lens that guides how maternal health policy should be made, priorities set, budgets made relevant, and programmes implemented.[26] In the context of resource strapped health services, a rights-based approach promotes systemic long term health system planning centred around a functioning health system necessary for sustained maternal mortality reduction.

What does a rights-based approach look like on the ground?

A rights-based approach should be evident in the coherent workings of government, development partners, international agencies and civil society. Examples of such actions include:

___ An integrated approach to implementation – as seen in Malawi's implementation of their national Road Map to Reduce Maternal Mortality. This includes scaling-up access to basic emergency obstetric care through an overall strengthening of the health system – aligning health worker training, infrastructure development, procurement of drugs and supplies and attention to improved referral and communication systems.

___ Health information systems that incorporate indicators to monitor both progress towards realizing access to emergency obstetric care and skilled attendance at birth, disaggregated according to social class, geographical regions, age and ethnicity.

___ A willingness to seek innovative solutions to the human resource crisis through the use of non-clinician physicians to expand access to comprehensive emergency obstetric care even in the most remote districts – a strategy successfully deployed over the past three decades in Malawi, Mozambique and Tanzania.[27]

___ Development of constructive accountability mechanisms that create an effective dynamic of entitlement and obligation between people and their government.[28] This requires not only the creation of spaces, both internal and external to government, for participation and engagement to occur, but also requires government to make more transparent its planning processes and priority setting criteria, and civil society to work together to translate available data into information that communities can use to hold government accountable.

We know that progress towards meeting MDG 5 is possible – countries such as Mozambique and Sri Lanka appear to be on track to meeting MDG 5. Hard experience tells us that technical interventions, while critical, are never enough. If the world is serious about reducing maternal deaths, that vision must be framed by a rights-based approach that guides hard political choices, setting priorities, confronting entrenched power interests, and a steadfast commitment to accountability.

1   O. M. R. Campbell and W. J. Graham, 'Strategies for reducing maternal mortality: getting on with what works' 368(9543) *The Lancet* (2006), at 1284–99.

2   World Health Organization (WHO) *The World Health Report 2005: Make Every Mother and Child Count* (Geneva: World Health Organization, 2005).

3   UNFPA, 'Stepping Up Efforts to Save Mothers' Lives 2007', available at http://www.unfpa.org/mothers/index.htm.

4   L. P. Freedman, W. J. Graham, E. Brazier et al., 'Practical Lessons from Global Safe Motherhood Initiatives: Time for a New Focus on Implementation' 370(9595) *The Lancet* (2007), at 1383–91.

5   A. Rosenfield, D. Maine, 'Maternal Mortality – A Neglected Tragedy: Where's the M in MCH?' 2 (8446) *The Lancet* (1985), at 83–5.

6   A. M. Starrs 'Safe Motherhood Initiative: 20 Years and Counting' 368(9542) *The Lancet* (2006) 1130–2.

7   United Nations, 'Report of the International Conference on Population and Development', 18 October 1994, UN Doc. A/CONF.171/13.

8   A. M. Starrs, *supra* note 6.

9   United Nations, *The Millennium Development Goals Report 2008* (New York: United Nations, 2008).

10 WHO, UNICEF, UNFPA, *Maternal Mortality in 2000: Estimates Developed by WHO, UNICEF and UNFPA* (Geneva: World Health Organization, 2004).

11 United Nations, *supra* note 9.

12 'Maternal Mortality Ratio Falling Too Slowly to Meet Goal', Joint News Release WHO/UNICEF/UNFPA/World Bank, available at http://www.who.int/mediacentre/news/releases/2007/pr56/en/print.html.

13 D. Maine and A. Rosenfield 'The Safe Motherhood Initiative: Why Has it Stalled?' 89(4) *American Journal of Public Health* (1999), at 480–2.

14 Ibid.

15 C. AbouZahr, 'Safe Motherhood: A Brief History of the Global Movement 1947–2002' 67 *British Medical Bulletin* (2003), at 13–25.

16 M. Koblinsky, 'Indonesia: 1990–1999', in M. Koblinsky (ed.) *Reducing Maternal Mortality: Learning From Bolivia, China, Egypt, Honduras, Indonesia, Jamaica and Zimbabwe* (Washington, DC: The World Bank, 2003).

17 Rosenfield and Maine, *supra* note 5.

18 H. de Pinho, 'Towards The "Right" Reforms: The Impact of Health Sector Reforms on Sexual and Reproductive Health' 48(4) *Development* (2005), at 61–8.

19 H. de Pinho, 'Conclusion: Towards the "Right" Reforms' in T. S. Ravindran and H. de Pinho (eds.) *The Right Reforms? Health Sector Reform and Sexual and Reproductive Health* (Johannesburg: Women's Health Project, School of Public Health, University of the Witwatersrand, 2005); L. P. Freedman, R. J. Waldman, H. de Pinho, M. E. Wirth, A. M. R. Chowdhury, A. Rosenfield, *Who's Got The Power? Transforming Health Systems For Women And Children* (New York: United Nations Development Programme, 2005).

20 Committee on Economic, Social and Cultural Rights (CESCR), *General Comment No. 14 on the right to the highest attainable standard of health*, 11 August 2000, UN Doc. E/C.12/2000/4.

21 Convention on the Elimination of All Forms of Discrimination Against Women (1979).

22 L. P. Freedman et al., *supra* note 19; A. E. Yamin, 'Will We Take Suffering Seriously? Reflections on What Applying a Human Rights Framework to Health Means and Why We Should Care' 10(1) *Health and Human Rights* (2008).

23 Yamin, *supra* note 22.

24 L. P. Freedman et al., *supra* note 19.

25 A. E. Yamin, *supra* note 22; L. London 'What Is A Human Rights-Based Approach to Health and Does It Matter?' 10(1) *Health and Human Rights* (2008).

26 L. P. Freedman, 'Using Human Rights in Maternal Mortality Programs: From Analysis to Strategy' 75 *International Journal of Gynecology and Obstetrics* (2001) 51–60; P. Hunt, J. Bueno de Mesquita, 'Reducing Maternal Mortality: The Contribution of the Right to the Highest Attainable Standard

Of Health' (New York: United Nations Population Fund and Human Rights Centre, University of Essex, 2007).

27 G. Chilopora, C. Pereira, F. Kamwendo et al., 'Postoperative Outcome of Caesarean Sections and Other Major Emergency Obstetric Surgery by Clinical Officers and Medical Officers in Malawi', *Human Resources for Health* (2007); C. Pereira, A. Cumbi, R. Malalane et al. 'Meeting The Need For Emergency Obstetrical Care in Mozambique: Work Performance and Work Histories of Medical Doctors and Assistant Medical Officers Trained For Surgery' 114 *British Journal Obstetrics Gynaecology* (2007), at 1253–1260.

28 L. P. Freedman, R. J. Waldman, H. de Pinho, M. E. Wirth, A. M. R. Chowdhury, A. Rosenfield, *Who's Got The Power? Transforming Health Systems for Women and Children* (New York: United Nations Development Programme, 2005).

Reframing the Right to Health: Legal Advocacy to Advance Women's Reproductive Rights

Luisa Cabal and Jaime M. Todd-Gher

Introduction

Historically, international human rights law was not effectively conceptualized or applied to address violations of women's human rights.[1] Women were also excluded from participating in the creation and early development of international human rights law.[2] It was not until after the 1979 United Nations (UN) General Assembly's adoption of the Convention on the Elimination of All Forms of Discrimination against Women (CEDAW), the "broad-based, comprehensive document [that] places women's rights at the centre of international legal discourse[,]" that women's human rights finally emerged and were given force under international human rights law.[3]

The human right to health was also narrowly interpreted to exclude women's needs and experiences, and failed to address obstacles faced by women in making decisions pertaining to health and obtaining health-related services. In this context, reproductive health was relegated to the fields of population and development, and notions of reproductive rights as human rights were non-existent. The blatant exclusion of the pillars of reproductive rights – the rights to reproductive health care and to reproductive self-determination[4] – from the human rights framework was revealing in that it exposed the biased lens with which human rights have traditionally been interpreted. As a result, violations occurring to women every day in the context of their families, the workplace and communities at-large were left unexposed and disregarded as human rights violations.

A new paradigm emerged in the 1990s, however, during two UN World Conferences held in Cairo and Beijing. Consensus documents that emerged from these conferences placed women's reproductive rights squarely within the human rights framework, and deemed those rights logically inclusive within the right to health.[5] This profound shift stemmed from the emerging international consensus that "reproductive rights embrace certain human rights that are already recognized in national law, international human rights documents and other consensus documents. These rights rest on the recognition of the basic right of all couples and individuals to decide freely and responsibly the number, spacing and timing of their children and to have the information and means to do so, and the right to attain the highest standard of sexual and reproductive health."[6] Since Cairo, there has been a strong movement to give meaning to and enforce Cairo's understanding of reproductive rights, leading to an expanded body of norms and jurisprudence that have broadened human rights interpretations and affirmed the notion that reproductive decision-making and access to reproductive health care services are protected by existing human rights law.[7]

This chapter seeks to highlight some of the key cases that, in the last decade, have laid the groundwork for human rights protections found in international human rights instruments to extend to reproductive rights. The successful outcomes of these cases hinged, in part, on advocates' ability to demonstrate the interdependence among human rights, thus making it possible for courts and treaty-monitoring bodies to deem reproductive rights integral to a larger constellation of human rights. This chapter also previews the next generation of legal advocacy initiatives that is building upon earlier successes, and aims to further clarify the scope of reproductive rights and their linkages to the right to health, as well as other fundamental human rights. It is precisely these linkages that will pave the way for the right to health to be recognized as a justiciable human right in an increasing number of jurisdictions. While litigation has its limitations and is but one strategy in a larger tool kit available to activists, it can be a highly effective means for furthering the understanding and enforcement of reproductive rights as basic human rights.

Landmark cases – setting the stage for the right to health to include women's reproductive health

Once a connection was made between human rights and women's reproductive health, advocates engaged in legal advocacy in an effort to address reproductive rights violations as human rights violations, under existing treaties. Below is a discussion of four recent human rights cases that serve as crucial entry points for advancements in women's reproductive rights, as premised on the right to health, among other human rights.

Criminal abortion ban overturned – Colombia – C-355/2006

In 2006, Colombia's Constitutional Court handed down an unprecedented case overturning the country's criminal abortion ban.[8] The petition before the Court argued that Colombia's Constitution required exceptions to the abortion prohibition to protect women's fundamental rights to life, health, privacy, and dignity.[9] It further argued that Colombia's refusal to permit abortion to save a woman's life, or protect her health, or in cases of rape or foetal impairment, was out of step with widely accepted norms that recognize minimum safeguards to protect women's basic human rights.[10]

The Court's decision to overturn the ban was groundbreaking in that it rested on an extensive analysis of Colombian constitutional law, as informed by the country's international legal obligations, including with respect to the right to health. The Court confirmed that "constitutional rights and obligations must be interpreted in harmony with international human rights treaties to which Colombia is a signatory[,]" and thus, international human rights treaties limit legislators' discretion, to some extent, over criminal matters.[11] The Court further affirmed that under international law, women's reproductive rights are rooted in the right to health, among other rights. Moreover, "[t]he right to health, which includes the right to reproductive health and family planning, has been interpreted by international bodies on the basis of international treaties, including CEDAW, to include the duty of all states to offer a wide range of high quality and accessible health services."[12] The Court stated that women's sexual and reproductive rights are considered fundamental rights: "Sexual and reproductive rights also emerge from the recognition that equality in general, gender equality in particular, and the emancipation of women and girls are essential to society. Protecting sexual and reproductive rights is a direct path to promoting the dignity of all human beings and a step forward in humanity's advancement towards social justice."[13]

After recognizing the firm grounding of reproductive rights within human rights doctrines, the Court held that "laws criminalizing medical interventions that specifically affect women constitute a barrier to women's access to needed medical care, compromising gender equality in the area of health, and amounting to a violation of states' international obligations to respect those internationally recognized rights."[14] Next, the Court turned to Colombia's constitutional law obligations. It held that while the right to health "is not expressly found in the Constitution as a fundamental right," it becomes fundamental when it is "in *close relation* to the right to life."[15] The Court went on to concede that foetuses pose competing interests during pregnancy (as they are accorded some protection under Colombia's constitutional law), but confirmed that the legislature's discretion to draft and implement criminal legislation to purportedly protect foetal interests is limited due to the likelihood of "seriously impair[ing] human dignity and individual liberties."[16] In the end, the Court held that "criminalization of abortion in all circumstances entails the complete pre-eminence of the life of the foetus and the absolute sacrifice of the pregnant woman's fundamental rights. This result is, without a doubt, unconstitutional."[17]

The Colombian Court's decision set a new standard for jurisprudence promoting and safeguarding women's reproductive rights. It reaffirmed a recognition of reproductive rights as human rights and demonstrated a progressive understanding of the interdependence of human rights and governments' responsibility to comply with both national and international law. The Court also found a right-to-health violation, despite this right not being considered a "fundamental" right in Colombia's constitution, based on the intricate connection between health and the right to life. In the end, the Court's decision was revolutionary in its recognition of the synergy between health rights and interests and other human rights, and its innovative application of international law at the domestic level.

Forced sterilization

While the Colombian Court safeguarded women's ability to terminate pregnancies in certain circumstances, other courts have advanced women's right to health in connection with their right to bear children and to make informed choices pertaining to their reproductive health. The two cases that follow – one before the Inter-American Commission on Human Rights and the other under the Optional Protocol to CEDAW – have led to marked success in terms of recognizing women's rights to health, physical integrity, equal protection of the law, freedom from gender-based violence, access to information and advice on family planning, appropriate services in connection with pregnancy, and to freely and responsibly decide the number and spacing of their children.

María Mamérita Mestanza Chávez v. Peru

María Mamérita Mestanza Chávez was a 33-year-old rural woman from Cajamarca, Peru, who was threatened by hospital officials with being reported to the police if she did not agree to undergo surgical sterilization.[18] Mestanza was coerced to submit to a tubal ligation, without a prior medical examination and without providing informed consent to the procedure, and was then discharged after the surgery, despite experiencing serious complications. Her health deteriorated over the next few days, but physicians refused to treat her and she died.

On 15 June 1999, advocates filed a petition on Mestanza's behalf with the Inter-American Commission on Human Rights, alleging violations of the rights to life[19] and personal integrity.[20] The petition further alleged that Mestanza's right to health[21] was violated when state agents put her physical health at risk by performing unnecessary surgery without her informed consent, and that health officials violated her rights to equality[22] and non-discrimination[23] when they gave her partner the sole authority to decide whether she should undergo the invasive sterilization procedure.

In Mestanza's case, her family members did not have access to an effective judicial remedy after her death[24] because state authorities refused to conduct an impartial investigation of her wrongful death. The parties signed a friendly settlement on 26 August 2003, recognizing violations of the rights to life, physical integrity and humane treatment, equal protection of the law, and freedom from gender-based violence. The agreement provided monetary damages to Mestanza's family and called for modifications to discriminatory legislation and policies. The agreement also mandated prompt implementation of the recommendations made by Peru's Human Rights Ombudsman, which included improving pre-operative evaluations of women being sterilized, providing better training for health personnel, creating a procedure to ensure timely handling of patient complaints within the health care system, and implementing measures to ensure that women give genuine informed consent, including enforcing a 72-hour waiting period for sterilization.[25]

The *Mestanza* case marks the first time that human rights advocates directly pressured a government in the Inter-American system, through human rights litigation, to concede to reproductive rights violations by state actors. Further, while the resulting agreement only conceded to violations contained in the American Convention, in which the right to health is not included, it positioned reproductive health violations within the regional human rights framework. It promoted women's health-related rights and sent a strong message to governments by validating the inherent connection between health and related human rights, rejecting coercive practices and mandating improvements in health care procedures and training for health personnel. Therefore, *Mestanza* supports the notion that health interests are integral to other related human rights, and that, over time, the right to health would be more prominent in the Inter-American context.[26]

A. S. v. Hungary

A similar case was recently brought before the CEDAW Committee against the Government of Hungary on behalf of a Hungarian Roma woman who was sterilized without her informed consent.[27] In *A. S. v. Hungary*, advocates relied upon CEDAW's explicit protection of women's right to health under Article 12.[28]

A. S. was a pregnant Hungarian woman of Roma origin, who, on 2 January 2001, was taken by ambulance to a public hospital because she was experiencing labour pain, her amniotic fluid had broken and she was bleeding heavily. When she arrived at the hospital, A. S. was dizzy, still bleeding heavily and in a state of shock. The attending physician informed A. S. that the foetus had died in her womb and that an immediate caesarean section was necessary. While on the operating table, A. S. was asked to sign a consent form, as well as a barely legible hand-written note that read: "Having knowledge of the death of the embryo inside my womb I firmly request my sterilization [a Latin term unknown to the author was used]. I do not intend to give birth again; neither do I wish to become pregnant."[29] Hospital records confirm that the caesarean, the removal of the dead foetus and placenta, and the sterilization occurred within seventeen minutes of A. S.'s arrival at the hospital.[30]

A. S. learned the meaning of the term "sterilization" only upon her departure from the hospital when she asked the doctor when she could have another baby. She later confirmed that she would never have agreed to the procedure. As a result of being sterilized, A. S. fell into a depression for which she was medically treated.[31]

After failing to obtain relief from the Hungarian courts, advocates submitted a communication to the CEDAW Committee, alleging violation of A. S.'s rights to access to information and advice on family planning,[32] to access health care services, including services in connection with pregnancy,[33] and to freely and responsibly decide on the number and spacing of her children.[34] The Committee found that Hungary had failed to provide, through hospital personnel, appropriate information and advice to A. S. on family planning.[35] It referred to General Recommendation 21, "which recognizes in the context of 'coercive practices which have serious consequences for women such as forced ... sterilization' that informed decision-making about safe and reliable contraceptive measures depends upon a woman having 'information about contraceptive measures and their use, and guaranteed access to sex education and family planning services.'"[36] In making its decision, the Committee considered the fact that given A. S.'s state of health when she arrived at the hospital, any counselling that might have been provided was given "under stressful and most inappropriate conditions."[37] CEDAW protects A. S.'s right to "specific information on sterilization and alternative methods for family planning in order to guard against such an intervention being carried out without her having made a fully informed choice."[38] Hungary failed to ensure this right.

The Committee also found that by failing to ensure that A. S. provided her "fully informed consent" to be sterilized, Hungary violated A. S.'s right to access health care services, including those in connection with pregnancy.[39] For A. S. to have been able to make a "well-considered and voluntary decision to be sterilized," hospital personnel were obligated to provide A. S. "with thorough enough counselling and information about sterilization, as well as alternatives, risks and benefits."[40] Examining the circumstances, the Committee determined that it was implausible that health personnel complied with the above requirements in the hurried seventeen-minute timespan between A. S.'s arrival at the hospital and the completion of the surgeries, especially given her compromised physical and mental state.[41] The Committee further noted that A. S. did not understand the Latin term for "sterilization", as evidenced by her question to the doctor about future pregnancies.[42] As such, under the circumstances, her signature on the consent form did not constitute consent.

Finally, the Committee found that Hungary violated A. S.'s right to freely and responsibly decide the number and spacing of her children.[43] By failing to obtain her full and informed consent to be sterilized, A. S. was "permanently deprived ... of her natural reproductive capacity."[44]

As a remedy, the Committee called for Hungary to provide A. S. compensation "commensurate with the gravity of the violations of her rights."[45] The decision also requires Hungary to take the following general measures: To ensure that health centre personnel are aware of and adhere to requirements for women's reproductive health under the Convention; to review and if necessary amend legislation regarding the requirement of informed consent for sterilization, as to ensure conformity with international human rights and medical standards; and to monitor health centres performing sterilizations to ensure that fully informed consent is obtained prior to carrying out the procedures and that, in cases of the breach of this requirement, sanctions be issued.[46] Finally, the Committee stated that the decision, including the above recommendations, should be translated into Hungarian and then "widely distributed in order to reach all relevant sectors of society."[47]

Similar to the *Mestanza* case, *A. S. v. Hungary* affirms the stark infringement of human rights associated with forced sterilization. The cases also demonstrate that the right to health can be promoted through varying strategies and regardless of whether the underlying source of law contains an explicit right to health, like Article 12 of CEDAW; or through making the linkage between one's health status and a constellation of human rights, as reflected in the Mestanza settlement.

Access to abortion – K. L. v. Peru

In October 2005, the United Nations Human Rights Committee handed down a landmark decision regarding women's access to abortion in *K. L. v. Peru*.[48] In considering an individual complaint submitted under the Optional Protocol to the International Covenant on Civil and Political Rights (ICCPR),[49] the Human Rights Committee held the Peruvian government in breach of its Covenant obligations for denying access to a therapeutic abortion permitted by its own domestic law. It ordered the state to provide the complainant with an effective remedy, including compensation, and to take steps to prevent the future occurrence of similar violations.

K. L. v. Peru involved a seventeen year-old Peruvian girl (K. L.) who became pregnant with an anencephalic foetus, which posed risks to her life and mental health if the pregnancy continued.[50] Despite medical recommendations to terminate K. L.'s pregnancy, Peru's state hospitals denied her request for an abortion because they claimed it fell outside the health and life exceptions to Peru's abortion ban, as there is no explicit exception for foetal impairment. She was compelled to give birth to the anencephalic girl and breast-feed her for the four days that she lived. After the baby's death, K. L. became severely depressed, requiring psychiatric treatment.

Three non-governmental organizations (NGOs) submitted a complaint to the Committee on K. L.'s behalf,[51] alleging that state authorities' denial of K. L.'s legal right to therapeutic abortion violated her right to have her rights ensured and respected,[52] along with her rights to equality and non-discrimination,[53] life,[54] freedom from torture and cruel, inhumane and degrading treatment,[55] privacy,[56] special measures for minors,[57] and equal protection of the law.[58]

The Committee found Peru in violation of several Covenant obligations.[59] The Committee reasoned that her depression and emotional distress were foreseeable and the state's omission in "not enabling [K. L.] to benefit from a therapeutic abortion was ... the cause of the suffering she experienced."[60] Therefore, the denial of an abortion that puts at risk a woman's physical and mental health can be deemed a violation of her fundamental right to be free from cruel, inhuman and degrading treatment, as recognized under the Covenant.[61]

Notably, when deciding K. L.'s right to privacy, the Committee relied on the World Health Organization's holistic definition of health to interpret therapeutic abortion as permitted under Peruvian law; it found that since K. L. was legally entitled to an abortion, "the refusal to act in accordance with the author's decision to terminate her pregnancy was not justified ..."[62] Infringing on K. L.'s rights in this regard, in turn, violated her right to privacy. The Committee also noted K. L.'s "special vulnerability" as a minor girl by recognizing the unique barriers and susceptibility to rights violations that adolescents face when attempting to access abortion.[63] Finally, the Human Rights Committee held that the state had a duty to provide a legal and administrative mechanism to prevent or redress rights violations.[64]

The significance of the *K. L.* case is immense because it marks the first time a UN human rights body has held a government accountable for failing to ensure access to reproductive health services to an individual. Under

K.L., the Human Rights Committee requires a broad reading of statutory health exceptions to include issues of mental health, the positive realization of a right to access abortion for states that permit abortions, necessary measures to guarantee adolescents' access to reproductive health services, and accessible, economically feasible procedures to appeal a doctor's refusal to perform a legal abortion.

Moreover, though the right to health is not enshrined within the ICCPR, the Human Rights Committee contributed to the understanding of this right by linking the denial of a reproductive health service that had devastating consequences for woman's health to violations of the rights to be free from cruel, inhumane and degrading treatment and to privacy, among others.

The value of the aforementioned cases cannot be overstated. These cases have expanded understandings of the meaning of human rights, laying the groundwork for further developments and interpretations of the right to health. They have also solidified international standards that have developed over the past ten years, confirming that women's reproductive rights are indeed human rights, and integral to the right to health. Finally, these cases highlight a new trend of women's rights advocates playing an active role in litigating within their own judicial systems to demand protection of reproductive health – and when their efforts fail, the willingness to seek redress within regional and international human rights systems.

The next generation – current advocacy initiatives expanding notions of the right to health while challenging restrictions on reproductive rights

Not only have there been advancements in the realm of the right to health, but a new generation of advocacy initiatives challenging reproductive rights violations is seeking to further bolster and clarify the human right to health. These initiatives include broader and more targeted allegations to further expand human rights interpretations and recognition of women's reproductive rights. They also seek to solidify a global understanding that access to quality reproductive health care is in fact a human right and one which is necessary to ensure protection of other rights such as the rights to life, health and equality and non-discrimination. Below is a brief discussion of recent initiatives to overturn a contraceptive ban, to hold a government accountable for its poor track record regarding maternal mortality, and to mandate that a government incorporate comprehensive, non-biased, science-based sexuality and reproductive health education into its national curriculum.

Challenge to Manila City's contraception ban before the Philippine High Court

On 30 January 2008, twenty women and men from Manila filed a case in a Philippine High Court against the Office of the Mayor of the City of Manila and the City Health Department of the City of Manila arguing that the city's eight-year ban on contraception has severely and irreparably damaged their lives and health, as well as that of the majority of women in Manila City.[65]

In 2000, former Mayor Jose "Lito" Atienza issued an Executive Order declaring that "[t]he City promotes responsible parenthood and upholds natural family planning not just as a method but as a way of self-awareness in promoting the culture of life while discouraging the use of artificial methods of contraception like condoms, pills, intrauterine devices, surgical sterilization, and others."[66] While this Order did not explicitly ban "artificial" contraception, in its application, the Order prohibits city hospitals and health centres from providing "artificial" family planning services. The fact that the majority of Filipinos rely on public facilities for health care services has exacerbated the irreversible and long-term effects of the ban on women and their families. Furthermore, the Order has chilled the provision of reproductive health information and services by private facilities and NGOs, despite the fact that they are not subject to the Order.

The sweeping Order violates the Philippine Government's national and international legal obligations to, among other things, protect and ensure the rights to health and well-being, dignity, due process, privacy and equal protection of the laws. It also violates the right of spouses to "found a family in accordance with their religious convictions and the demands of responsible parenthood,"[67] the right of families to "participate in the planning and implementation of policies and programmes that affect them,"[68] as well as the obligation of local governments to ensure the availability of all methods of family planning.[69]

When the new Mayor, Alfredo S. Lim, took office in July of 2007, local NGOs called upon Mr. Lim on various occasions to revoke the ban. Local organizations Likhaan and ReproCen also partnered with the Center for

Reproductive Rights to publish a fact-finding report entitled *Imposing Misery: The Impact of Manila's Contraception Ban on Women and Families*, documenting the devastating impact of the ban on women and their families, and calling upon the local government to take action.[70] Nevertheless, after it became clear that the Mayor would not take action, ReproCen filed *Osil v. Office of the Mayor of the City of Manila, City Health Department of the City of Manila*, on behalf of twenty petitioners directly affected by the contraceptive ban.[71] The petition called upon the Philippine Court of Appeals to cease implementation of the Order while the case is pending and to ultimately issue a writ annulling the Order.[72]

The Philippine Court of Appeal recently dismissed the Petition on two procedural grounds: (1) the litigants failed to submit tax declarations to prove they were pauper litigants; and (2) the litigants should have first filed the petition before the Regional Trial Court of Manila. Soon thereafter, the petitioners filed a motion for reconsideration, asserting that the dismissal was unfounded as they had paid the necessary court filing fees, thus negating any obligation to prove that they were pauper litigants seeking exemption from fee payment. Moreover, legal precedent confirmed that both the Court of Appeal and the Supreme Court can determine petitions that have not been first adjudicated in a lower court, when there are no questions of facts but simply questions of law, specifically constitutional law. The Court of Appeal again dismissed the motion, yet it is currently unclear on what grounds. The petitioners are now strategizing what step to take next; however, if they are unable to obtain redress at the national level, recourse may be sought within the UN human rights system.

The fact that treaty-monitoring bodies have increasingly issued interpretations and jurisprudence protecting and promoting reproductive rights over the past ten years has provided groups such as ReproCen with the tools to argue, with increased credibility and force, that an order such as this one violates the human rights of women and girls. It also enables NGOs, as in this instance, to directly challenge the city government. If successful, the *Osil* case will be another example of a national forum enforcing human rights at the domestic level, while also strengthening human rights as a whole.

Challenge to Brazil's high incidence of preventable maternal mortality
before the CEDAW Committee

On 30 November 2007, the Center for Reproductive Rights and Citizens'
Advocacy for Human Rights (ADVOCACI) filed a complaint before the
CEDAW Committee on behalf of Alyne da Silva Pimentel Teixiera (Alyne), a
pregnant Afro-Brazilian woman who died of preventable maternal mortality.[73] Pregnant with her second child, Alyne arrived at a hospital on 11 November 2002, complaining of nausea. Without being admitted or examined,
she was sent home with anti-nausea medication, vitamins and cream. Two
days later, she learned that there was no foetal heartbeat, and after a long
delay, doctors assisted her in giving birth to the stillborn foetus. Following
the surgery, Alyne began to haemorrhage and her symptoms worsened, but
doctors neglected to perform any tests diagnosing her illness. She died five
days after her initial visit to the health centre.[74]

For four and a half years, Alyne's family sought recourse within Brazilian courts, to no avail. Human rights advocates then took up Alyne's cause
by initiating international litigation before the CEDAW Committee.[75] The
petition alleged that the Government violated Alyne's rights to life, health,
and redress in Brazilian courts. These rights are grounded in both Brazil's
constitution and international human rights treaties, CEDAW in particular.[76] The petition also highlights the racial and socio-economic factors that
contribute to treatment disparities in Brazil, as indigenous, poor, single
and Afro-descendent women are disproportionately affected by the country's high rates of pregnancy-related deaths. In the end, the petition requests that the Brazilian Government compensate Alyne's family, including
her nine year-old daughter, prioritize the reduction of maternal mortality,
including training providers and establishing and enforcing protocols, and
improve care in vulnerable communities.

The *Alyne* case is significant in that it is the first petition to be filed
against a Latin American country before the CEDAW Committee. Furthermore, it is the first case that has the potential to build from the CEDAW
Committee's analysis and recommendations regarding preventable maternal mortality as a violation of human rights – and in so doing, confirms
that there is strength behind treaty-monitoring body interpretations and
jurisprudence. If successful, the *Alyne* case will lead to recognition of government accountability for preventing maternal deaths and state obligations to promote women's health.

Challenge to Croatia's biased, inaccurate sexuality education programme before the Council of Europe

On 10 October 2007, the first international legal challenge to a biased, non-science-based sexuality education programme was brought before the European Committee of Social Rights.[77] Interights, in collaboration with the Center for Reproductive Rights and the Center for Education and Counselling of Women, filed a collective complaint against the Croatian Government for its sponsorship of Teen STAR, an extra-curricular educational programme that draws from Catholic ideology to promote abstinence, to the exclusion of all other alternatives such as contraception. The complaint also challenges the Government's proposed implementation of the nearly identical GROZD (Glas Roditelja Za Djecu [Parents' Voice for Children]) programme into the country's national curriculum.

Both Teen STAR and the GROZD programme promote abstinence only, discourage contraceptive use, discount the effectiveness of condoms, disparage relationships outside of a traditional family model, analogize lesbian, gay, bisexual and transgender (LGBT) relationships to socially "deviant" phenomena, and reinforce stereotypes such as the notion that stay-at-home mothers make for better families. Despite research and public outcry criticizing the Teen STAR and GROZD programmes, including pleas by Croatia's own Ombudspersons for Children's Rights and Gender Equality, the Croatian Government has continued to promote inaccurate, biased education for the country's youth.

As a signatory of the European Social Charter, Croatia has agreed to protect the social and economic rights of its citizens, including providing young people with accurate and comprehensive sexuality education. Article 11 of the Charter requires states to take appropriate measures "to provide advisory and educational facilities for the promotion of health and the encouragement of individual responsibility in matters of health."[78] This commitment has been interpreted by the Committee to include the provision of sexual and reproductive health education throughout the whole period of a young person's education and as part of the school curricula. As such, human rights advocates are attempting, through international litigation, to hold the Croatian Government responsible for failing to protect the health and well-being of its citizens, and more specifically, for creating a generation of youth ignorant of the dangers of HIV/AIDS and other sexually transmitted infections, which can have devastating health consequences. This recent endeavour is groundbreaking because if the Committee decides against Croatia, it would be the first time an international human rights body reinforced the principle that failing to provide comprehensive, science-based, non-discriminatory sexual and reproductive health education violates young people's human rights, including their right to health.

Conclusion

Over the past ten years, treaty-monitoring bodies' interpretations and jurisprudence regarding women's human rights have led to a marked expansion in recognition of the right to health, particularly as it relates to women's reproductive health. With this foundation, advocates have been given a platform to further reinforce the right to health and protections of health by making linkages to other human rights. As such, they have pressured governments to comply with their international human rights obligations related to health through litigation, as in the Colombian Constitutional Court Case C-355/2006 and *A. S. v. Hungary;* pressed for positive realization of women's reproductive health and autonomy rights through friendly settlements, as in *María Mamérita Mestanza Chávez v. Peru;* and supported an understanding and connection of a woman's health status and the broader human rights frameworks, through the lens of the ICCPR, as in *K. L. v. Peru.* In turn, all of these cases have sought to affirm the interdependence between the right to health and related fundamental human rights.

As the first phase of advocacy has led to increased recognition of the right to health, advocates must continue to devise creative strategies and pursue them in multiple fora to further promote the right to health as an independent, justiciable right, while still recognizing the intricate interdependence between all human rights. In the process, advocates should also ensure that women's experiences are addressed and redressed within the human rights framework. In the end, it is the synergy between human rights that makes the dynamic advancement of the human right to health possible.

1   See Rebecca Cook, 'Women's International Human Rights Law: The Way Forward', in R. Cook (ed.), *Human Rights of Women: National and International Perspectives* (Philadelphia: University of Pennsylvania Press, 1994) at 10.

2   See B. E. Hernandez-Truyol, 'Human Rights Through a Gendered Lens: Emergence, Evolution, Revolution', in K. D. Askin and D. M. Koenig (eds.), *Women and International Human Rights Law* (Vol.1, Ardsley, NY: Transnational Publishers, 1999) at 3. Even today, women continue to be underrepresented in key international courts and tribunals. See Christine Chinkin et al., 'Feminist Approaches to International Law: Reflections from Another Century', in D. Buss and A. Manji (eds.), *International Law: Modern Feminist Approaches* (Oxford: Oxford University Press 2005) at 20.

3   See Hernandez-Truyol, *supra* note 2, at 4; see also Convention on the Elimination of All Forms of Discrimination against Women (1979) (CEDAW).

4   For a detailed description of these principles and their grounding in human rights law, see Center for Reproductive Rights, *Gaining Ground: A Tool for Advancing Reproductive Rights Law Reform* (New York: Center for Reproductive Rights, 2006) at 14–16.

5   The advancements made during Beijing and Cairo were preceded by the 1993 Vienna World Conference on Human Rights, in which women's rights in general were positioned as human rights, thanks to the dedicated efforts of women's rights activists. See C. Romany, 'On Surrendering Privilege: Diversity in a Feminist Redefinition of Human Rights Law' in M. Schuler (ed.), *From Basic Needs to Basic Rights: Women's Claim to Human Rights* (Washington, D. C., 1995) at 544–547.

6   Programme of Action of the International Conference on Population and Development, Cairo, Egypt, 5–13 September 1994, U. N. Doc. A/CONF.171/13/Rev.1, at para. 7.3.

7   For a summary and analysis of UN treaty-monitoring body interpretations of reproductive rights, see Center for Reproductive Rights, *Bringing Rights to Bear: An Analysis of the Work of U.N. Treaty Monitoring Bodies on Reproductive and Sexual Rights* (New York: Center for Reproductive Rights, 2008.

8   See Sentencia C-355/06, Constitutional Court of Colombia (2006). Cited in Women's Link Worldwide (ed.), *C-355/2006: Excerpts of the Constitutional Court's Ruling that Liberalized Abortion in Colombia* (Spain: Women's Link Worldwide, 2007). For more information on the case, visit www.womenslinkworldwide.org.

9   See ibid. at 14–15.

10 See ibid. at 15–16.

11 See ibid. at para. 8.4, at 45.

12 See ibid. at para. 7, at 28

13 See ibid. at para. 7, at 32.

14 See ibid. at para. 7, at 29.

15 See ibid. at para. 8.3, at 41. Justiciable rights are generally deemed to be the group of rights that can be demanded before a tribunal and therefore are regarded as enforceable rights. In Colombia, these are adjudicated through the writ of protection of fundamental rights. The writ of protection of fundamental rights is found in Article 86 of the Colombian Constitution that states that through this action any individual whose fundamental rights are threatened or breached can request any judge to protect these rights. Citizens can present their claims in an informal way without the need of a lawyer. Judges have a strict term of ten days to rule on each case. Every case is sent to the Constitutional Court who can choose on a discretional basis to revise the ruling. Article 49 of Colombia's Constitution protects the right to health, which belongs to the chapter that recognizes economic, social and cultural rights in Colombia's Constitution. Therefore, it is not considered as a justiciable right by itself. Nevertheless, the Constitutional Court in Colombia has determined that there are other rights, generally the ones addressed as social rights, i.e. the right to health that can be protected by a constitutional tribunal when they have an intrinsic or close connection with fundamental rights, as the right to life or dignity.

16 See ibid. at para. 10.1, at 49.

17 See ibid. The Court found disproportionate the criminalization of abortion when the continuation of the pregnancy implied a risk to a woman's life or health because it is excessive to demand the sacrifice of a formed life to protect a developing life. It also affirmed that the prohibition of abortion under the stated circumstances would constitute a breach of the State's international obligations under different human rights' treaties. The Court explicitly acknowledged that the risk to a woman's health included mental health in accordance with Article 12 of the International Covenant on Economic, Social and Cultural Rights.

18 See *María Mamérita Mestanza Chávez v. Peru,* Case 12.191, Inter-American Commission on Human Rights, Report No. 66/00, OEA/Ser. L/V/II.111, Doc. 20 (2000) (hereinafter Friendly Settlement, *María Mamérita Mestanza Chávez v. Peru*).

19 See American Convention on Human Rights (1978), Article 4 (American Convention); Inter-American Convention on the Prevention, Punishment and Eradication of Violence against Women (1994) (Convention of Belém do Pará), Articles 3, 4.

20 See American Convention, *supra* note 19, at Article 5; Convention of Belém do Pará, *supra* note 19, at Articles 1, 4, 7.

21 See Additional Protocol to the American Convention on Human Rights in the Area of Economic, Social and Cultural Rights (Protocol of San Salvador) at Article 10; Convention of Belém do Pará, *supra* note 19, at Article 2; CEDAW, *supra* note 3, at Article 12.

22 See Convention of Belém do Pará, *supra* note 19, at Article 4.

23 See American Convention, *supra* note 19, at Article 1.

24 See Friendly Settlement, *María Mamérita Mestanza Chávez v. Peru, supra* note 18, at section IV.

25 See ibid.

26 Another case that reinforced the connection between the right to health and other fundamental rights is *Villagrán Morales et al. v. Guatemala,* in which the Inter-American Court of Human Rights concluded that the right to life includes "not only the right of every human being not to be deprived of his life arbitrarily, but also the right that he will not be prevented from having access to the conditions that guarantee a dignified existence." Such conditions include the right to health. In addition, the Court's Advisory Opinion *Juridical status and human rights of the child,* issued three years later in 2002, defines the notion of a "decent life" as including protection of the right to health, among others. See M. F. Tinta, 'Justiciability of Economic, Social, and Cultural Rights in the Inter-American System of Protection of Human Rights: Beyond Traditional Paradigms and Notions' 29(2) *Human Rights Quarterly* (2007) at 446–7.

27 See *A. S. v. Hungary,* United Nations Committee on the Elimination of Discrimination against Women, Communication No. 4/2004, U. N. Doc. CEDAW/C/36/D/4/2004 (2006) (hereinafter *A. S. v. Hungary*).

28 Article 12 of CEDAW establishes that states parties must "take all appropriate measures ... in the field of health care in order to ensure ... access to health care services, including those related to family planning." In interpreting this provision, the Committee has established that provision of services has to guarantee women's dignity and informed consent. See Committee on the Elimination of Discrimination against Women, *General Recommendation No. 24 on Women and Health,* U. N. Doc. A/54/38 (1999) (confirms that "acceptable services are those that are delivered in a way that ensures that a woman gives her fully informed consent, respects her dignity ...").

29 *A. S. v. Hungary, supra* note 27, paras. 2.2, 2.3.

30 See ibid. at para. 2.3.

31 See ibid.

32 See CEDAW, *supra* note 3, at Article 10(h).

33 See ibid. at Article 12.

34 See ibid. at Article 16(1)(e).

35 See *A. S. v. Hungary, supra* note 27, at para. 11.2.

36 Ibid. at para. 11.2 (citing CEDAW, *supra* note 3, at Article 10(h) (emphasis added) and *General Recommendation No. 21*).

37 Ibid. at para. 11.2.

38 Ibid. at para. 11.2.

39 See ibid. at para. 11.4; see also, CEDAW Committee, *General Recommendation No. 24, supra* note 28.

40 Ibid. at para. 11.3.

41 See *A. S. v. Hungary, supra* note 27, at para. 11.4.

42 See ibid.

43 See ibid.

44 Ibid.; See also, Committee on the Elimination of Discrimination against Women, *General Recommendation No. 19 on Violence against Women*, U.N. Doc. A/47/38 (1993) at 1.

45 *A. S. v. Hungary, supra note 27*, at para. 11.5.

46 Ibid. at para. 11(5).

47 Ibid. at para. 11(6).

48 See *K. L. v. Peru*, Human Rights Committee, Communication No. 1153/2003, Doc. No. CCPR/C/85/D/1153/2003 (2005) (hereinafter *K. L. v. Peru*).

49 See International Covenant on Civil and Political Rights (1966) (ICCPR).

50 See *K. L. v. Peru, supra* note 48, at para. 2(2). Anencephaly is a foetal anomaly characterized by the absences of major portions of the brain; such foetuses are either stillborn or die soon after birth.

51 The organizations include Peruvian organizations Estudio para la Defensa de los derechos de la Mujer (DEMUS) and Latin American and Caribbean Committee on the Defense of Women's Rights (CLADEM), and the United States organization the Center for Reproductive Rights.

52 See Civil and Political Rights Covenant, *supra* note 49, at Article 2.

53 See ibid., Article 3.

54 See ibid., Article 6.

55 See ibid., Article 7.

56 See ibid., Article 17.

57 See ibid., Article 24.

58 See ibid., Article 26.

59 See *K. L. v. Peru, supra* note 48, para. 6(3). The rights violated included: Article 2 (respect and ensuring rights), Article 7 (freedom from torture and cruel, inhumane and degrading treatment), Article 17 (right to privacy), and Article 24 (special measures

for minors). Alternatively, the Article 3 (equality and non-discrimination) claim was deemed substantiated and the Committed found it unnecessary to make an Article 6 (right to life) finding based on the finding of an Article 7 violation.

60 Ibid.

61 Notably, the Committee's finding did not depend on the lawfulness of the procedure, as there is no derogation from the right, which thus opened the possibility for both the legal and practical inaccessibility of a therapeutic abortion.

62 *K. L. v. Peru*, supra note 48, at para. 6.4.

63 Ibid. at para. 6.5.

64 See ibid. at para. 6.6.

65 Local NGO Reproductive Health, Rights and Ethics Center for Studies and Training (ReproCen) is serving as counsel. Attorneys with the Center for Reproductive Rights are serving as legal advisors in this matter.

66 Declaring Total Commitment and Support to the Responsible Parenthood Movement in the City of Manila and Enunciating Policy Declarations in Pursuit Thereof, Executive Order No. 003 (2000).

67 Constitution of the Philippines (1987), Article XV, section 3(1).

68 Ibid. at Article XV, section 3(4).

69 For more information on the devastating impact of the ban on women and their families, see Center for Reproductive Rights, *Imposing Misery: The Impact of Manila's Contraception Ban on Women and Families* (New York: Center for Reproductive Rights, 2007) available at http://www.reproductiverights.org/pdf/Philippines%20report.pdf.

70 See ibid.

71 See *Osil v. Office of the Mayor of the City of Manila*, Philippines Court of Appeals (filed 30 January 2008).

72 See ibid. at para. 1(1).

73 See *Alyne da Silva Pimentel v. Brazil*, United Nations Committee on the Elimination of Discrimination against Women (filed 30 November 2007).

74 Ibid. at paras. 2–21.

75 See ibid. Advocates relied on research indicating that approximately 4100 Brazilian women die a year due to pregnancy-related complications, 98% of which could be prevented at a low cost, and on statistics confirming that Brazil accounts for one-quarter of Latin America's maternal mortality rate combined. See United Nations Population Fund (UNFPA), *Maternal Mortality in 2005: Estimates Developed by WHO, UNICEF, UNFPA, and The World Bank,* 23 (annex 3), available at http://www.unfpa.org/upload/lib_pub_file/717_filename_mm2005.pdf; see Latin American and Caribbean Committee for the Defense of Women's Rights (CLADEM), *Monitoring Alternative Report on the Situation of Maternal Mortality in Brazil to the International Covenant on Economic, Social and Cultural Rights,* available at http://www.cladem.org/english/regional/monitoreo_convenios/descMMbrasili.asp.

76 Petitioners relied heavily on the CEDAW Committee's jurisprudence around Article 12, which requires that governments "take all appropriate measures to eliminate discrimination against women in the field of health care," and specifically requires that governments ensure access to "appropriate services in connection with pregnancy, confinement and the post-natal period, granting free services where necessary, as well as adequate nutrition during pregnancy and lactation."

77 See *International Centre for the Legal Protection of Human Rights (INTERIGHTS) v. Croatia,* Complaint No. 45/2007, European Committee of Social Rights (filed 10 October 2007).

78 European Social Charter (revised), Article 11(2).

Supporting Women Subjected to Sexualized Violence: Health and Human Rights Challenges and Approaches in War and Post-War Areas

Monika Hauser

Sadly, the worldwide violation of the human rights of women and girls to physical and emotional integrity – irrespective of social class or ethnic background, is all too common. Sexualized violence,[1] including physical and psychological experiences of violence, is still part of the lives of women, even in times of peace. For many women this violence ends with death.[2] In war and crisis zones, social bonds and cultural norms concerning acts of violence are even weaker or completely ignored, so much so that there is even an assumption that such acts are widespread. From Mexico to Afghanistan, from Bosnia to the Democratic Republic of the Congo, women and girls know they are more likely to have their rights to integrity trampled on than being able to have their rights respected. In too many countries we are forced to speak of an insidious femicide committed by men raised within a male-dominated "culture" that completely disregards the rights of women.[3] In order to counter this process with feminist professional support and political awareness, *medica mondiale* was founded 15 years ago as a reaction to the rape of women in the war in Bosnia.

This chapter will present the working methods of *medica mondiale*, followed by a review of the political implications of sexualized violence in the context of war and its consequences on the physical and individual well-being of the women involved, with examples from Afghanistan. It will then compare the human rights guaranteed by international conventions with current realities. It will conclude with a discussion of the fields of action that are most important to advocates working to provide long-term support to the survivors.

The organization *medica mondiale* has been assisting and supporting girls and women traumatized by war for 15 years. Projects were originally developed in Bosnia and Herzegovina, Kosova, Albania, Afghanistan and Liberia. Today, *medica mondiale* supports partner projects in Uganda, the Democratic Republic of the Congo (DRC), Indonesia, Sierra Leone, India and other places around the world. The programmes aim at combining trauma-related work with human rights activities and focus on the consequences of, and strategies to deal with, the trauma of the survivors within the particular cultural context.

Projects led by *medica mondiale* are based on long term interdisciplinary concepts focussing on the establishment of therapy and counselling centres, as well as on community-based approaches. After a reasonable period of time, the projects on the ground are usually handed over to local colleagues. This means that – from the very beginning of a project – services and assistance are provided to women affected by violence, while simultaneously long-term strategies are developed for capacity-building activities for *medica mondiale* staff members and other professionals or organizations (such as health personnel in hospitals or non-governmental (NGO) activists). A holistic concept is employed combining gynaecological and psychosocial care with legal counselling. These activities are always linked to political education, awareness-raising activities at the local and at the international level.

Sexualized violence in war and post-war areas, and patriarchal structures in health services: Impacts on women's health[4]

Sexualized violence against women is part and parcel of every war. It is a gross violation of human rights and often neglected in the public debate. The consequences of sexualized violence have to be borne by the survivors in addition to further war-related disturbances and loss. Sexualized violence is an attack on the innermost self of survivors and causes feelings of extreme helplessness, loss of control and dehumanization among the victims. Sexualized violence harms the sexual identity of women and fundamentally violates women's position in society.

The impact of war rape is particularly destructive and effective since the control over female sexuality in patriarchal societies is entirely in the hands of men. Accordingly, the value of a woman is judged by the degree of submission to this control. Naturally, this message is understood among the defeated men within the enemy group. But the message is also understood by the survivors of sexualized violence. This, in turn, means that women do not only fall victim to rape but they become victims of the intent to destroy; a message that is fully understood within their society. This leads to extreme violations of the individuals themselves and their position within society, i.e. one consequence of sexualized violence is the confirmation of the – assumed – degradation of women within their society and social environment.

This deliberate destruction of women and girls has grave and often long-term consequences for the physical and mental well-being of the survivors. These consequences include physical and genital injury, sexually transmitted diseases, unwanted pregnancy and acute symptoms of shock, as well as long-term anxiety disorders in connection with flashbacks and severe depressions – just to name some symptoms. In the long run, these symptoms often transform into a variety of physical, psychosomatic and mental disorders from which survivors will suffer for the rest of their lives.[5]

It is not only the symptoms that make girls and women feel that they have changed. The violation of their most intimate boundaries forces them to experience the destruction of their identity. The social dimension of the mental injury is of the utmost importance in this context since the individual interpretation and the way of dealing with sexualized violence always depends on the traditional, religious and cultural standards within a society. The notion of shame and disgrace is attached to the women – and not to the perpetrators. Thus the aim pursued by sexualized violence is achieved: Women are disparaged and treated with contempt in their society and, as a consequence, consider themselves to be of little value. This results in exclusion and stigmatization.

As a result of the strongly patriarchal structures in many conflict regions, the conditions for medical care are not at all women-friendly. In the Balkan states, for example, it means that few pro-women or women-centred medical services are available. Polyclinics and hospital departments are often poorly equipped and staff are often overstressed. One frequently encounters unfriendly staff, and often personnel lack the necessary sensitivity during initial patient interviews and medical examinations. Their attitude towards termination of pregnancy or sterilization is for the most part discriminatory. Verbal (and on occasions even physical) attacks on patients are not uncommon, for example, during childbirth if the women are not as "easy to manage" as the staff would like.

Throughout male-dominated societies there are still few medical services designed for women. Where they do exist, they are usually mother-and-child health services. Women only go to hospitals in emergencies and for crisis intervention in connection with giving birth. Prenatal care is usually only offered in private clinics, and is too expensive for most women.

In the case of Afghanistan, the majority of women give birth at home, alone, and as a result, the maternal mortality rate is one of the highest in the world.[6] Many women are totally exhausted and anaemic, and their immune system fails; the danger of infection or severe blood loss is greatly increased in multiparous women (i.e. women who have given birth to more than two children). Women can even be denied life-saving operations such as a Caesarean section in the event of an emergency, such as for example a ruptured uterus, if the husband or another male member of the family refuses to give permission for the operation.[7]

According to tradition, after a surgical operation a woman is regarded as "soiled" or "besmirched" and children born under these circumstances are regarded as "born under a bad sign". Other reasons are that, in the event of death, doctors are accountable and may, for example, have to fear blood revenge of "badal" (the exchange of women and girls in blood feuds between tribes or families). If the woman dies without surgical intervention, this is considered "the will of God". Here, the combination of lack of education, the misogynous attitude of family members and hospital staff (which is also supported and promoted by the structures of the health service and the legal system), have a very negative effect on women's health.

Medical professionals of *medica mondiale* in Kabul repeatedly witnessed the deaths of women who had been hospitalized in emergencies. Deaths occurring under such circumstances are only rarely investigated. However, thanks to *medica mondiale's* persistent advocacy work at the Ministry of Health in Kabul, a decree was issued in 2002 stipulating that medical professionals have to carry out emergency operations even without permission of male family members.

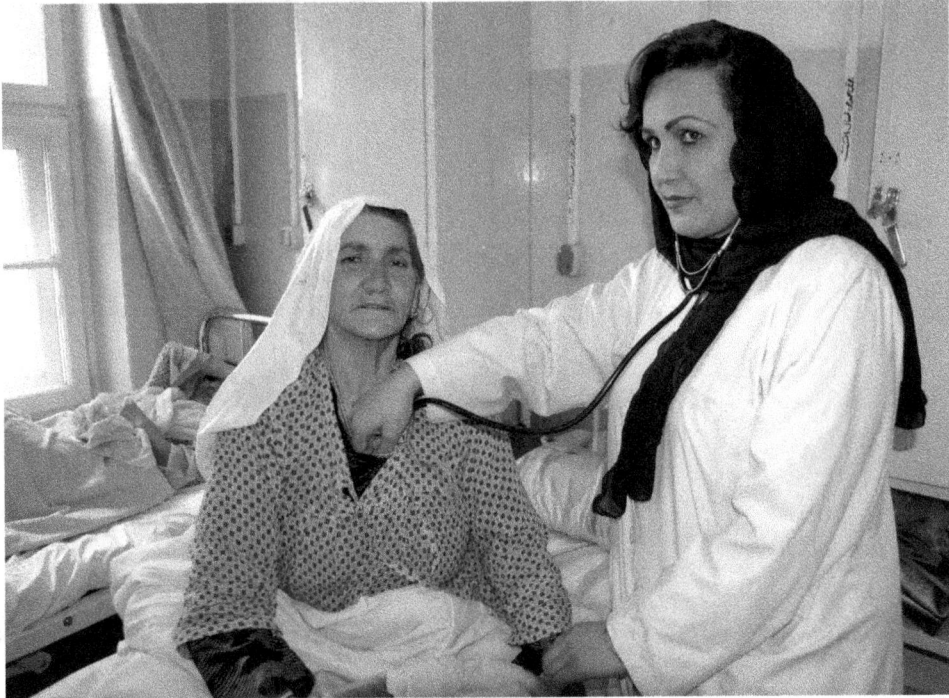

01

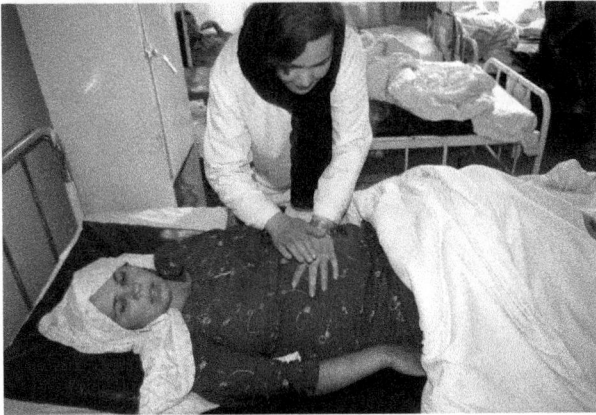

02

01
02
Afghan doctor examining patients at Rabia
Balkhi Maternity Hospital, Kabul, April 2008.

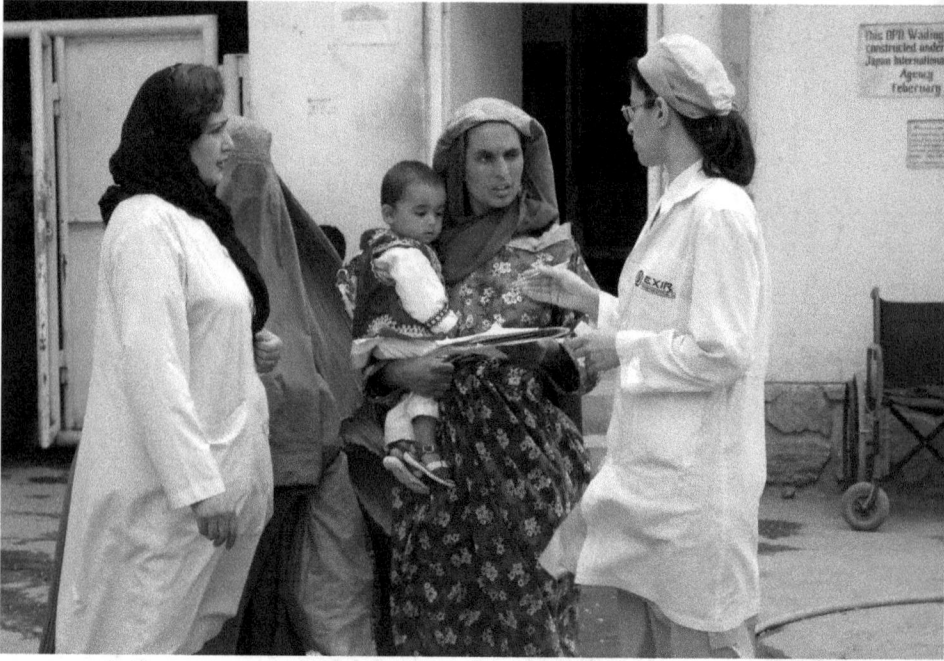

03

Afghan doctors with patients at Rabia
Balkhi Maternity Hospital, Kabul, April 2008.

Another act of violence is child and forced marriage: 57% of girls under the age of 16 years, recently abolished as the legal marriage age in Afghanistan, are married and 70–80% of women in the country are obliged to marry.[8] Traumatized women and girls have no safe place in this society – violence against women is accepted as "normal". Nor do they have any chance of receiving support within this system. Often women and girls themselves perceive violence as "normal" and have no knowledge about the fact that violence against women is a violation of human rights and could be punished. Their survival depends above all on how well they function. In most cases, they will be penalized or excluded at the first sign of resistance or rebellion, and punishment can culminate in the killing of the woman. Girls and young women who, for example, want to escape from a forced marriage, or women who oppose family violence perpetrated by their husband or mother-in-law, must fear punishment in the form of mental or physical violence. Only too frequently, they will be put in isolation, either by being sent to prison or by being imprisoned in a barn, cellar or dungeon.[9] This situation led to a horrific number of self-immolation among especially young women in the last year.

Reproductive rights

In a significant number of countries women have no rights whatsoever as regards pregnancy and family planning. But even in somewhat less patriarchal countries like Croatia or Bosnia-Herzegovina, liberal laws, which dated from the pre-war period, were some of the first to succumb to the "new" policies in the immediate post-war period, when more rigid regulations were introduced.[10] Reproductive rights or their denial, respectively, are always a mirror of the general political atmosphere; in the aftermath we see mostly a more restrictive and gender stereotype attitude.

After the war in Bosnia-Herzegovina, the permit granted previously to Medica Zenica to perform abortions in its modern clinics was withdrawn on the unsubstantiated grounds that there was not enough emergency equipment. Apart from the financial aspect – since the Centre was in competition with the state-run clinics – the notion of control naturally played a role, as the state now wanted to be solely in charge. In the post-war period it was hoped that the birth rate would rise. The individual experiences and needs of women were not taken into account at all. After the war there were certainly women for whom pregnancy was a positive expression of life – and also a sign that they had survived and overcome the insanity. But on the other hand, there were others who had only just survived the horrors of war, who felt more dead than alive, and who needed time to rebuild their lives – all of which was difficult to do with an unwanted pregnancy.

Human rights conventions and the reality of women on the ground

In view of the discriminatory attitudes in many countries, women do not expect protection from the law. What use is the right to physical integrity when the majority of the female population is not aware of their rights or does not believe they will be protected? And who would help to make them aware of their rights and seek remedy for violations should this not be in the interest of the dominant group, i.e. men? What should a woman who is effectively completely dependent on a husband, father or uncle do? How can cultural norms, which dictate that women have no say in deciding anything related to their bodies, be changed?

For the health and wellbeing of women, it is indisputable that they must be in charge of their reproductive rights and thus have access to gynaecological facilities. The more patriarchal the society, the more endangered is the health and wellbeing of the female population. Returning to the example of Afghanistan, married women and girls are forced to have as many pregnancies as possible and if they do not function in the expected manner (bearing boys, diseases during pregnancy, etc.), husbands would rather take a second or third wife than spend money on the cost of an expensive treatment. For a 14–15 year old girl, birth control can be life-saving.

When speaking about reproductive rights we mean the right to family planning, to spacing pregnancies, to safe motherhood, to effective abortion and post-abortion care and sterilization, to prevention of sexually transmitted diseases such as HIV, to treatment of persistent gynaecological problems, to freedom from psychological problems, to discouragement of harmful traditional practices (early and forced marriages, "honour" killings, badla, female genital mutilation (FGM), etc). The trap women find themselves in is inescapable: On the one hand, the conditions of their child-bearing are, in all probability, fraught with pathological implications; on the other hand, the women's access to adequate medical care is extremely limited. Health education would be helpful as a key to better self-care and self-determination over one's body.

The right of women to their physical and emotional integrity is thus violated through innumerable misogynistic forms of violence, through the usually very limited access to health care, through additional violence in the health care structures as well as through the lack of possibilities to know their own rights and to enforce them.

Health should be seen both as a need and as a right of all women. Health as a human right is grounded in national and international law, in several Conventions, in the World Health Organization (WHO) Alma-Ata declaration[11] from 1978 and in treaties addressing women's rights specifically such as the 1979 Convention on the Elimination of All Forms of Discrimination Against Women (CEDAW), Article 12.[12] According to these, governments must take appropriate measures to, inter alia:

___ **Eliminate discrimination against women in the field of reproductive rights and provide services for pregnancy, childbirth.** The 1993 World Conference on Human Rights affirmed in the Vienna Declaration and Programme of Action in paragraph 41:[13] "Woman's right to accessible and adequate health care, including to the widest range of family planning services ..."

The 1994 International Conference on Population and Development (ICPD) in Cairo adopted a set of principles affirming, inter alia, that:[14] "... Women are entitled to universal access to ... reproductive health care, which includes family planning and sexual health ... and that reproductive health care programmes should provide the widest range of services without any form of coercion."[15]

But the complete denial of all these rights is reality for many women, as said in the words of a participant in a *medica mondiale* training (Kabul 2005): "A woman has a right to decide about her life, if she wants to have children or not. The families don't support the implementation of the law. Men force women to bear children and often they say that it says in the Koran that women must have children."

Fields of action for long term support and change

___ **Developing a multisectoral response.** The consequences of sexualized violence have to be seen in the mental and physical health, social, economic and legal fields. In order to support women holistically and react appropriately to their needs, it is necessary to offer them interdisciplinary professional support and expertise. For *medica mondiale* this includes the psychosocial, medical and legal fields as well as raising the awareness of relevant professional groups. In order to become effectively involved in this context, it is vital to develop adequate strategies. That is why the first step to any strategy must be an assessment of the living conditions as well as of the political and cultural context in which these are embedded. This approach means to adjust always the professional work to the political and social context.

___ **Creating safe places for immediate and midterm support.** Creating easy access to medical support can be vital for survivors. By taking into account the current security situation in the respective country (this includes the cultural and social security of the female population) the necessity to create a safe place is more than obvious. This is shown, for example, by the poor culture of reporting rapes, even in peaceful times. But we should always bear in mind that the term "vulnerability" would not be necessary if men behaved and reacted differently: The women are neither "wrong" nor the "problem"; rape is not the problem of the women, but the behaviour of men.

Example: Afghanistan, 2007. A gynaecologist made contact with a 15 year old pregnant girl in a prison. The girl initially refused any contact, but the midwife was able to gain her confidence and learned that she had been raped by a neighbour. When her mother discovered the pregnancy, she wanted to report the perpetrator to the police. But the police accused the daughter of having had premarital intercourse and put her in prison. After the delivery, the young mother experienced great disturbances as the baby reminded her of the rapist. She was eventually released from prison but her father didn't want her to return home. One option for the girl would have been to marry an old man – but the gynaecologist helped her to find a place in a shelter, which she preferred.

In countries and societies where war rape is regarded as an attack on the honour of the family or the husband, women are under immense pressure not to let anyone know about what they have been through. This can prevent them from seeking gynaecological care in the first place or may lead to them not confiding their specific problems and symptoms resulting from their experience of violence to the gynaecologist. Also, women and girls who are either not of reproductive age, unmarried, or widows, are often denied permission to see a gynaecologist (e.g. in Kosova, Afghanistan etc.). This is why it is important to conduct a needs assessment in order to develop the necessary structures so that the women in question can be reached. *Medica mondiale* has built up a repertoire of suitable approaches for different situations and settings. Easy access to medical care via gynaecological support has proven to be an ideal approach. The gynaecological mobile unit is particularly helpful in offering medical care to women in rural areas as well as in pursuing a strategy of destigmatizing survivors of sexualized violence.

Best practices of Medica Kosova

The team of gynaecologists and nurses carry out their work in an outpatient department which is integrated into the therapy centre and also in a fully equipped mobile unit. The approach focuses on psychosomatic symptoms and offers access to the complex range of symptoms shown by severely traumatized patients.

Psychological consequences of trauma result in a variety of somatic functional disorders. The team is experienced in the diagnosis and treatment of these symptoms. By taking a thorough social case history and adopting a sensitive approach, the staff offers the women a safe environment in which they can talk about the violence they have experienced. The very fact that medical staff can convey to the patients that they have knowledge of what has happened – for example, sexualized violence during war or in a domestic context – and that they are there to help and offer them the opportunity to come to the therapy centre and/or to refer them to the psychosocial or legal teams opens up entirely new opportunities for the women to become active themselves.

This is often the first time that survivors speak about the seemingly unspeakable. In this respect, the thorough social case history that is based on a screening, including routine questions on violence, has been a helpful tool for documentation. Through the case history, medical professionals gather valuable information on violence experienced during war, flight and aftermath as domestic violence. In many cases, this information is essential to diagnose the presented symptoms more clearly. As a matter of course, questions about physical symptoms relating to PTSD (Post Traumatic Stress

Disorder) and susceptibility to suicide were also included in the question-naire. In the test phase during 2002, the case history format and its appli-cation was constantly modified. Questions concerning sexualized violence are asked in a systemized manner; however, the questions have to corre-spond to the mental constitution of the patient. If necessary, the medical staff can arrange a special appointment with the patient to talk about her problems. The reactions of the patients have been positive. For most, hav-ing a consultation lasting more than three minutes and being treated as a human being was already a completely new experience.

Defined quality criteria have been established including areas that deserve particular attention in connection with gynaecological care. For further information on the subject, see the *medica mondiale* handbook available at www.medicamondiale.org.

—— **Qualifying local staff as a crucial step in development and capacity building.** The aim of *medica mondiale* is to make all staff aware of, and sensi-tive to, trauma and the special needs of survivors of sexualized violence and to convey expert knowledge to them. Apart from medical knowledge, this also includes the psychosomatic approach and background information on how to avoid retraumatization of the patient and vicarious traumatization of the medical professionals themselves. When dealing with the subject, it is also important to bear in mind that many local colleagues of *medica mondiale* have made their own experiences with (sexualized) war violence. This is why intensive training, which encompasses elements of self-experi-ence and self-reflection, is indispensable for medical and other staff to be-come aware of their own triggers.

The transfer of knowledge concerning human rights violations and violence against women is a top priority for all project activities which are carried out in an atmosphere partial to women. For this type of training, specific modules have been developed which integrate and mainstream quality cri-teria: The holistic view of women and their resources; the empowerment of women to decide themselves on how to lead their lives; regaining control and safety by respecting the patient's personal boundaries; building up a re-lationship of trust by taking the women's side; and reducing stress and fear by creating the appropriate setting.

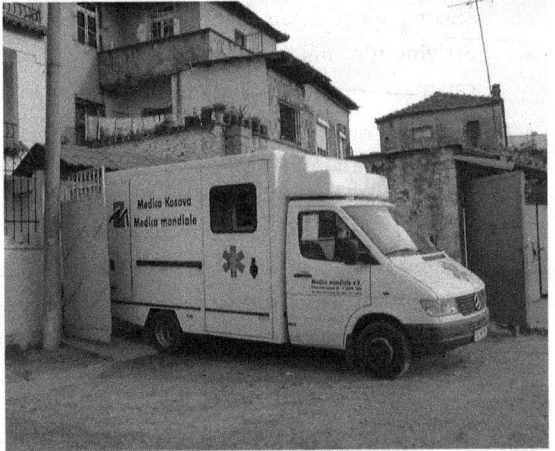

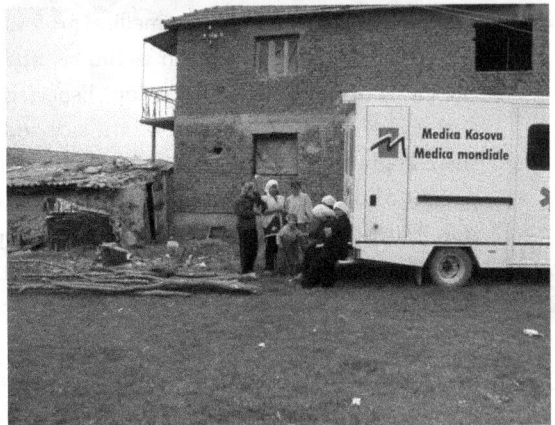

05
Medica Kosova's mobile gynaecological unit.
06
The mobile gynaecological unit regularly tours villages in
order to provide treatment or counselling to women.

The implementation of these principles represents a demanding challenge. Striving for empathic attitudes as medical or psycho-social professionals can make those providing care susceptible to the destructive pull of trauma including all interrelated emotions and defence mechanisms. This might make the assessment of one's own resources and those of the patient even more challenging. With regard to training, it is crucial that the staff members of all disciplines learn from each other and acquire basic knowledge of trauma and the medical and legal implications of sexualized violence. This is important to coordinate interdisciplinary work more efficiently and to better assess the impact of one's own intervention.

A primary goal: Avoiding retraumatization

Particularly as members of the medical profession, we need to be aware that our patients might have fallen victim to rape and that this entails a high risk of iatrogenic retraumatization. Especially in gynaecological and obstetric care which touches upon intimacy and embarrassment thresholds, there are numerous moments, which – even subconsciously – remind the patient of the traumatic experiences and can thus trigger a retraumatization. Having to get undressed, the examining position on the gynaecology chair, vaginal and rectal examinations, a catheter insertion into the bladder can re-awaken feelings of extreme helplessness. Additionally, actions such as applying gel for a sonogram can stimulate associations with sperm, or the initial patient interview and case history might be associated with an interrogation. Even standard medical examinations such as having an electrocardiogram (ECG) can arouse associations with torture simply by attaching the electric cables. Also ear, nose and throat and dental examinations can function as a trigger for women who have experienced oral rape.

Such triggers can transport the patient's conscious thoughts back to the place, time and circumstances of the traumatic event. As a result, a woman can start to panic, or have cramps and pain, and may show a lack of emotion, start trembling or freeze. She may also suffer from a circulatory collapse or become dissociated. In these situations, it is indispensable that the medical professional has the necessary expertise on how to support women in the reorientation process.

Documenting human rights violations in situations of humanitarian crisis

It is not always possible to ask for detailed information, particularly during the first contact with the patient. In many cases, the link between symptoms, diagnosis, behaviour and general background information only becomes apparent from the overall context. This is particularly evident when medical professionals are sensitive to the topic and have received special training. Documentation and the recording of forensic results is of the utmost importance not only for legal actions to be taken at a later point in time but also as an official proof that sexualized violence is the cause of the presented symptoms and disorders. Due to the fact that trauma patients suffer from a loss of memory, many women are not able to see the connection between the traumatizing experience and their symptoms anymore. Additionally, survivors of sexual gender-based violence often tend to blame themselves for what happened. Naturally, there is an obvious contrast between this behaviour and the statement that the symptoms and disorders are the consequences of crimes.

It goes without saying that, in everyday work, it is often extremely difficult to pursue a psychosomatic approach and to build a relationship of trust and a friendly atmosphere in view of the given circumstances and surroundings. Maintaining such an approach under difficult circumstances represents one of the greatest challenges those working in the field face. But striving to do so, even partially, is critical. If not, the permanent contradiction between personal expectations and reality will inevitably result in cases of burnout for those seeking to offer this kind of care and treatment. New projects of *medica mondiale* are also measured against this standard.

Conclusion

When working with survivors of war-related sexualized violence it is essential to try to relate to the very individual situation of the women and girls involved. The very fact that staff are aware of their specific situation is a first, important step. This means for us confronting the issue of violence, the extent to which it is perpetrated against women worldwide and the lack of gender democracy. This work demands reflecting one's own thoughts and feelings on those issues. The willingness to confront yourself with this painful topic is the precondition for any constructive work with traumatized women or women refugees. The early, intensive reflection of this issue increases one's general awareness and also reduces the danger of being overwhelmed by one's own undealt-with feelings. Above all, we should always keep in mind that we may be the first – and perhaps the only – empathetic and unconditionally supportive specialists the patient may have encountered in her life. We must give her the security that she needs. In the provision of gynaecological and medical care for survivors of war-related sexualized violence, interdisciplinary collaboration and close cooperation with different specialist areas have proved invaluable for *medica mondiale*.

There is still a lot to be done, particularly in terms of improving health care for women who have experienced war-related sexualized violence – not only on an individual or specialist level, but also on a political level.

1   Sexualized violence, as sociologist Ruth Seifert once put it, is "not an aggressive expression of sexuality but rather a sexual expression of aggression." Seifert, Ruth. *War and Rape. Analytical Approaches*. Women's International League for Peace and Freedom, 1992. The term "sexualized violence" shifts the emphasis from the sexual aspect to the violent act. Sexualized violence is a form of violence intentionally directed against a person's most intimate sphere and which aims to demonstrate power and superiority by humiliating and debasing the other person. Sexualized violence describes not only rapes, but rather all attacks and violations, aimed against another person's intimate sexual sphere.

2   Worldwide, an estimated 40–70% of homicides of women are committed by intimate partners, often in the context of an abusive relationship. World Bank, *Violence against Women: The Hidden Health Burden* (Washington: World Bank, 1994).

3   According to Amnesty International, 1188 women were killed in Guatemala between 2001 and 2004. See further, Amnesty International, *Guatemala:* *No Protection, No Justice: Killings of Women in Guatemala*, AI Index Number AMR 34/017/2005, 9 June 2005. See also www.focus.de/politik/ausland/irak-die-frauenmorde-von-basra_aid_315 921.html.

4   Ibid., at 24–26.

5   For detailed information on trauma work and symptoms, see *medica mondiale* (ed.), *Violence against Women in War* (Frankfurt: Main, 2nd edition, 2008).

6   According to the UNDP (WHO) there were 1600 maternal deaths per 100 000 live births in Afghanistan in 2004. WHO Afghanistan. Report on major achievements 2003 and priorities for 2004. Kabul 2003, available at www.who.int/disasters/repo/11782.pdf.

7   See the case study from Kabul on the *medica mondiale* website: http://www.medicamondiale. org/index_e.html.

8   Charlemagne Gomez, *Afghan Perspectives on Child Marriage: Causes, Consequences and Solutions* (unpublished report on file at *medica mondiale*, 2008).

9 Rachel Wareham, *Trapped by Tradition* (Cologne: *medica mondiale*, 2003), available at http://www. medicamondiale.org/_en/bibliothek/eigene/doku /index.html.

10 The attitude towards terminations was fairly liberal and pragmatic before and during the war (terminations were permitted up until the twelfth week of pregnancy).

11 World Health Organization, Alma-Ata Declaration, available at http://www.paho.org/English/ DD/PIN/alma-ata_declaration.htm.

12 Convention on the Elimination of All Forms of Discrimination Against Women, available at http://www.un.org/womenwatch/daw/cedaw/text /econvention.htm.

13 Vienna Declaration and Programme of Action, available at http://www.unhchr.ch/huridocda/hu ridoca.nsf/(Symbol)/A.CONF.157.23.En?Open Document.

14 See further UNFPA, Summary of the ICPD Programme of Action, available at http://www.unfpa. org/icpd/summary.htm#chapter2.

15 ICPD Programme of Action, Principle 8, available at http://www.unfpa.org/icpd/icpd_poa.htm.

For having kindly permitted us the use of their photographs, we thank:

p. 143, 144: Lizette Potgieter/*medica mondiale*

p. 151: *medica mondiale*

THE RIGHT TO HEALTH IN EMERGENCIES

The Right to Health in Armed Conflict

Pierre Perrin*

Introduction

The effects of war on health are multifaceted and range from striking effects such as the wounded, the dead, the epidemics and famine, to less visible ones including the disorganization of health services and, in some cases, their total annihilation. Both types of effects may result in humanitarian tragedies which affect whole populations.

Health services react to these situations, however, the implementation of the response strategies encounters constraints that limit their effect, especially when violence is established as a war strategy against the civilian population. Such tactics of hostilities run counter to the humanitarian logic.

Health professionals are not only responsible for proposing technical solutions to resolve health problems, but they also must use legal means, in particular through international humanitarian law (IHL) and international human rights, to effectively protect the right to health. In this regard, the role and responsibilities of health professionals in identifying the effects of weapons with the view to applying IHL rules on means and methods of warfare is a telling example of such a role, as well as of the complexity of addressing health issues in the context of war.[1]

In times of armed conflict, both international humanitarian law and international human rights law offer important protections for the right to health. Given the various components of this right, the applicable legal framework entails interaction between those two bodies of norms. When considering IHL, it is worth noting that protection goes beyond specific provisions related to health and health services. It also encompasses norms that indirectly contribute to protecting the right to health, such as the principles and rules governing the means and methods of warfare.

While one may primarily think of civilians as persons whose health is affected by war, combatants are affected too. Indeed, IHL rules first developed by focusing on ways to alleviate the suffering of wounded combatants on the battlefield and to ensure access by health services to those persons.

This chapter first seeks to look at the legal bases of the right to health in armed conflict to show that IHL provides for a broad protection. Second it offers a brief overview of the protection of this right in practice. Finally it gives elements on the underlying humanitarian and political background to understand the current evolution with respect to the protection of the right to health in armed conflict.

The legal bases of the right to health

The right to health

The right to health is understood as the right to have access to health services. However, it is not an absolute right, as such, to be in good health.[2]

The WHO defines health services as all activities intended to restore and maintain health.[3] One therefore has to include vaccinations, medical care, but also sanitary services related to water and hygiene, and a clean environment under this heading, as well as all activities ensuring access to food resources. Those "underlying determinants of health"[4] imply consideration of the right to health in a broader perspective, which is the basis of Article 25 of the Universal Declaration of Human Rights.[5]

The corollary of this right is the idea that states are responsible for adopting appropriate sanitary and social measures for the populations to have effective access to health services.[6] Such obligations are found in several legal instruments, including the International Covenant on Economic, Social and Cultural Rights (Articles 12, 24), the International Convention on the Elimination of All Forms of Racial Discrimination (Article 5), the Convention on the Elimination of All Forms of Discrimination Against Women (Articles 10, 12, and 14), the Convention on the Rights of the Child (Article 24).

While all these legal instruments are applicable at all times, including during armed conflict, this chapter will focus primarily on the provisions of international humanitarian law. Having defined the right to health as the right to access to health care, it applies to all persons whether they are wounded or not. As this chapter covers situations of armed conflict however, it will address mainly the right to health for persons, be they combatants or non-combatants, who are injured.

The right to health in armed conflict

Within possible limits, medicine has always responded to the needs of injured persons and tried to limit the means and methods of warfare, including through describing and providing expertise to better understand the effects of weapons. In his work 'On The Physician', Hippocrates refers to war injuries as an area of surgical specialization.[7] Based on reports of the consequences on health of the use of nuclear weapons, two physicians, a Russian and an American, launched the idea of an association of medical doctors to prevent a nuclear war. This idea was the origin of the creation of the organization called International Physicians for the Prevention of Nuclear War in Geneva. In 1985, this association received the Nobel Peace Prize for making people aware of the catastrophic consequences a nuclear conflict would entail.

The development of IHL, in particular through the First Geneva Convention,[8] was aimed at protecting and caring for persons injured during armed conflict, firstly combatants. This constituted a major turning point in modern humanitarian thinking and offered a legal framework for providing assistance to the wounded in wars.[9]

In parallel, various legal instruments were elaborated with a view to limiting the means of warfare, and to forbid the use of certain weapons. In 1863, during the American Civil War, the Lieber Code[10] was elaborated, limiting the military's means of warfare. Several international instruments were later adopted, prohibiting the use of expanding bullets,[11] biological[12] and chemical weapons.[13] Such regulations are relevant when considering health issues in armed conflicts. Although the International Court of Justice, following a request by the World Health Organization on the legality of the use of nuclear weapons, ruled in its 1996 advisory opinion that such request did not relate to a question which arises within the scope of WHO activities,[14] this finding was limited to the purpose of assessing the conditions to file a request for an advisory opinion. It does not mean that IHL norms regarding means and methods of warfare are not relevant rules offering a protection of the right to health against the effects of certain weapons.

This dual approach – to provide care and to prevent the effects of weapons – has been consistent throughout the development of the law of armed conflict.

Protecting the right to health through international humanitarian law

Numerous aspects of international humanitarian law address the protection of the right to health in armed conflict; they concern the protection of the right to be given care and the protection of essential services to maintain health. The 1977 Additional Protocol I states that:

> "... all the wounded, sick and shipwrecked, to whichever Party they belong, shall be respected and protected. In all circumstances they shall be treated humanely and shall receive, to the fullest extent practicable and with the least possible delay, the medical care and attention required by their condition. There shall be no distinction among them founded on any grounds other than medical ones."[15]

Several articles in the Geneva Conventions and their Additional Protocols protect medical structures and medical personnel. It is forbidden to attack hospitals, and medical staff must be able to perform their work without any discrimination whatsoever.[16]

Protection is also required for essential services aimed at maintaining health, namely food, drinking water, hygienic measures, and habitat. To ensure such protection, it is forbidden to attack or destroy these services, or to render them inoperable. With respect to access to food, it is forbidden to attack food stocks, agricultural zones, harvests, cattle, and irrigation installations.[17]

International humanitarian law also contains rules regarding the responsibilities of the parties to the conflict. For instance, in case of occupied territories, the occupying power has the duty to ensure and maintain the medical and hospital establishments and services, public health and hygiene in the occupied territory in cooperation with the national authorities.[18]

Restrictions on the means and methods of warfare

Restrictions on the means and methods of warfare, be they through general principles or through specific rules covering particular weapons, are also relevant when considering the protection of the right to health in armed conflict. These restrictions affect a range of aspects, from the effects of weapons that may impact upon the health of combatants, to the indirect effects on civilians.

It is for example forbidden to use famine as a weapon of war.[19] Pillaging, and poisoning of water supplies, is also prohibited.

The development and use of weapons is an area where the interface between the law and health is particularly important. In this regard, the health impact of a weapon is used in order to assess the effects of a weapon when determining whether it causes superfluous injury or unnecessary suffering. This rule also requires medical considerations to be applied in order to identify the nature of the effects of a means of warfare. Moreover, the quality and availability of hospitals and health services in the enemy area may be an element to take into account when assessing the superfluous or unnecessary character of the effects of a weapon compared to its military utility, depending on the peculiarity of the effect. For example, if a party to a conflict has no means to treat a particular type of injury, it may be relevant in applying the prohibition of superfluous injury or unnecessary suffering rule.

Recently, several humanitarian organizations[20] have shown that civilian populations are particularly affected by the use of cluster munitions.[21]

"Cluster munitions are weapons that spread hundreds of tiny explosive devices over wide areas and leave hidden unexploded bomblets that keep on killing for many years. In modern wars, civilians pay a high price from the use of such weapons."[22]

In May 2008, 107 states adopted a draft Convention on Cluster Munitions which effectively prohibits the use, production and transfer of all existing types of cluster munitions. The draft Convention establishes important commitments regarding assistance to victims, clearance of contaminated areas and destruction of stockpiles. Further, the adoption of the Protocol on Explosive Remnants of War in 2003 obliges the parties to the conflict to remove all explosive remnants. This is a step forward in the protection of the populations in the post-conflict phase, but the essential issue here is to protect the civilian population during the conflict. More and more, governments and other actors are committing to prohibitions on such weapons, since their use goes against the principle of distinction between military objectives and the civilian population/objects.[23]

The problem of landmines and explosive remnants of war shows the difficulties encountered in the efforts to ban weapons having harmful post-conflict effects, particularly when they are already being widely used. It is preferable to adopt a strategy of primary prevention, with a view to prohibiting the development of certain weapons right from the initial concept, if their potential effects violate the principles of international humanitarian law. This approach had been successfully adopted for banning the use of blinding laser weapons.[24]

International humanitarian law and human rights law is expressed in a variety of legal instruments that are applicable in armed conflicts. These situations are often accompanied by displacements of the populations to a country other than that of their origin. These populations may be specifically protected by extra protections under the 1951 Refugee Convention and its Protocol of 1967, which define the responsibilities of states vis-à-vis refugees, and the Guiding Principles on Internal Displacement, which sets out the situation vis-à-vis internally displaced persons (IDPs).[25]

Health staff can also have recourse to the recommendations of the World Medical Association (WMA). While these are not binding legal instruments in the strict sense of the term, they outline the position of the medical profession on difficult problems such as torture,[26] or economic embargoes,[27] which are sometimes encountered in armed conflicts. Moreover, a certain number of recommendations concern armed conflict directly.[28] For instance, the WMA defines the position of health personnel in the case of surgical triage,[29] which may result in limited access to care for certain groups of wounded.

This ethical framework complements the legal framework, so as to help health staff "to work for the highest possible standards of ethical behaviour and care by physicians, at all times".[30]

These examples give a general overview of the legal framework that exists to ensure the protection of the right to health in armed conflict. The enjoyment of this right depends on the willingness of the parties involved in these situations to carry out their responsibilities in this regard.

In practice: Protection of the right to health in armed conflict

For the right to health to be respected, health services must function correctly and populations must have access to them.

The responsibilities within health services

Providing appropriate care to persons affected by armed conflict is the responsibility of national (military and civilian) authorities.

Depending on the willingness and capacity of the authorities to face this responsibility, humanitarian organizations concerned with health care should adopt a strategy that combines the following various approaches:

—— Reminding the authorities of their responsibility by referring to the rules of international humanitarian law and human rights law, in particular when the authorities appear insufficiently concerned about populations that are affected by the conflict, specifically the ones at the highest risk, such as prisoners and detainees.

—— Supporting national health services with a view to assisting them in responding to the needs of the civilian population. Of course, the authorities still need to have a minimum functional capacity and be willing to cooperate with humanitarian organizations.

—— Providing direct care to the populations concerned. This approach must not contribute to relieving the authorities from their responsibility.

The last approach is required when the capacity of the national health services is overtaxed by the increase in demand for health services (for example, through massive displacements of people), deterioration due to structural problems (dysfunctional government or insufficient budget allocations for health services), health personnel fleeing for security reasons, or the refusal of authorities to provide health assistance to certain groups of people based on ethnic, political, religious or other criteria.

> "... if circumstances cause it to provide services to the affected populations, the ICRC does not have the vocation to substitute the responsibilities of the authorities. It will continue its efforts towards the latter so that they take care of these services and thus fully fulfil their obligations."[31]

The interface between the authorities and humanitarian organizations depends on the applicable legal frameworks; thus, in non-international armed conflicts, humanitarian organizations may offer their services to the authorities based on the right of initiative,[32] and on the political willingness of the authorities to give access to the people to humanitarian organizations.

The good functioning of health services is a first, necessary stage for obtaining respect for the right to health, but health services must also be accessible to all persons without discrimination.

Responsibilities for protecting access to health services

In many armed conflicts, people no longer have access to health services for different reasons, such as:

—— Insecurity which limits the access to health facilities:

"[The] Mortality rate was higher in unstable eastern provinces, showing the effect of insecurity. Most deaths were from easily preventable and treatable illnesses rather than violence. Regression analysis suggested that if the effects of violence were removed, all-cause mortality could fall to almost normal rates".[33]

—— Discrimination at the point of access to health facilities, based on ethnic, religious, political, or other factors:

"... these conflicts are often characterized by rampant and gross disrespect for the principle of medical neutrality, which guarantees the provision of health care without discrimination to all injured and sick combatants and civilians in time of conflict".[34]

Access to health services depends on whether the parties to the conflict take all measures required to ensure free access to health facilities. The role of humanitarian organizations is to assess whether people do have access to health services and, if necessary, to identify the obstacles which hinder such access. Based on this analysis, humanitarian organizations should initiate the following:

—— Dialogue with all parties concerned:

With the parties to the conflict, to remind them of their responsibilities and to request that measures be taken with a view to ensuring the security of the population. Respecting the principles of international humanitarian law requires that all those bearing arms be informed of the applicable standards. Teaching the basic rules of international humanitarian law is therefore a first step.

With health staff, to remind them of the rules of international humanitarian law and of the ethical recommendations applicable to the medical profession.

—— Mobilizing the international community by means of declarations, reports, interventions with multiple players (states, media, non-governmental organizations ...) who have influence in a given context, with the objective of exerting pressure on the parties to the conflict and to encourage them to guarantee access to health services.

—— Humanitarian organizations can sidestep the prerogatives of authorities and offer health services without the approval of the latter. This approach has been at the origin of the "without borders" movements.

As one observes a radicalization of violence in armed conflicts,[35] there follows a certain "radicalization" in the protection of the right to health, which is integrated into the strategies that include protection by armed means to ensure the direct protection of persons. For example, the "humanitarian intervention" approach is used, or *"le droit d'ingérence"*, based on ethical considerations regarding the obligation to provide care to people in emergency health situations. Such interventions may serve to maintain peace or to restore peace.

> "Most United Nations multi-dimensional peacekeeping operations are therefore mandated to promote and protect human rights by monitoring and helping to investigate human rights violations and/or developing the capacity of national actors and institutions to do so on their own."[36]

The decisions to establish peacekeeping forces to protect populations are based on political and humanitarian factors. Whatever the share of one or the other may be, health considerations will play an important role. In a study on mortality in the Democratic Republic of the Congo (DRC), the authors recommended an increase of the UN peacekeeping forces to fight insecurity, which is the main factor that prevents populations from accessing health services in times of armed conflict.[37]

This type of epidemiological study has a positive impact on political decisions, especially when they are conducted with a high degree of professionalism. Following a study on mortality in Iraq,[38] the respective political players tried to discredit the results of the study by criticizing the method used to gather data.[39] There is a risk of focusing the discussion on the methods, instead of on the recommendations to overcome the problems encountered.

There is an interaction between humanitarian and political activities. In the short term, this tendency may have repercussions on the perception of the responsibilities of the players in armed conflicts.

The protection of the right to health in armed conflict: What is its evolution?

Two factors have to be considered:

—— Integration of the right to health in the general concept of "human security"; and
—— The search for some consistency between the political and humanitarian management of armed conflicts.

The right to health and human security

The right to health and other fundamental human rights are interrelated. The different violations of the physical and mental integrity of persons (torture, ill treatment, sexual violence, mutilations, etc.), and attacks on the social integrity of populations (ethnic purges, forced resettlements, breaking up of families, etc.), all have dramatic consequences for health. In more general terms, health professionals feel that it would be unethical to care for people without also taking into account the serious violations of human rights and IHL, of which they could also be victims.

For some years now, this global approach to human rights has been found in the concept of human security, which allows for the integration of all dimensions of human rights.[40]

The search for coherence between the political and humanitarian approaches to armed conflict

The political management of armed conflicts, and their humanitarian consequences, are increasingly considered to be an exercise that needs to be conducted in a coordinated manner.

The current trend is to search for coherence between the handling of armed conflict and its humanitarian consequences:

> "The original concept of coherence envisioned a collective rallying of military, political, economic and humanitarian assets to support peace and security. It assumed a common understanding of the nature and dynamics of conflict between these different domains, and a shared vision of the means of resolving such conflict and of the nature of peace."[41]

In practice, this global strategy designed to ensure the protection of human security will require interventions from several angles:

> "Civilians are the main casualties in conflicts. Both norms and mechanisms to protect civilians should be strengthened. This requires comprehensive and integrated strategies, linking political, military, humanitarian, and development aspects."[42]

This integration has repercussions on the specific strategies for protecting the right to health. For instance, preventing health problems in the context of massive population resettlements primarily rests on making the zones where these populations live safe, in order to prevent them from having to move for reasons of insecurity. If, in spite of everything, evacuations are unavoidable and people find themselves in camps, ensuring their safety is an essential element for the prevention of violations of their fundamental rights, and also to allow for the regular organization of medical assistance.

Integration also has repercussions for the sharing of responsibilities between the parties involved in armed conflict. To guarantee access to health services, we find ourselves in a two-way flow of responsibilities between civilian organizations (NGOs, specialized UN organizations), and the military either under a UN mandate (peacekeeping forces), or acting within the framework of agreements with national authorities (for example, the United States in Iraq).

The integration of political and humanitarian activities within a common strategy is not without risk.

Humanitarian organizations will have difficulty in distinguishing themselves from the political actors, who are parties in this strategy, and consequently to comply with the principle of neutrality vis-à-vis the parties to the conflict. The financing of humanitarian interventions by donor countries runs the risk of being conditioned by the progress achieved in the political handling of the armed conflict. A certain confusion may arise in the minds of the population regarding the perception of the mandates.

For instance, in Afghanistan the International Security Assistance Force (ISAF)[43] mission is to assist the Afghan government and the international community in maintaining security. In practice, this means that there will be joint interventions between ISAF forces and the Afghan police, and the Civil Military Cooperation (CIMIC)[44] projects concerning education, health, and drinking water.[45]

This mix of activities creates some confusion relating to the perception of the mandates, both among the population and the authorities. OXFAM notes: "As a result of the U.S. engaging in 'aid for information', Oxfam was forced to close its program in Kandahar in 2003 ... Communities that we work with have become confused as the lines between aid agencies and the military have become blurred in Afghanistan."[46]

In an attempt to avoid this confusion, some coherence will have to be sought, both at the political and the humanitarian levels. In the political handling of armed conflicts, the United Nations Organization plays this role with regard to bilateral interventions. In the handling of humanitarian matters that arise as a consequence of armed conflict, the current reforms of the UN system have the objective of achieving greater coherence in the realm of humanitarian action.

In the more specific area of health, the emergence of the World Health Organization (WHO) as a player in emergency situations, including those arising from armed conflicts, has given it a certain formalized credibility due to its status as head of the health cluster.

In 2008, the declaration of the WHO concerning the situation in the Gaza strip not only indicates that the WHO takes part in the analysis of health problems in situations of armed conflict, but also that it tries to achieve some coherence with its political management:

"WHO urges and requests:

1. Access of all urgent patients to specialized medical care outside the Gaza strip, without unnecessary delays which reduce their possibility of surviving;
2. Free and unhindered passage into Gaza of all necessary medical equipment, drugs, and consumables;
3. Provision of sufficient amounts of fuel and electricity for the Gaza strip to ensure the full functioning of hospitals, ambulances, generators, water and sanitation systems, and other vital infrastructures;
4. Availability of primary and secondary health care, water and food for people living under curfew within the Gaza strip.

WHO advocates for all parties concerned to bring to an immediate end all military operations and resume peace negotiations. Furthermore, WHO calls all parties involved to abide by and conform with the International Humanitarian Laws and the Human Rights Treaties including the respect and fulfilment of the right to health."[47]

Conclusion

The protection of the right to health in armed conflict requires reliance on a legal framework that recognizes the many facets of this right. While IHL integrates specific considerations, striking a balance between humanitarian considerations and military necessity, human rights law remains relevant to complement IHL in order to fill the potential gaps.

Considering the current and future evolution of armed conflicts and their impact on health, it is no longer a matter of thinking in terms of managing the humanitarian consequences of war, but rather of having to choose between war or health, because the consequences of war on the right to health will no longer be manageable for the medical corps.

Health professionals are also responsible for participating in the elaboration of a true strategy for the prevention of conflicts. In practice, they can contribute to this goal by:

—— Rationally using the epidemiological tools to promote health concerns in the context of current and future armed conflicts.

—— Exercising their ability to influence political players.

—— Controlling research and biotechnological work, for example through ethical committees, to ensure such research will not be applied towards developing new weapons.

—— Paradoxically, one major risk may derive from medical research: The use of genetically engineered germs, or even germs produced by nanotechnology, would have effects on the population, which would extend beyond any therapeutic capacity.

Only a strategy of preventing armed conflicts will allow us to safeguard the right to health for future generations.

---

* This chapter was originally written by the author in French and translated into English by Salomé Hangartner. The author would like to acknowledge with gratitude Theo Boutruche for his contribution to this chapter.

1 See, for example, Robin Coupland, 'The effects of weapons and the Solferino cycle' 319(7214) *British Medical Journal* (1999), at 864–865.

2 Committee on Economic, Social and Cultural Rights (CESCR), General Comment No. 14 on the right to the highest attainable standard of health, 11 August 2000, UN Doc. E/C.12/2000/4, at paras. 9 and 11.

3 See further http://www.who.int/topics/health_services/en/.

4 CESCR, *supra* note 2.

5 Article 25 of the Universal Declaration of Human Rights reads:

1. Everyone has the right to a standard of living adequate for the health and well-being of himself

and of his family, including food, clothing, housing, and medical care and necessary social services, and the right to security in the event of unemployment, sickness, disability, widowhood, old age or other lack of livelihood in circumstances beyond his control.

2. Motherhood and childhood are entitled to special care and assistance. All children, whether born in or out of wedlock, shall enjoy the same social protection.

6 Preamble of the Constitution of the World Health Organization (WHO) (1946), available at http://www.who.int/gb/bd/PDF/bd46/e-bd46_p2.pdf.

7 Hippocrates, *On The Physician,* 14: "Surgery concerning the injuries by war weapons is related to our topic, insofar as it has to do with the extraction of arrows."

8 First Geneva Convention for the Amelioration of the Condition of the Wounded in Armies in the Field (1864).

9 The IHL rules for protecting non-combatants in armed conflicts are contained in the four Geneva Conventions of 1949 and their two Additional Protocols of 1977. IHL depends on classifying a conflict as either an international armed conflict or a non-international conflict. International armed conflicts are those in which at least two states are opposing each other. These conflicts are ruled by a vast range of rules, among them the ones stated in the Geneva Conventions of 1949 and the additional Protocol I of 1977. In non-international armed conflicts, dissident armed forces are confronting each other on the territory of a single state, or armed groups are fighting each other. More limited rules, overall, are applicable to this type of conflict.

10 Instructions for the Government of Armies of the United States in the Field (1863).

11 Declaration (IV, 3) concerning Expanding Bullets (1899), available at http://www.icrc.org/ihl.nsf/FULL/170?OpenDocument.

12 Convention on the Prohibition of the Development, Production and Stockpiling of Bacteriological (Biological) and Toxin Weapons and on their Destruction (1972), available at http://www.icrc.org/ihl.nsf/FULL/450?OpenDocument.

13 Convention on the prohibition of the development, production, stockpiling and use of chemical weapons and on their destruction (1993), available at http://www.icrc.org/ihl.nsf/INTRO/553?OpenDocument.

14 *Legality of the Use by a State of Nuclear Weapons in Armed Conflicts,* I. C. J. Reports (1996), para. 31.

15 Article 10, First Additional Protocol to the Geneva Conventions (1977).

16 Article 12, paragraph 1, and Article 15, paragraph 1 of the First Additional Protocol to the Geneva Conventions; Article 19 of the Fourth Geneva Convention, Article 15 of the First Additional Protocol and Article 11 of the Second Additional Protocol.

17 "Starvation of civilians as a method of combat is prohibited. It is therefore prohibited to attack, destroy, remove or render useless, for that purpose, objects indispensable to the survival of the civilian population, such as foodstuffs, agricultural areas for the production of foodstuffs, crops, livestock, drinking water installations and supplies and irrigation works": Article 14, Second Additional Protocol to the Geneva Conventions.

18 Article 56 of the Fourth Geneva Convention.

19 Article 14, Second Additional Protocol to the Geneva Conventions.

20 International Committee of the Red Cross (ICRC), Handicap International, Human Rights Watch, United Nations Mine Action Service.

21 Cluster munitions are defined as "all ammunitions or explosive charges designed to blow up at a specific moment after having been launched or ejected from a parent cluster munition": 10th Session of the Group of Government Experts of the Parties to the 1980 Convention on Certain Classical Weapons, 8 March 2005.

22 Human Rights Watch, *Cluster Weapons: Scourge of Civilians,* 23 September 2008.

23 ICRC, *Cluster Munitions: Decades of Failure, Decades of Civilian Suffering* (Geneva: ICRC, 2008), available at http://www.icrc.org/web/eng/siteeng0.nsf/html/p0946.

24 Protocol on Blinding Laser Weapons, Protocol IV of the 1980 Convention on Certain Conventional Weapons (1995).

25 See further http://www.unhchr.ch/html/menu2/7/b/principles.htm.

26 Tokyo Declaration of the World Medical Association Directives for physicians concerning torture and other punishments or cruel, inhumane or debasing treatments in the context of detention or imprisonment.

27 World Medical Association Resolution on Economic Embargoes and Health (1997).

28 World Medical Association Regulations in Times of Armed Conflict (1956).

29 World Medical Association Statement on Medical Ethics in the Event of Disasters (2006).

30 World Medical Association Mission Statement, available at http://www.wma.net/e/about/index.htm#mission.

31 ICRC, 'Assistance Policy', reproduced in 855 International Review of the Red Cross (2004), at 677–693.

32 Common Article 3 of the four Geneva Conventions.

33 Benjamin Coghlan, Richard J. Brennan et al. 'Mortality in the Democratic Republic of the Congo: A Nationwide Survey' 367 The Lancet (2006), at 44–51.

34 World Health Organization (WHO), 25 Questions on Health and Human Rights (Geneva: WHO, 2002), available at http://www.who.int/entity/hhr/NEW37871OMSOK.pdf.

35 Report of the Secretary-General of the United Nations on the Protection of Civilians in Armed Conflict, 28 November 2005, UN Doc. No. s/2007/643.

36 Jean-Marie Guéhenno, Under-Secretary-General for Peacekeeping Operations, United Nations Peace Keeping Operations: Principles and Guidelines, March 2008.

37 Coghlan, supra note 33.

38 Gilbert Burnham, Riyadh Lafta, Shannon Doocy, Les Roberts, 'Mortality after the 2003 invasion of Iraq: A cross-sectional cluster sample survey', 368(9546) The Lancet (2006), at 1421–1428.

39 U.S. President George Bush dismissed the methodology as "pretty well discredited": CNN,

'Study: War Blamed for 665 000 Iraqi Deaths', 11 October 2006. Australian Prime Minister John Howard said: "It's not plausible, it's not based on anything other than a house-to-house survey ...": Australian Broadcasting corporation, 'Report reignites debate over human cost of Iraq war', The World Today, Tuesday, 27 March 2007.

40 Perrin Pierre, 'Santé publique et sécurité dans les urgences complexes' 25 Refugee Survey Quarterly (2006), at 35–41.

41 Humanitarian Policy Group, 'The Politics of Coherence: Humanitarianism and Foreign Policy in the Post-Cold War Era', Briefing Paper 1, July 2000, available at www.odi.org.uk/hpg/papers/hpgbrief1.pdf.

42 Commission on Human Security, Human Security Now (New York: Commission on Human Security, 2003), available at http://www.humansecurity-chs.org/finalreport/index.html.

43 The International Security Assistance Force (ISAF) is NATO's first mission outside the Euro-Atlantic area. ISAF operates in Afghanistan under a UN mandate and will continue to operate according to current and future UN Security Council resolutions.

44 Civil Military Cooperation (CIMIC) Projects are developed by NATO to reinforce cooperation between NATO and the civilian authorities of the population.

45 NATO, 'NATO in Afghanistan: Factsheet', July 2007, available at http://www.nato.int/issues/afghanistan/040628-factsheet.htm.

46 Caroline Green, OXFAM spokesperson, comments reported by International Inter Press Service, August 2004.

47 WHO, 'Statement on the situation in Gaza', 3 March 2008, available at www.who.int/entity/hac/crises/international/middle_east/WHO%20statement%20on%20situation%20in%20Gaza.pdf.

The Right to Health in Emergencies: Natural or Man-Made Disasters

Obijiofor Aginam*

Introduction: Overview of natural disasters

Recent emerging and re-occurring natural and man-made disasters around the world reinforce the potency of the forces of humanity's destruction as depicted by 'The Four Horsemen of the Apocalypse – Conquest, War, Famine/Pestilence/Drought/Mass Starvation, and Death.'[1] Examples of the devastation caused by disasters abound in every region of the world. The Hanshin Earthquake ("Kobe earthquake" as it is commonly known outside of Japan) of 17 January 1995 with its epicentre in the Awaji Island, Japan, claimed over 6000 lives, and devastated the city of Kobe. This was the worst earthquake in Japan since the Kanto earthquake of 1923 that claimed 140 000 lives. The Indian Ocean tsunami of December 2004, with its epicentre off the west coast of Sumatra, Indonesia, triggered a series of devastating tsunamis on the Indian Ocean coasts killing over 200 000 people. As one of the deadliest natural disasters in history, it caused massive damage and claimed thousands of lives in Indonesia, Sri Lanka, India, and Thailand. In August 2006, hurricane Katrina, one of the deadliest hurricanes in the history of the United States, devastated the city of New Orleans, caused extensive damage along the entire Mississippi coast, and led to the loss of over 1500 lives. In May 2008, cyclone Nargis flattened buildings, claimed over 100 000 lives, and rendered over 1 million people homeless in Myanmar. The recent earthquake in China, past and recurring hurricanes and tornadoes in the Americas and the Caribbean, flood, famine and drought in parts of Africa, have brought in their wake complex questions about realizing the right to health in emergencies.

Natural or man-made disasters: Cyclone, tornado, hurricane, flood, tsunami, earthquake, volcanic eruption, forest fire, chemical spills, and climate change-induced drought, famine, rainfall variations, and the shrinking of fresh watercourses, result in unimaginable human suffering, mass starvation, and unquantifiable humanitarian catastrophe. These are crises that often bring together the two components of human security: "freedom from fear" (as in the case of Myanmar) where the state constitutes an impediment to humanitarian assistance from the international community, and "freedom from want" where disasters lead to mass starvation, breakdown of public health infrastructure, hunger, and lack of the essential necessities of life.[2]

This chapter assesses the challenges of promoting and realizing the right to health in natural and man-made disasters, and suggests practical ways of achieving the "right of everyone to the highest attainable standard of health" in emergencies. The promotion of the right to health in natural or man-made disasters is of particular concern to the international community, especially in the light of recent disasters such as the Indonesian tsunami, the earthquake in China, and the cyclone Nargis in Myanmar. Both in normal times and during disasters, the overwhelming burden of health problems, disease, hunger, starvation, and death lies on vulnerable groups who are least able to afford medical treatment and preventive measures, and whose governments have the least capacity to meet these urgent needs. Simultaneously, the human cost of climate change and related natural disasters is especially severe in developing countries. Disasters raise serious human security questions for the international community. In situations like the Indonesian tsunami, although international humanitarian response was remarkable, serious problems were encountered in distributing humanitarian aid. So where does the right to health fit in emergencies?

Overview of the right to health in international legal instruments

International legal instruments, including human rights treaties, contain numerous provisions that protect and promote the right to health. This chapter highlights, as examples, a few of the key international legal instruments that codify the right to health. First, early in the history of the United Nations, the Universal Declaration of Human Rights (1948) affirmed that:

> "Everyone has the right to a standard of living adequate for the health and
> well-being of himself and of his family, including food, clothing, housing,
> and medical care and necessary social services, and the right to security
> in the event of unemployment, sickness, disability, widowhood, old age or
> other lack of livelihood in circumstances beyond his control."[3]

Second, the Constitution of the World Health Organization (WHO), one of the first specialized agencies to be established within the United Nations system provides that:

> "[T]he enjoyment of the highest attainable standard of health is one of the
> fundamental rights of every human being without distinction of race, re-
> ligion, political belief, economic or social condition."[4]

Third, Article 12(1) of the International Covenant on Economic, Social, and Cultural Rights (ICESCR) 1966 recognizes the "right of everyone to the enjoyment of the highest attainable standard of physical and mental health", and lists the steps to be taken by States Parties to the ICESCR to achieve the full realization of this right. With respect to other health-related economic and social issues, especially food and housing, Article 11 of the ICESCR recognizes "the right of everyone to an adequate standard of living ... including adequate food, clothing and housing, and to the continuous improvement of living conditions." Everyone has a fundamental right to be free from hunger.

Fourth, in the specific context of children, the Convention on the Rights of the Child (1989) provides that "States Parties recognize the right of the child to the enjoyment of the highest attainable standard of health and to facilities for the treatment of illness and rehabilitation of health. States Parties shall strive to ensure that no child is deprived of his or her right of access to such health care services."[5]

Although normative provisions on health abound in international legal instruments, realizing, protecting, enforcing, and promoting the right to health both in ordinary times, and in emergencies, has proved exceedingly complex. As the outgoing United Nations Special Rapporteur on the Right to Health Paul Hunt rightly observed, the key next step is to foster an understanding "... that the right to the highest attainable standard of health is not just a rhetorical device, but a tool that can save lives and reduce suffering, especially among the most disadvantaged."[6] And the most powerful tool it provides is that of accountability – accountability that does not seek to blame and punish, but one that sets standards and seeks to discover what works and what can be improved.[7]

Accountability for the right to health in emergencies

In an emergency situation of a natural or man-made disaster, the right to health can be used to monitor the humanitarian response by local, regional, national and international actors. Every international legal instrument that provides for the right to health stresses the need for "international assistance and cooperation". This is because disasters often overwhelm local capacity and infrastructure for health-care delivery. A disaster, as observed by the WHO Collaborating Centre for Research on the Epidemiology of Disasters (CRED), is "... a situation or event, which *overwhelms local capacity*, necessitating a request to national or international level for *external assistance*."[8] As unforeseen and often sudden events, disasters cause "great damage, destruction and human suffering."[9] The key questions remain: is there an obligation on the affected state to accept external "humanitarian" assistance without delay where a significant percentage of its population is vulnerable to starvation, unnecessary suffering, and imminent death? Do other states have an obligation to offer humanitarian assistance to a state hit by a disaster?

The Guiding Principles for the provision of humanitarian assistance, as set out in UN General Assembly Resolution 48/182 (1991), affirm that "the sovereignty, territorial integrity and national unity of States must be fully respected in accordance with the Charter of the United Nations. In this context, humanitarian assistance *should be provided with the consent of the affected country and in principle on the basis of an appeal by the affected country*."[10] However, even though "[e]ach State has the responsibility first and foremost to take care of the victims of natural disasters and other emergencies occurring on its territory,"[11] what happens if that State cannot or does not take care of its own population? Here the international community has to grapple with the tension between state/territorial sovereignty, and humanitarian intervention which has now been addressed in the emerging norm of the "Responsibility to Protect".[12] This scenario, as exemplified in the attitude of the government of Myanmar towards international humanitarian assistance after cyclone Nargis, presents a difficult conundrum in realizing the right to health in emergencies. In the wake of cyclone Nargis, opinions were sharply divided on whether the norm of Responsibility to Protect should be invoked to deliver food, medicine and other essential supplies to the affected population in Myanmar.

The French Foreign Minister and co-founder of the humanitarian non-governmental organization, Médecins sans Frontières, Bernard Kouchner, and Lloyd Axworthy, former Canadian Foreign Minister and now President of the University of Winnipeg, strongly called for the invocation of the Responsibility to Protect norm to protect the people of Myanmar who were at risk, not only from natural disaster, but also from their government's neglect by wilfully blocking the delivery of humanitarian aid: Food, medicines, and other essential supplies. According to Axworthy, "there is no moral difference between an innocent person being killed by machete or AK-47, and starving to death, or dying in a cholera epidemic that could have been avoided by proper international response."[13]

Gareth Evans, former Australian Foreign Minister and now head of the International Crisis Group, and Ramesh Thakur, former Senior Vice Rector, United Nations University and now distinguished fellow at the Centre for International Governance Innovation (CIGI), Waterloo, Canada, were ambivalent about invoking the Responsibility to Protect in the Myanmar case. Both Evans and Thakur were part of the Canadian-sponsored International Commission on Intervention and State Sovereignty (ICISS) that put forward the Responsibility to Protect norm. Thakur points out that, while the original Responsibility to Protect concept included issues surrounding natural disasters, the need to build international consensus on the concept at the UN World Summit in 2005 restricted the circumstances for invoking the norm to large scale killings and ethnic cleansing, not death caused by natural disasters.[14] According to Evans, the norm is about protecting vulnerable populations from genocide, war crimes, ethnic cleansing and crimes against humanity. Even in such cases, the norm allows the use of military force only with the authorization of the UN Security Council.[15]

Calling for some form of action, Knight and Popovski advocated for the categorization of the (in)action of the government of Myanmar as a crime against humanity. Doing so would have bolstered the case for discussion in the UN Security Council about invoking the norm in the Myanmar case. To do otherwise would portray the international community as more concerned about preserving the norm than protecting the vulnerable Myanmar people.[16] As the case of Myanmar has demonstrated, the international community must find ways to deal with "overwhelming natural and environmental catastrophes" within the Responsibility to Protect doctrine. While there is little room for shuttle diplomacy in emergency situations, simply because people are dying by the minute, in situations like Myanmar, where the government wilfully blocks humanitarian aid, it is imperative that the use of good offices of top diplomats, even at the level of the UN Secretary-General as Ban Ki-moon did with his visit to Myanmar, could persuade the government to shift its position.[17] In other emergency situations, where governments accept external humanitarian assistance, difficult questions remain on the coordination and implementation of humanitarian assistance.

The role of the international community in promoting the right to health in emergencies

The question whether one state owes an obligation to promote the right to health of populations in another state, albeit complex in the context of state sovereignty, seems to find support in Article 2 of the ICESR which contemplates that states do have obligations to those in other countries. Although this question reflects the realities of the state-centric international system, Professor Louis Henkin, one of the most influential human rights scholars of our time, has rightly argued that:

> "[A]nother state can help to give effect to some economic-social rights – the right to food, education, health-care and an adequate standard of living – without forcible intervention, merely by financial aid to the local government ... and as the Third World has insisted on its campaign for a new International Economic Order ... wealthy states are therefore morally obligated and should be legally obligated to help the poorer states."[18]

Despite this persuasive view, difficult questions still need to be answered. As Gostin and Archer queried, "... if States have the capacity to assist less developed States (while continuing to fulfil their obligations to the health of their own citizens), to what extent do they have a well-defined legal or ethical responsibility to do so?"[19] The problem remains that while states' responsibilities to assist other states may derive from law, political commitments, ethical values, and national interests, international human rights law currently does not provide clear direction to states in order to operationalize this responsibility.[20] This is partly because of the weak enforcement mechanisms for international human rights treaties. But there is no reason why the principle of sovereignty should not give ground to human need in order to, as Gostin and Archer argue, "enlarge the political space for developing a forum of consensual international cooperation."[21] At the moment, as pointed out by Hardcastle and Chua, there exists no multilateral treaty like the Geneva Conventions (applicable in times of armed conflict) that provides for the right of victims of national disasters to receive humanitarian assistance.[22]

Because of the lack of a political space to operationalize the responsibilities of states during disasters, it becomes extremely difficult to determine the scope of such responsibilities. This is also complicated by the real challenges that the right to health in international law faces: Definition, scope, benchmarks for identification of a violation, and enforcement. In order to deal with such problematic issues, and give meaning to the language of the ICESCR, the Committee on Economic, Social and Cultural Rights (CESCR) has produced a number of General Comments which were intended to, and indeed do, have significant normative force. In 2000, the CESCR clarified that under Articles 12(1) and 2(1), states do have an international legal obligation to be active in respect of the right to health (and its violations), and where resources are available, they "should facilitate access to essential health facilities, goods and services in other countries, wherever possible and provide the necessary aid when required."[23] This is particularly relevant in the context of disasters, where "State parties have a joint and individual responsibility, in accordance with the Charter of the United Nations and relevant resolutions of the United Nations General Assembly, and of the World Health Assembly, to cooperate in providing disaster relief and humanitarian assistance in times of emergency ..."[24] In fact, the CESCR went so far as to state:

> "[For] the avoidance of any doubt, the Committee wishes to emphasize that it is particularly incumbent on States parties and other actors in a position to assist, to provide 'international assistance and cooperation, especially

economic and technical' [Article 2(1) ICESCR] which enable developing countries to fulfil their core and other obligations ..."[25]

While there are still instances where states do refuse external humanitarian assistance, most notably North Korea, Iran after the 1990 earthquake, Afghanistan after the 1998 earthquake, and most recently Myanmar after cyclone Nargis, the CESCR has emphasized that in order to comply with its core obligations under the ICESCR, a state must demonstrate not only that it is using the maximum of its own available resources, but that it has attempted to use the maximum of the international community's available resources.[26]

National sovereignty is indeed an increasingly weak defence against intervention when a government is failing to fulfil its responsibilities to its own people. In this context, some legal scholars have expressly called for a significant shift towards recognizing the right to health in emergencies, especially during natural and man-made disasters within the emergent Responsibility to Protect norm.[27] Perhaps the broader issue is whether or not a legal enforcement mechanism would be helpful at all. There is a strong case to suggest that were it actually possible to create such a mechanism, it would not improve the current effectiveness of pressuring governments to rectify individual privations and to provide humanitarian assistance or to accept it in times of disaster.[28]

Towards a better disaster response framework: The way forward

"Intervention", even when its overwhelming mission is to deliver humanitarian assistance in times of emergency, can be extremely politicized. Because of "national interests" and ideological and other differences, the governments of Iran, Myanmar, and Afghanistan under the Taliban, for instance, would flatly refuse any humanitarian assistance from the United States and the major powers in Europe. With the end of the Cold War, the world moved away from hard state security issues, like nuclear threats, to soft human security issues, like infectious diseases, hunger and environmental threats. Despite this transformation, differences still remain. Humanity will continue to live with natural disasters: Cyclones, tornados, hurricanes, floods, tsunamis, earthquakes, volcanic eruptions, forest fires, chemical spills, and other climate-change-induced calamities. The question is how to cope with and mitigate their impact on vulnerable populations within the territories of nation-states.

As a basic first step, the international community must re-think how to improve the effectiveness of humanitarian assistance and how to better coordinate response to disasters. Academic and policy debate, thus far, has narrowly focused on the impediments of state sovereignty to the right to health provisions in international legal instruments, as well as the right to intervene to deliver humanitarian assistance. The right of access to victims of natural disasters has operated on a patchwork of laws and frameworks. In a recent exhaustive and insightful study, the International Federation of Red Cross and Red Crescent Societies comprehensively articulated the law and legal issues in international disaster response.[29] This ambitious work points the way forward on most of the difficult issues that impede the delivery of humanitarian assistance: Problems with visas and work permits for doctors, nurses, and other humanitarian workers, customs procedures for clearance of relief materials and essential supplies like medicines, food and water, transportation and movement of equipment, as well as how to balance sovereignty and humanitarian concerns using both hard law and soft law approaches. The study also includes a survey of the relevant treaties and soft-law provisions that aid humanitarian work and the challenges of using these mechanisms in various regions of the world, given each region's specific social and economic context. The study also highlighted lessons learned from responses to past disasters as a way to improve future responses by the international disaster response community. All of these issues have to be addressed holistically by all actors: States, international organizations, and non-state actors that work on response to natural disasters.

* The author would like to acknowledge the excellent research assistance provided by David M. H. Stranger-Jones in the writing of this chapter.

1 Brian D. Vos, 'The Four Horsemen of the Apocalypse', *The Outlook*, June 2006 vol. 56 no. 4, at 16–20; Four Horsemen of the Apocalypse, available at http://en.wikipedia.org/wiki/Four_Horsemen_of_the_Apocalypse.

2 Commission on Human Security, *Human Security Now* (New York: Commission on Human Security, 2003); Report of the UN Secretary-General, Kofi Annan, *In Larger Freedom* (New York: United Nations, 2005).

3 Article 25(1) of the Universal Declaration of Human Rights (1948).

4 Preamble, Constitution of the World Health Organization, signed on 22 July 1946, and entered into force on 7 April 1948.

5 Article 24.

6 Paul Hunt, 'Poverty, Malaria and the Right to Health: Exploring the Connections', Annual Lecture on Malaria and Human Rights, 10 December 2007, at 6, available at http://www.malaria consortium.org/data/files/10_dec_2007_malaria_paper_with_footnotes__18_dec_07_.pdf.

7 Ibid., at 5.

8 CRED's 'EMDAT: International Emergency Disasters Database' website, http://www.emdat.be/ExplanatoryNotes/glossary.html.

9 Ibid.

10 'Strengthening of the coordination of humanitarian emergency assistance of the United Nations', General Assembly Resolution A/RES/46/182, 19 December 1991, Annex, para. 3 (emphasis added), available at http://www.un.org/documents/ga/res/46/a46r182.htm.

11 UN Resolution 46/182, para. 4.

12 See *The Responsibility to Protect*, Report of the International Commission on Intervention and State Sovereignty (Ottawa: IDRC, 2001)

13 Lloyd Axworthy, 'It's time to Intervene', *Ottawa Citizen*, Ottawa, 13 May 2008.

14 Ramesh Thakur, 'Should the UN Invoke the "Re-

sponsibility to Protect"', *The Globe and Mail*, Toronto, 8 May 2008.

15 Gareth Evans, 'Facing up to Our Responsibilities', *The Guardian*, London, 12 May 2008.

16 W. Andy Knight and Vesselin Popovski, 'Putting People Ahead of Protocol', *The Edmonton Journal*, Edmonton, 4 June 2008.

17 On the use of the good offices of the UN Secretary General, and his role as a norm entrepreneur, see Thomas Franck, 'The Secretary General's Role in Conflict Resolution: Past, Present, and Pure Conjecture' 6 *European Journal of International Law* (1995), 360–387; T. M. Franck and G. Nolte, 'The Good Offices Function of the UN Secretary-General' in Adam Roberts and Benedict Kingsbury (eds.), *United Nations, Divided World* (Second edition, New York: Oxford University Press, 1993) 143–182; Simon Rushton, 'The UN Secretary-General and Norm Entrepreneurship: Boutros Boutros Ghali and Democracy Promotion' 14(1) Global Governance (2008), 95–110.

18 Louis Henkin, *The Age of Rights* (New York: Columbia University Press, 1990) 4.

19 Lawrence O. Gostin and R. Archer, 'The Duty of States to Assist Other States in Need: Ethics, Human Rights, and International Law', *Journal of Law, Medicine & Ethics* (2007) 526–533, at 530.

20 Ibid.

21 Ibid., at 531.

22 Rohan Hardcastle and Adrian Chua, 'Humanitarian Assistance: Towards a Right of Access to Victims of Natural Disasters' 38 *International Review of the Red Cross* (1998), at 589.

23 Committee on Economic, Social and Cultural Rights (CESCR), *General Comment No. 14*, UN Doc. E/C.12/2000/4, 4 July 2000, at para. 39, available at http://www.unhchr.ch/tbs/doc.nsf/(symbol)/E.C.12.2000.4.En?OpenDocument.

24 Ibid., at para. 40.

25 Ibid., at para. 45.

26 CESCR, *General Comment No. 12 on the right to adequate food*, UN Doc. E/C.12/1999/5, 26 April – 14 May 1999, at para. 17, availableat http://www.

unhchr.ch/tbs/doc.nsf(symbol)/CESCR+General+comment+3.En?OpenDocument.

27 See C. Stahn, 'Responsibility to Protect: Political Rhetoric or Emerging Legal Norm?' 101 *American Journal of International Law* (2007) 99–120, at 101.

28 Michael J. Dennis and David P. Stewart, 'Justiciability of Economic, Social and Cultural Rights: Should There Be an International Complaints Mechanism to Adjudicate the Rights to Food, Water, Housing and Health?' 98 *American Journal of International Law* (2004), at 462–515.

29 See the recently released study by the International Federation of Red Cross and Red Crescent Societies, *Law and Legal issues in International Disaster Response: A Desk Study* (Geneva: International Federation of Red Cross and Red Crescent Societies, 2007).

04

PEOPLE AND GROUPS AT RISK

The Right to Health in Prisons: Implications in a Borderless World

Slim Slama, Hans Wolff and Louis Loutan

Introduction

The right to health in prison[1] has been recently subject to increased attention, at both national and international levels, with many standards, rules and codes of practice having been defined in order to guarantee the fundamental rights of prisoners and make prisons healthier places for both detainees and staff.

It is now generally recognized that prisoners have a right to health care and to protection against inhumane and degrading treatment. Regardless of the nature of their offence, prisoners are entitled to all fundamental human rights, including the right to the highest attainable standards of physical and mental health. More specifically, they retain the right to a standard of medical care which is at least equivalent to that provided in their broader community.

However, despite some improvements in the conditions of detention, in too many parts of the world rhetoric does not match reality.[2] Minimal standards of living conditions and access to health care for prisoners are often inadequate, if not totally inexistent. Prisons and jails in even the richest and most developed countries are still plagued by severe overcrowding, decaying physical infrastructure, a lack of medical care, security abuses and

corruption, and prisoner-on-prisoner violence. Rates of infection with regards to tuberculosis, HIV and hepatitis are much higher than in the general population, and chronic diseases, especially psychiatric conditions, are
often neglected.[3]

International monitors

Various international and regional oversight bodies concerned with human rights systematically investigate and document the living conditions
of prisoners. Two UN Human Rights bodies are particularly important to
mention: The UN Committee Against Torture (CAT) and the Special Rapporteur on Torture, both of which monitor the implementation of the Convention against Torture and Other Cruel, Inhuman or Degrading Treatment
or Punishment, and the Working Group on Arbitrary Detention which in-
vestigates cases of deprivation of liberty imposed arbitrarily and monitors
compliance with the relevant international standards. Since 2006 and the
entry into force of the Optional Protocol to the Convention against Torture
and other Cruel, Inhuman or Degrading Treatment or Punishment, an international visiting mechanism for the prevention of torture has been set
up. To date, 37 of the 62 countries that have signed the Optional Protocol
have also ratified it,[4] allowing regular visits on their territory.

Similar mechanisms have been implemented at a regional level, within
the member states of the Council of Europe, with the European Committee for the Prevention of Torture and Inhuman or Degrading Treatment or
Punishment (CPT). The Committee, composed of independent and impartial experts from various backgrounds, exerts its control by means of regular visits to different places of detention (e.g. prisons and juvenile detention centres, police stations, holding centres for immigration detainees and
psychiatric hospitals). It surveys the conditions of detention and recommends, if necessary, improvements to the states visited.[5]

The work of these international oversight bodies is also supported by a
wide range of international non-governmental organizations and civil society actors. Many, like Amnesty International or Human Rights Watch, are
engaged in advocacy and raising awareness about human rights violations
in places of detention. Others, like the Association for the Prevention of
Torture, advocate for legislative reform, ratification and implementation
of relevant international treaties. Many of them work closely with states
through regular visits to places of detention. Rarely acknowledged, the In-

ternational Committee of the Red Cross (ICRC), under the Geneva Conventions, has developed a long-standing practice of visiting prisoners of war and civilian internees.

The role of health workers

Primary care physicians and front-line workers (nurses) play a central role in prisons and share a direct responsibility to ensure that detainees can exert their right to health as they do for other patients outside the penitential setting.[6] Although medical workers in general do not require knowledge of human rights and law, their ethical duties require them to assume the role of advocates on behalf of their patients. This is particularly true in the closed and isolated environment of prisons, where human rights abuses occur with impunity and where health workers are sometimes the first witnesses of such violations.

This said, health professionals are often unaware of the ethical and human rights framework in which their activity takes place. Moreover, they tend to underestimate the use of legal instruments and litigation as a way to enforce the right to life and to health. Developing an understanding of the right to health does not necessarily entail adopting a different way of working. On the contrary, the right to health could be a practical tool for health professionals that are confronted with human rights issues in their daily clinical practice.[7] Practising medicine in prison requires that clinical competence, which guarantees quality of care, be linked with a sharp awareness of deontology codes and international ethical standards. Innovations and improvements in health services are often the result of interactions between end users, health care providers and policy makers. Protecting the rights of the prison population imposes innovative thinking inspired first by patients' needs and expectations. The accumulated experiences of prison medicine could play a complementary role in documenting situations that could lead to health policy reforms. The systematic screening of violence at prison entry – which explores violence experienced by detainees during arrest or incarceration (violence expert testimony evaluation) – is a good example of how organized epidemiologic and clinical information collection could be used to defend prisoners' rights and improve prison practice.[8] Such operational research, using equity as its conceptual "lens", offers a means of monitoring the relevance and responsiveness of clinical activities in such settings.

This chapter will not review legal instruments or expert recommendations. International human rights standards and legal instruments are used as a reference point that serves as a guide to translating what may be considered abstract theory into practical application in the day-to-day work of health professionals involved in prisons.[9] One of the aims of this chapter is to discuss how front line health care professionals, working in prisons, can contribute to protecting and improving prisoners' rights to health by using medical evidence collected from their daily clinical experiences.

While conditions of detention vary substantially from country to country, and despite the fact that the cases presented here are based on real situations in a remand prison of Switzerland, one of the richest and most developed countries in the world, many of the issues addressed illustrate some important aspects of promoting good health in prisons worldwide.

The chapter will first describe the trajectory of an inmate entering the prison of Champ-Dollon, the remand prison of the State of Geneva, Switzerland, highlighting some important issues that could hamper access to health in prison. We will then use two short stories inspired from our local practice to illustrate some of the daily challenges encountered. The last section will concentrate on the growing number of prisoners worldwide, and, more specifically on the increase of foreign populations in Swiss and European prisons, which constitutes one of the greatest challenges for prison management in Europe. We will discuss the impact of the political environment upon prisoners' health and rehabilitation opportunities. Some recommendations will be proposed in conclusion.

Setting the scene: The medical unit at the remand prison of Champ-Dollon, Geneva, Switzerland

The remand prison of Champ-Dollon is Switzerland's largest prison. Its organization is the result of an interesting legal framework that has been subject to several adaptations.[10]

A special state decree, in force since September 2000,[11] describes the obligations and organization of medical care in prisons. It follows the recommendation of the Committee of Ministers of the Council of Europe (No. R (98) 7 on the Ethical and Organizational Aspects of Health Care in Prison).[12] The total separation of power between the judicial system and health care providers has been central to responding to detainees' health-related rights. Indeed, all medical units responsible for the care of detainees are independent of the prison administration and the Cantonal Department of Justice and Police. All are part of the University Hospitals of Geneva, which is under the responsibility of the Cantonal Department of Health.

The prison health services comprise outpatient primary care clinics (one for adult and one for juvenile detainees) as well as inpatient units (one for psychiatric patients, located on the prison grounds, and a second medico-surgical unit, located at the main site of the University Hospital), the overarching mandate being to ensure comprehensive somatic and psychiatric health care.

Prison health staff consist of university-trained rotating physicians and nurses. The interdisciplinary team, comprised of general practitioners, nurses, psychiatrists, psychologists and various specialists, engages in more than 14 500 consultations per year, offering curative and preventive interventions.[13]

Champ-Dollon prison population

Champ-Dollon is sadly notorious for being the country's most overcrowded prison.[14] In 2007, for a normal capacity set at 270, an average of 456 detainees (169% capacity) were incarcerated. 95% were male, and the average age was 30.1 years. Of the 108 national origins, 10.6% were Swiss, 18.7% Eastern European, 18.5% Western European, 18.8% North African, 18.9% sub-Saharan African, 10% Asian and 4.5% American (North and South). In terms of legal status, 62% were undocumented migrants. The length of stay in the prison was less than 1 week for 33% of those incarcerated, less than 1 month for 50% and less than 90 days for 71% of the detainees. In January 2008, Geneva authorities opened La Brenaz, a modern prison on land adjacent to Champ-Dollon, designed to help ease the situation at the neighbouring facility.

Beyond principles: Access to health care in Champ-Dollon prison

The right to health in prison begins with the recognition that, despite having been deprived of their liberty, people in prison retain their fundamental right to good health – both physical and mental – and can expect to receive health care that is at least equivalent to that provided in the wider community. This principle of equivalence is cited in numerous national and international directives and recommendations, the most explicit being the

Recommendation (No. R (98) 7, of 8 April 1998)[15] of the Committee of Ministers of the Council of Europe, and the recent Recommendation (No. R (2006) 2)[16] updating the European Prison Rules.[17]

Along with the principle of equivalence, three other governing principles of the European instrument form the ethical pillars of health care in prison: Confidentiality, informed consent and independence.

Prison medicine in Geneva strives to apply these guiding principles. Effective implementation requires a constant battle to overcome several barriers.

The equivalence of care in prison is a measure of the extent to which a society practices the principle of equality of citizens by providing the same quality and range of care as in the wider community.

The application of this principle also responds to the values of justice and solidarity. However, the characteristics of the prison population and the settings in which care is provided are far from being equivalent to what is provided to the general population. As shown by Niveau, the principle of equivalence is often insufficient to take into account the adaptation of the organization of health care essential to the correctional setting.[18]

Providing care in prison involves working with men and women who have been deprived of their liberty. Many of them are likely to be mentally disturbed, suffer from addictions or other chronic conditions, have poor social and educational skills, and come from marginalized groups in society.[19] Prisoners are more likely to be in a bad state of health when they enter prison and have therefore more health-related needs, and higher consumption of health services, than the general population.[20]

Moreover, assessing health needs is often difficult. Uncertainty regarding judicial decisions, security or disciplinary measures, overcrowding, dirty or depressing environments, poor food, lack of activity, availability of illicit drugs, promiscuity, power struggles and intimidation between inmates and guards, all tend to affect the health of prisoners and their ability to express their needs.

Health evaluation therefore must be more systematic and proactive than in a conventional primary care setting. For this transient, high risk, vulnerable population, medical services offered free of charge offer a unique chance to express a health concern and seek care. Prison health services provide an opportunity to screen and diagnose neglected conditions or symptoms that, if left untreated, may lead to life-threatening conditions (chronic viral hepatitis, insulin-requiring diabetes) and/or may be a cause of public health concern when the detainee returns to the community (e.g. tuberculosis). Common problems encountered in health care practice are listed in box 01.

Box 01: Common problems in prison health care practice

Physical illness includes:

1. Dependence (drugs, alcohol, tobacco);

2. infections;

3. dental disease;

4. chronic disorders (lung disease, heart disease, diabetes, epilepsy, diseases of the reproductive system, cancer).

Mental health problems include:

1. Low mood or self-confidence (self-esteem and dependence: Drugs or alcohol);

2. anxiety;

3. depression;

4. severe mental disorders.

Co-occurring problems include:

1. "Vulnerable" people (learning disability, brain injury, learning difficulty, for instance resulting from autistic spectrum disorder or Asperger's syndrome or dyslexia; and

2. the nature of the sentence (harm against women, offences against children, bullying or recollection of being a victim of abuse).

Poor general condition includes:

1. Hygiene;

2. nutrition;

3. mobility;

4. personality disorder;

5. physical and mental trauma and stress.

Source: Lars Møller, Heino Stöver, Ralf Jürgens, Alex Gatherer and Haik Nikogosian (eds.) *Health in Prisons: A WHO Guide to the Essentials in Prison Health* (Copenhagen: WHO Regional Office for Europe, 2007), at 26, available at http://www.euro.who.int/document/e90174.pdf. (with permission).

On the other hand, while providing access to health care to all detainees, health professionals working in prisons need to regulate health demands and avoid manipulation by both detainees (overuse) and security staff (limiting access by the regulation of escorts, for example). Moreover, all aspects of health care provision (prevention, diagnosis and treatment) need to be grounded in good medical evidence. This implies integrating evidence-based medicine and the concept of equivalence, rationalizing and taking into account the resources available.

The Champ-Dollon prison offers a wide range of curative and preventive services, some of which were implemented early in comparison to other neighbouring cantons and countries. The prison was one of the pioneer institutions in some pilot projects regarding harm reduction (e.g. methadone substitution, condom distribution, syringe and needle exchanges). On entry to prison, all prisoners are briefly seen by a nurse in order to evaluate their health status and assess whether an urgent medical consultation is necessary. Screening for contagious infections is conducted, as well as screening for violence, mental health problems, and drug and alcohol addiction. The initial assessment also includes medical history, risk factors for communicable infectious diseases (which are more prevalent in this population) such as HIV, hepatitis B and C, and sexually transmitted diseases, and the checking of vaccine status. A general physical examination is performed which includes an appraisal of active signs of drug withdrawal (see case 2) that may warrant a substitutive treatment (e.g. benzodiazepines, methadone maintenance therapy). All health services and screening tests are offered on a voluntary, confidential basis and are free of charge.

Detainees can send a confidential written request to the medical service. In addition, the need for a medical consultation can be assessed by nurses who have regular and direct contact with inmates during their daily rounds while distributing drugs or controlling health parameters (fever, blood pressure, sugar levels). Security staff also relay detainees' health requests and regularly inform the prison health team of health complaints.

All consultations are reported in a personal medical record kept in the medical health unit. According to the same rules as apply in the community, information about medical status, diagnosis or therapeutic measures are not divulged to a third party without the informed consent of the patient. Once a detainee is released, efforts are made to ensure continuity of care with community health services or with a former family doctor. This is particularly important for methadone maintenance therapy or when chronic treatments for conditions such as HIV or hepatitis infection have been initiated (case 2). Figure 1 summarizes the clinical trajectory of a given detainee entering the Champ-Dollon prison. Table 01 highlights some of the medical conditions that may warrant prompt interventions after the first medical assessment.

In spite of a legal framework that strongly protects the rights of the detainees, Champ-Dollon still remains a prison which, as such, is a hostile environment for both prisoners and staff, rendering health care and promotion difficult. As in any prison, health is not the primary concern, and the need for security and discipline can cut across a perception of the individual (prisoner) as patient. Consequently, individual movement is restricted and subject to strict rules. In a study on space, place and movement in prison, Stoller describes, through prisoners' narratives, how the spatial organization and structure of the prison can impede movement, and, as such, restrict access to health care.

The study highlights that the "spatial organization and structure of the prison reflect management goals in opposition to the putative goals of a

Table 01. Examples of conditions that may warrant urgent health intervention on entry into prison

Condition	Intervention
Contagious infectious disease ex. active tuberculosis	Isolation, transportation to the relevant hospital, treatment started, measures to prevent the propagation of the infection to other inmates and staff
Mental health or addiction problems	Psychiatric evaluation, substitution therapy for addiction (methadone), or transfer to mental health unit (risk of suicide, self-harm)
Trauma during arrest	Allegations of violence are reported, specific exams are performed (x-rays, pictures), treatments are given (stitches for a wound, pain killers)

Figure 01: Trajectory of a given detainee entering the prison of Champ-Dollon

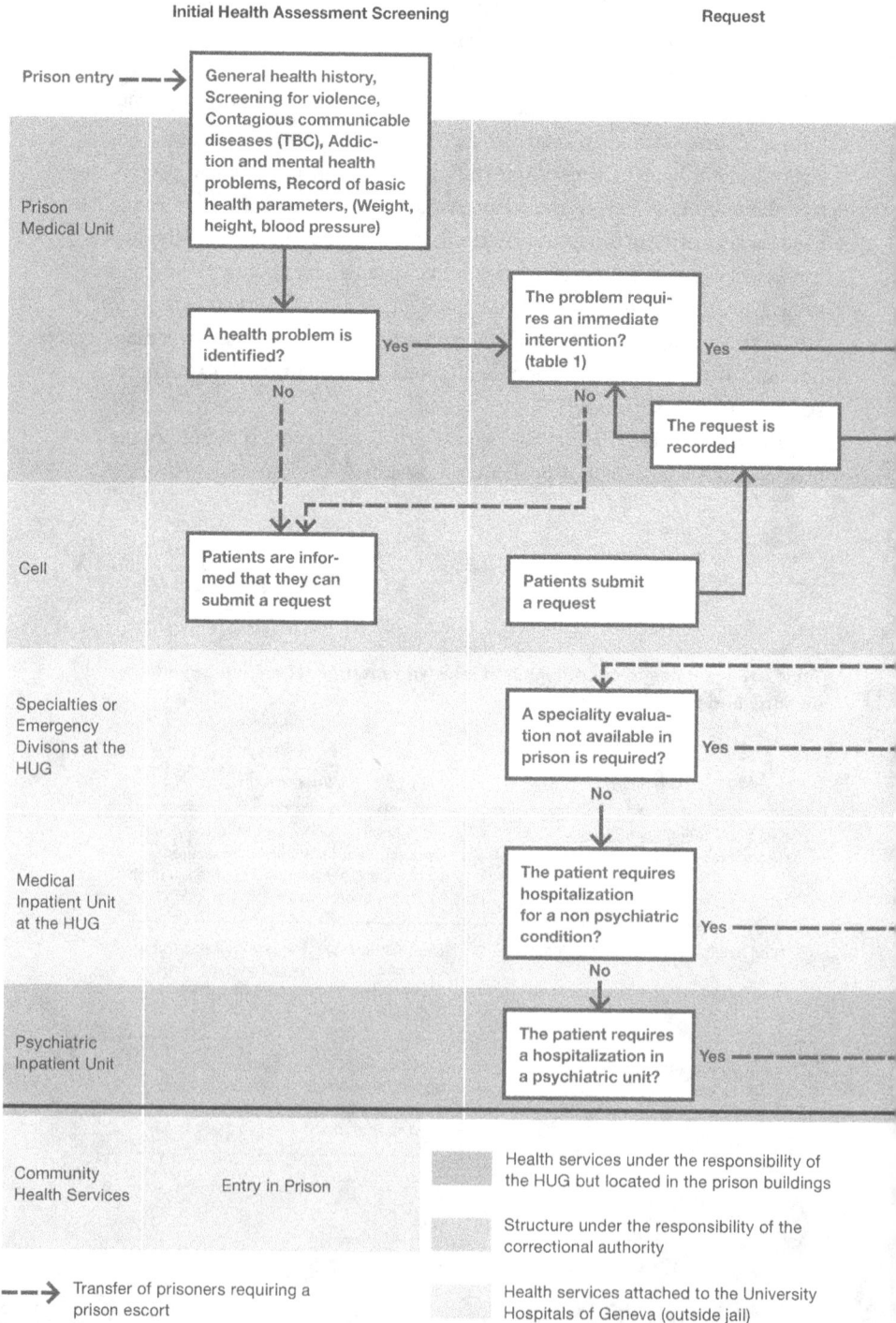

Initial Health Assessment Screening — Request

Prison entry - - -> General health history, Screening for violence, Contagious communicable diseases (TBC), Addiction and mental health problems, Record of basic health parameters, (Weight, height, blood pressure)

Prison Medical Unit

A health problem is identified? — Yes —> The problem requires an immediate intervention? (table 1) — Yes

No — No

The request is recorded

Cell

Patients are informed that they can submit a request

Patients submit a request

Specialties or Emergency Divisons at the HUG

A speciality evaluation not available in prison is required? — Yes - - -

No

Medical Inpatient Unit at the HUG

The patient requires hospitalization for a non psychiatric condition? — Yes - - -

No

Psychiatric Inpatient Unit

The patient requires a hospitalization in a psychiatric unit? — Yes - - -

Community Health Services — Entry in Prison

Health services under the responsibility of the HUG but located in the prison buildings

Structure under the responsibility of the correctional authority

- - -> Transfer of prisoners requiring a prison escort

Health services attached to the University Hospitals of Geneva (outside jail)

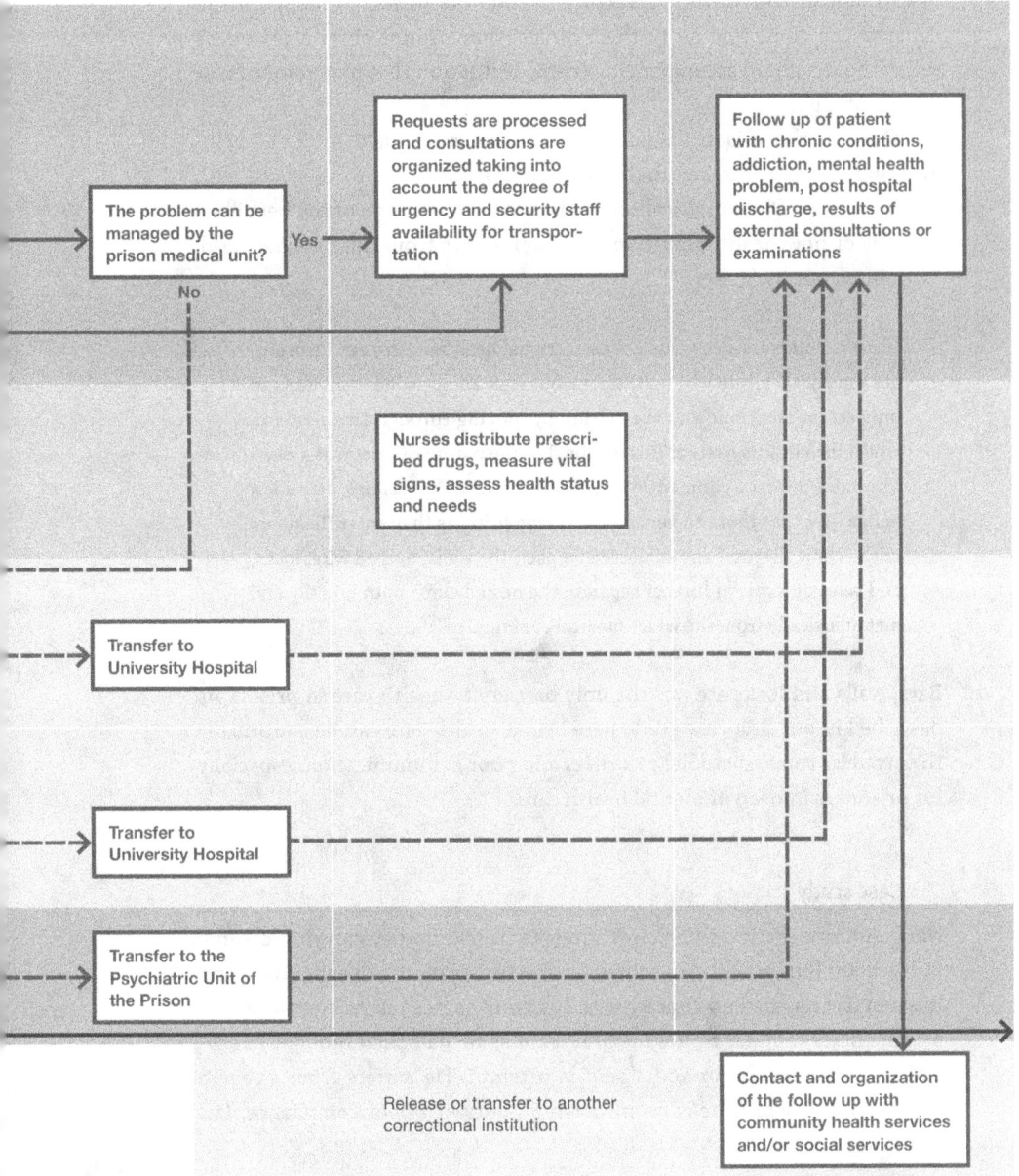

Request

Ongoing Interventions

Follow up

The problem can be managed by the prison medical unit?

Yes

No

Requests are processed and consultations are organized taking into account the degree of urgency and security staff availability for transportation

Follow up of patient with chronic conditions, addiction, mental health problem, post hospital discharge, results of external consultations or examinations

Nurses distribute prescribed drugs, measure vital signs, assess health status and needs

Transfer to University Hospital

Transfer to University Hospital

Transfer to the Psychiatric Unit of the Prison

Release or transfer to another correctional institution

Contact and organization of the follow up with community health services and/or social services committed health care provider. Where humanistic health practice requires an acknowledgment of interconnectedness, prisons are based on principles of exclusion, separation, and confinement."[21]

Figure 01 (dotted arrows) shows that any medical act in Champ-Dollon can only take place if the detainee is brought out of his cell to the medical health unit or to a medical structure outside the prison. Although medical staff can come and go to their clinics, they cannot enter a prisoner's cell without a guard accompanying them, a situation that may compromise confidentiality.

Once in the prison medical unit, detainees are held in closed cells, awaiting their turn to see the health staff, or to return to their cell with other inmates. These physical constraints are perhaps one of the best illustrations of how health provision in prison differs from the outside world. As pointed out by Stoller:

> "Prison clinics are also nested. A correctional health service can incorporate a medical culture within its doors, but staff and prisoner/patients can only access the clinic and the culture by moving through the prison in which the clinic is nested. This means that the nature of prison as a place inevitably affects a clinic within it, if only through the feelings, attitudes, and beliefs that those traversing the prison bring as they enter the doors of the clinic. Beyond any subjective impact, the walls, barbed wire, locks, and rules of a prison further separate the nested clinic both literally and metaphorically from the wider medical community."[22]

Bars, walls and locks are not the only barriers to health care in prison. As described in our first case study here below, health care can be continually thwarted by rules, custodial priorities and poor communication, especially for prisoners in need of mental health care.

Case study 1

Natig Amirov (fictive name) was arrested at the border carrying cocaine in his body (bodypack). He comes from Azerbaijan and speaks Azeri and Russian. He has had no contact with his family since his incarceration. He became quite familiar to the medical team as he had been brought in several times for self-harm and a suicide attempt. He suffers from a severe depression for which he is on medication, but with poor compliance. His detention was marked by incidents involving security staff, who registered him as being a "hard to handle" with "an oppositional behaviour". His self-aggression contributed to his further isolation in the prison, other inmates being reluctant to share a cell with him. Condemned to three years imprisonment, he was about to be transferred to another prison to serve his sentence when he was brought again to the medical unit after a scarring of his right forearm. Mumbling words in Azeri, the detainee was escorted by two guards who showed obvious signs of irritation. On this busy Monday afternoon with numerous prison escorts to the medical unit, Amirov's repeated self-injury exacerbated the tensions due to the workload among the medical and the security staff who do not understand why Amirov was not on "a good medication that would calm his pathological self–aggressive tendencies".

As none of the staff spoke Azeri or Russian, the doctor and the nurse, after taking care of the wound, tried to explain to the patient, in German, that in order to protect him from any further attempt to self-injure during the night (as there was only one nurse on duty for more than 450 inmates), he would be transferred to the prison psychiatric unit where closer observation would be possible. Filled with anxiety, the prisoner started shouting and crying. He was brought forcefully to a closed cell in the medical unit to await his transfer to the psychiatric unit. Once in the closed cell, he knocked repeatedly at the door before being tartly called to order by the guards who opened the cell, shouting at him, and finally pushed him back violently to the floor. Nobody from the medical team dared to intervene or say a word. The patient was then transferred to the psychiatric unit.

Case discussion

This case study illustrates how prisoners with mental illness, poor literacy or facing language barriers, are more prone to fail to access effective health care and may be subject to isolation, abusive acts, racism or indifference by medical and security staff.

Mental health problems and suicide are known to be more prevalent among prison inmates.[23] Before entering prison, prisoners with mental health conditions often belong to the most vulnerable groups of society. Unemployment, low levels of education and homelessness are frequently associated social conditions. Substance abuse is also common before and in prison, and many of the offences that lead to imprisonment are drug related. In addition, substance abuse and dependency are frequently associated with known mental illnesses or personality disorders, creating an additional challenge for their management. Moreover, a review of the medical history of mental health offenders often reveals traumatic life events (e.g. violent or sexual assaults, living in disaster or conflict areas, and previous history of imprisonment). This is particularly true for prisoners who are migrants, who may have experienced significant stressful events and may have related pathologies often left undiagnosed before their incarceration (e.g. post-traumatic stress disorder[24] or Ulysses syndrome[25]).

Psychosis, major depression, and antisocial personality are the most common mental disorders encountered in prisons. A systematic review of 62 surveys from 12 different western countries reviewed the prevalence of psychiatric disorders among the prison population.[26] A total of 22 790 prisoners (mean age 29 years, 81% men) were included. Of the male prisoners reviewed, 3.7% had a psychotic illness, 10% major depression and 65% a personality disorder. Of the female prisoners reviewed, 4% had a psychotic illness, 12% major depression and 42% a personality disorder. These disorders are often chronic and do not lend themselves easily to therapeutic interventions.

The prison environment also creates new mental problems and further exacerbates previous ones. While in prison, nearly all prisoners experience depressed moods or stress symptoms. Anxiety and sleep disorders are the most frequent complaints, for which psychotropic drugs are requested.

At an individual level, all aspects of life in prison affect the mental health of prisoners. Prison takes away liberty, autonomy, breaks familial ties and damages self-esteem. Rules and regulations within prisons do not marry well with mental disorders. Breaches in discipline by prisoners experiencing an acute psychiatric deterioration or a nervous breakdown are often the source of incidents and create tensions among staff, as illustrated by the case discussed above.

Depressive patients, or those experiencing impulsive or aggressive behaviour due to their illness, suffer the most from the monotony of the daily routine, the restrictions imposed on their movement, and the lack of activities available. Self-harm becomes a stereotypical way of reducing tension and symbolically restores a sense of control over one's self. This is particularly true when language barriers reduce the ability of the detainees to express themselves, as was the case with the Azeri patient in the case study above.

In this regard, intercultural communication, both verbal and non-verbal, is the backbone of all facets of everyday life in prison. Optimal communication between the three actors involved in the triangular relationship formed by the patient-detainee, the security guard and the health care worker constitutes a prerequisite to good health in prison. In this case study, the language barrier hampered basic communication, created tension and fear among inmates and staff, and further exacerbated the medical condition (self-harm episodes, violence perpetrated by staff). The final violent event is the result of poor communication by both security and medical staff. Providing the necessary translation/interpretation services at the times they are needed is often problematic. The inability of the medical team to provide understandable information to the patient contributed to his anxiety and agitation, and indirectly contributed to the violent measures taken by the guards.

As will be discussed further, the presence of large groups of foreign inmates in Swiss and European prisons creates an additional challenge for both health professionals and prison administration to deliver appropriate healthcare and respond to the health needs of this population.

Achieving health care continuity is another important objective of health professionals working in prison. It requires that a prisoner with a given health problem or disability achieves continuity of health care as he or she moves back to the community. The second case study illustrates the difficulty of meeting this objective.

Case study 2

M. B. K. originally from North Africa, an undocumented migrant, 28 years of age, has sent a written request to the medical unit (see illustration 01):

> "Je trop mal-mal-mal-mal-mal ... [I'm too ill-ill-ill-ill-ill ...]"

M. B. came to Geneva 6 years ago "because living was too difficult in Algeria". Since then, he earns money from dealing heroine and cocaine, lacks health care insurance, and sleeps frequently in shelters for the homeless. His drug dependency started in Algeria. In the past, he required admission to the emergency department several times, once even to the intensive care unit for a drug-related coma. When entering the prison, he was seen by the nurses who suspected a withdrawal syndrome, and asked a general practi-

DEMANDE DE CONSULTATION MÉDICALE :

NOM : *B*

Prénom(s) : *K*

Date de naissance : *16 09 87*

N° de cellule : *163*

Motifs : *Je trop Mal - Mal - Mal - Mal - Mal Mal - Mal - Mal - Mal - Mal - Mal Mal - Mal - Mal - Mal - Mal - Mal - Mal Mal - Mal - Mal - Mal - Mal - Mal*

Date : *08 - 01 - 2007*   Signature :

▶ Dès réception de votre demande, celle-ci est enregistrée et vous serez reçu(e) à l'Unité médicale dès que possible.

Formulaire développé par l'Unité médicale & la prison de Champ-Dollon – [WordO/edm.inun/formulaires/dendeconsult]

01

tioner (GP) to see him immediately. The GP confirmed a withdrawal syndrome with irritability, diffused muscular pain, secretions of the nose and goose-pimples. He received a substitution therapy (methadone). As prisoners with heroine withdrawal are at high risk of overdose after release, the GP convinced the detainee to keep up the substitution therapy during incarceration. He also recieved information about withdrawal clinics in town where he could go after release.

Furthermore, an active Hepatitis C infection was diagnosed during the first two weeks of incarceration. As the sentence of M. B. was not yet known, no antiviral treatment was prescribed. This treatment (2000 CHF/month) has to be taken for at least 6 months and his sentence was likely to be less than 4 months. M. B. was released a few days later. Time did not allow for contact to be established with the health care centre for undocumented migrants or with the withdrawal centre.

Case discussion

Today's migratory trajectories are becoming more complex and diversified. In Switzerland, scientific studies have shown that various aspects of the health of members of the migrant population are worse than that of the local population. Whatever the reason and type of migration (voluntary migration, forced or economic), migrants are exposed to greater health risks and find it harder to access the services of our health care system.[27]

01
Written request sent by an inmate to the medical
unit of the remand prison of Champ-Dollon, Geneva
"I am too ill, ill, ill, ill…".

This is particularly true for undocumented migrants or failed asylum-seekers, who are often reluctant to seek assistance in public health services due to lack of financial means or fear of the immigration authorities.[28] Despite the fact that undocumented migrants residing in Switzerland can receive insurance from the public health insurance system if they fulfil the general conditions (residence in Switzerland and payment of premiums), many of them are not aware of their rights and do not use public health services unless there is an emergency.

For this vulnerable population, access to health services is, paradoxically, easier while in prison. Imprisonment offers an opportunity to screen and diagnose what are often severe physical and mental illnesses that contribute to their precarious social situation.[29] The neutral space of the medical consultation allows migrants to express past sufferings related to their migratory trajectory, often marked by harsh living conditions, difficult losses and grief.

Medical services offered free of charge represent an additional incentive for these individuals to seek care, many of them being generally unable to pay medical fees or medicines in the outside world.

Providing health care to this population necessitates a close collaboration with many actors of the community health services. A good knowledge of the network and a comprehensive health and social needs assessment plan allows for a correct orientation of the patient during his incarceration and after release.[30] Pre-existing relations with community health services or health professionals that are based simultaneously in the jail and in the community can enhance such collaboration.[31]

Continuity of health care is only possible when a discharge plan is set up well in advance.[32] This is a condition that is rarely met in remand prisons where most inmates are released on short notice without a set medical appointment. Even when release can be anticipated, costly treatments and the lack of health insurance can further impede access to health care.

Furthermore, in Switzerland, the recent tightening of immigration laws has reduced the social security benefits and emergency aid that failed asylum-seekers could once claim.

Since sentenced undocumented migrants or failed asylum-seekers can be repatriated after release under immigration law and/or penal law, continuity of care for this group is often difficult to maintain. This discontinuity may lead to poor health outcomes, overuse of emergency health services and recidivism (drug trafficking).[33]

In the last case described, the interruption of treatment (methadone maintenance therapy) will most likely be followed by a relapse with drug injection and a risk of overdose.[34] Indeed, the risk of death from overdose may
be greater for injecting drug users who resume drug use after a period of abstinence, during which their tolerance may have declined. Overdose is the
leading cause of death in the immediate period after release from prison.[35]

These selected case studies depict two foreign prisoners. Our choice
was not made by chance or only to illustrate a deprived and vulnerable
group. With a proportion of around 70%, Switzerland is among those European countries with the highest rates of foreign prisoners. This trend is not
unique to Switzerland, and many other countries see their prisons filled
with foreign nationals. The reasons behind this phenomenon are complex
and far beyond the scope of this chapter. Improvements in communication
and travel possibilities, increased transnational trade activities, migration
accentuated by economic crises or conflicts, are all factors that contribute
to globalized criminalization. As we will discuss in this last section, the global prison population worldwide is increasing and becoming more hetero-
geneous. This continuously changing body of inmates constitutes one of
the most challenging issues prison facilities will have to manage in the coming years.

The prison population grows

Prisons are no longer at the margins of our society. Over 9 million people are held in penal institutions throughout the world, mostly as pre-trial
detainees (remand prisoners) or having been convicted and sentenced. Almost half of these are in the United States (over 2 million), China (1.5 million) or Russia (0.9 million).[36] According to the World Prison Population
List (2007), prison populations are growing in many parts of the world.
In comparison with the 2005 and 2006 figures, the Prison Population List
shows that prison populations have risen in 64% of the countries in Africa,
84% in the Americas, 81% in Asia, 66% in Europe and 75% in Oceania. Key
facts on Swiss prisons are summarized in box 02. This increase in the numbers of detainees and the use that we make of imprisonment poses several
questions for the kind of society that we aim to be, as well as the role given
to any criminal justice system to best serve society. If the main purposes
of prisons are to punish criminals, as well as to rehabilitate them, we still
need to make sure that this should only be done for the most serious crimes

and when there is no reasonable alternative. Yet in all countries prisons are filled with marginalized groups: The poor, the unemployed, the homeless, the mentally ill or ethnic minorities.

Box 02: Swiss prison population-key facts

In September 2007, 5715 people were in prison for a total capacity of 6654 places. 1653 people were being held in detention. A further 3586 were serving time, while 403 were waiting to be expelled from the country. The 73 others were being held for a variety of reasons. Prisons were 86% full, with the vast majority of detainees being adult males. Women accounted for 6% of the prison population, and teenagers 1%.

Source: Federal Statistics Office, Prisons' census, September 2007.

The confusion between really dangerous criminals and those offenders who have a mental illness, a history of drug abuse, or marginal lifestyle, contributes to maintaining, both in government planning and in the eyes of the public, the perception that the best response to insecurity is more emphasis on imprisonment.

Speaking in December 2004 at the launch of the report by the UK Parliamentary Joint Committee on Human Rights into Deaths in Custody, the Chairperson, Jean Corston MP, noted:

> "Crime levels are falling but we are holding more people in custody than ever before. The misplaced over-reliance on the prison system for some of the most vulnerable people in the country is at the heart of the problems that we encountered ... Extremely vulnerable people are entering custody with a history of mental illness, drug and alcohol problems and potential for taking their own lives. These people are being held within a structure glaringly ill-suited to meet even their basic needs."[37]

At a time when many countries, including Switzerland, are engaged in reforms to limit the use of imprisonment as a measure of punishment, the general tendency to emphasize questions of security and migration control tends to restore the original notion of prison as a place for the exclusion of specific subgroups of individuals.

Particularly alarming is the overrepresentation of particular groups in society, especially detainees of foreign origin or ethnic minorities. For example, a 2000 report of Human Rights Watch[38] revealed that out of a total population of 1 976 019 incarcerated in adult facilities in the United States, 1 239 946 (or 63%) are African-American or Latino, though these two groups constitute only 25% of the national population. In the UK, between 1999 and 2002 the prison population increased by 12%, while the number of black prisoners increased by over 54%.

Foreign nationals: A new marginalized group in prison populations

In recent years, a new marginalized group has emerged that contributes to the increase of prison populations: Foreign nationals. This phenomenon has become a worrisome reality for several European countries. In 2006, there were more than 100 000 foreign prisoners in European countries.[39] Their numbers vary greatly per country. In Switzerland, around 70% of all prisoners are foreign nationals. In Austria, Belgium, Cyprus and Greece there are over 40%, while in Estonia, Italy, Malta and the Netherlands the proportion is over 30%. The average percentage of foreigners in the prison population of the countries of the European Union is over 20%.

Over the last decades, in addition to the considerable growth of the EU prison population, populations have also changed significantly. Prison populations throughout Europe are characterized by a wide variation of nationalities, religions and cultural backgrounds. In many countries, over 100 different nationalities are represented in prison. This shift of composition remains a major challenge for prison staff in their daily interactions with prisoners, notably with regard to issues such as the multiplicity of languages, religious practices, or food preferences. This raises fundamental questions concerning the capacity of these institutions to provide culturally adapted information regarding rules, obligations and rights.

Until recently, the causes of this growing proportion of foreign nationals in prisons and the impact of this growing heterogeneity on the professionals involved (prison employees, decision-makers in administration and politics) have not received much attention.[40]

Particularly revealing is a one-year project on foreign prisoners in European penitentiary institutions co-funded by the European Commission in 2005. Based on the collaboration of several experts working in the field, the objective of this project was to address the issue of social exclusion of prisoners who are detained in the EU outside their country of origin. Its aim was to study and analyse their situation in 25 European Union (EU) Member States, to exchange information among experts, to identify innovative approaches and to develop recommendations to combat their social exclusion.[41]

Despite the diversity of the criminal systems and penitentiary services studied, the report underscores the overrepresentation of foreign prisoners in European penitentiaries and reports several common trends:

1.   EU national laws and immigration control regulations tend to lead to a concentration in prison of individuals with foreign citizenship, and, increasingly, undocumented immigrants, resulting in a higher application of deprivation of liberty, at the level of both remand custody and sentencing for this population.

The combination of criminal and administrative procedures tend to create a "double sentence" where foreign prisoners have a greater tendency to be incarcerated, spend more time in prison, benefit less from non-custodial measures or other forms of sentence alleviation (prison leave, conditional release) and have less access to measures of reintegration (work, professional training).[42] This is particularly true for undocumented immigrants. This issue has recently been recognized by the European Directors of Prison Administration, as one of the most pressing challenges faced by prison administrations in Europe. During an international conference organized in Vienna, in November 2007, under the theme of "Managing Prisons in an increasingly complex environment", two representatives of the Austrian Penitentiary Administration made the following remarks:

> "A growing part of prisoners consist of non-citizens in an elementary sense, of scantly tolerated displaced persons who lack rights of asylum but cannot be repatriated. They are affected by a number of measures of aliens police, ranging from ban of residence and custody pending deportation to deportation. Legal procedures including the proceedings for the enforcement of deportation usually take a long time. Pending proceedings mean insecurity for all parties, for prisoners as well as for the administration, they render prisoners incalculable and hamper a prison regime which approximates normal life conditions. In fact these prisoners live in a legal no man's land and they remain – whatever the nature of their offence – in double custody. First in prison and in addition under an alien's

police regime that adheres to a quite different logic than that of imprisonment on remand or penal custody with its perspectives of rehabilitation
and reintegration."[43]

**2. The lack of social integration for many foreign prisoners is often
seen by actors of the criminal justice system to enhance the risk of criminality or recidivism, resulting in a higher application of deprivation of
liberty.**

The absence of legal status and residence for many foreign prisoners is
seen by the judiciary apparatus as enhancing both the risk of absconding
and the risk of recidivism.[44] The risk of escape often being taken for granted, foreign prisoners – particularly those without residence permits – are
incarcerated in closed prisons. The poor socioeconomic and financial situation of many foreign or ethnic minority offenders, as well as a higher
prevalence of mental health disorders and drug dependency in this population, are again seen as enhancing the risk of recidivism.

**3. Foreigners or ethnic minorities face different problems during de-
tention, ranging from severe language and communication problems, to
religious or cultural conflicts or racism.**

Daily interactions between prisoners and staff are seriously hampered if prisoners do not speak any of the local or common languages (case
study 1). These communication constraints are the source of tensions or
conflicts among inmates sharing cells or with security staff.

A lack of migrant-friendly health care contrasts with the current efforts
put in place in the community. Indeed, providing culturally adapted health
care has, in recent decades, become a priority for many countries. In 2002,
for instance, the EU Commission created the European migrant-friendly
hospitals (MFH) pilot project, which invites all European hospitals to develop into transculturally competent organizations. In Switzerland, several
strategies have been developed since the early 1990s. Based on a vision of
equal opportunity, the Federal Office of Public Health launched, in spring
2007, the "Migration and Public Health Strategy: 2008–2013", the second
phase of the national strategy. Among the achievements of the first phase,
500 interpreters were trained and certified according to defined standards.
They are now employed in health institutions throughout the country. Despite these improvements, having translation available in prison is still a
challenge in practice. Even when available, many interpreters are reluctant

to offer their services in the prison environment, where security rules make any external intervention difficult. International telephone companies who offer translation/interpretation services in more than 100 languages and dialects could be an alternative. Internet-based translation software might provide some help too.

Health care provision in prison also has cultural connotations, which could be hampered by inadequate communication. As presented by De Viggiani:[45]

> "Prisoners 'import' values, attitudes, beliefs and social norms from their respective communities (...) Today's prisons are not completely closed systems. They have permeable boundaries and transient populations and represent microcosms of the wider society. Prisoners' backgrounds and biographies, therefore, contribute to their abilities to cope with and survive imprisonment."

Intercultural misunderstandings, prejudices and stereotypes, which see certain national groups as representing a higher risk of criminality, are common in prison.

Summary and recommendations

Various forms of action are being taken by the international community to address health care and social justice issues in prisons. This chapter is not exhaustive. Drawn from our daily practice, the issues and examples described illustrate only a few of the critical aspects of health care provision in these particular environments. We have presented some of the guiding principles regulating health care in prison, showing the daily challenges we face in implementing them. We have also highlighted how health professionals working in prisons face problems that are different from those faced by colleagues that work with the ordinary population. In the last section on foreign prison populations in Europe and Switzerland, we have illustrated the growing challenge of meeting the right to health in a globalized world.

Whatever diverse prisons may be worldwide, health professionals involved in prisons share a direct responsibility to make sure that the right to health is properly enjoyed. Adhering to standards of good practice, they should first provide quality health care in a manner that is independent and equivalent to what is prevalent in the community. For this to take place, continual professional training, adapted to the exercise of the profession in prison settings, and including courses on human rights and ethics in prisons, should be encouraged. Pre-graduate and continuous medical education, using concrete situation-based learning, like the case studies presented, could serve to better integrate the human rights and ethical framework into the daily practice of health professionals.

In addition to their clinical tasks, health professionals working in prisons should demonstrate the capacity to diversify their roles to better meet the health needs of the vulnerable prison population with which they are in contact on a daily basis. This could include taking part in the policy debate to make prison health a public health priority, and/or being involved in collaborative research. Systematic data collection on the health situation in prisons could be an important contribution, and a means to inform prison administrations and policy makers. Where possible, professional associations should work to ensure that health professionals are aware of the channels through which they can draw attention to the information they have identified and documented. Professional associations also need to provide doctors with the support and legal backing to speak out against incidences of abuse, neglect or torture whenever its members encounter such situations and provide support in case of litigation with the prison authorities. Increased and closer collaboration with prison administrations, civil society organizations and community health services could help health professionals working in prisons to raise awareness about the human rights issues encountered and to better coordinate and plan the provision of health care in prison.

1   The term prison is usually applied to an institution holding convicted felons who are serving sentences of more than one year. In this chapter the term "prison" refers to all places of detention including police stations, remand prisons (in the United States (US): jails), or penitentiaries (US: prisons). Remand prisons (or jails in US) ordinarily hold both detainees and persons convicted of misdemeanours who are awaiting trial or serving sentences of less than one year.

2   Human Rights Watch, Global Report on Prisons: 1993 (New York: Human Rights Watch, 1994), available at http://hrwpubs.stores.yahoo.net/globrep onpri.html. Human Rights Watch's most recent reports relating to prison conditions, prison abuses, and the treatment of prisoners, are available at http://www.hrw.org/advocacy/prisons/ hrw-reports.htm; European Institute for Crime Prevention and Control, World Prison Population: Facts, Trends and Solutions (Helsinki: European Institute for Crime Prevention and Control, 2001), available at http://www.heuni.fi/uploads/ 6mq2zlwaaw3ut.pdf.

3   Lars Møller, Heino Stöver, Ralf Jürgens, Alex Gatherer and Haik Nikogosian (eds.) Health in Prisons: A WHO Guide to the Essentials in Prison Health (Copenhagen: WHO Regional Office for Europe, 2007), available at http://www.euro.who. int/document/e90174.pdf.

4   The status of ratification of the Optional Protocol to the Convention against Torture and Other Cruel, Inhuman or Degrading Treatment or Punishment is available at http://www2.ohchr.org/ english/bodies/ratification/9_b.htm.

5   Under the European Convention for the Prevention of Torture and Inhuman or Degrading Treatment or Punishment, CPT delegations have unlimited access to places of detention. They also have the right to unrestricted access inside secure units and can interview detainees in private. The last periodic visit (5th visit) to Switzerland took place in autumn 2007. It was one of 11 that the CPT undertook in 2007. Other countries include Spain, the Netherlands, Croatia and Moldova. Af-ter each visit, the CPT sends a confidential report containing its conclusions and recommendations to the country concerned. Preliminary observations by the CPT after its last visit to Switzerland are accessible at http://www.cpt.coe.int.

6   Roger Watson, Anne Stimpson, Tony Hostick, 'Prison Health Care: A Review of the Literature' 41(2) International Journal of Nursing Studies (2004) 119-28; Louise Condon, Gill Hek, Francesca Harris, 'A Review of Prison Health and Its Implications For Primary Care Nursing in England and Wales: The Research Evidence' 16(7) Journal of Clinical Nursing (2007), at 1201-1209; Watson, supra note 6; Dave Beer, Bruno Gravier, 'Primary Care in a Detention Environment' 2(88) Revue Médicale Suisse (2006), at 2690-2696; Bertrand D, Niveau G (eds.) Médecine, Santé et Prison (Chêne-Bourg: Editions Médecine & Hygiène, 2006).

7   Rick Lines, 'The Right to Health of Prisoners in International Human Rights Law' 4(1) International Journal of Prisoner Health (2008), at 3-53; Judith Asher, Danielle Hamm, Julian Sheather, The right to health: A toolkit for health professionals (London: British Medical Association, 2007), available at: http://www.bma.org.uk/ap.nsf/Content/Right tohealthtoolkit; Andrew Coyle, 'A Human Rights Approach to Prison Management' 13(2) Criminal Behaviour and Mental Health (2003), at 77-80; Jerome Amir Singh, Michelle Govender, Edward J. Mills, 'Do human rights matter to health?' 370 The Lancet (2007), at 521-527.

8   Dominique Bertrand, Laurent Subilia, Daniel S. Halpérin, Romano La Harpe, Jean-Marc Reymond, Donatella Bierens de Haan, Louis Loutan, 'Victims of Violence: Importance of Medical Testimony for the Practitioner' 87(12) Praxis (1997), at 417-420.

9   Prisoners, whatever the nature of their offence, retain all those fundamental rights to which they are entitled as human persons, including the right to enjoy the highest attainable standards of physical and mental health. Specific international instruments set out more clearly what this implies in terms of the healthcare provision to be

made by prison administrations. These instruments include: The International Covenant on Economic, Social and Cultural Rights, Article 12; the Basic Principles for the Treatment of Prisoners, Principle 4; the Basic Principles for the Treatment of Prisoners, Principle 9; the Body of Principles for the Protection of All Persons under Any Form of Detention or Imprisonment, Principle 24; the Standard Minimum Rules for the Treatment of Prisoners, Rule 22; Standard Minimum Rules for the Treatment of Prisoners, Rule 25; the Standard Minimum Rules for the Treatment of Prisoners, Rule 62; the UN Principles of Medical Ethics relevant to the Role of Health Personnel, particularly Physicians, in the Protection of Prisoners and Detainees against Torture and Other Cruel, Inhuman or Degrading Treatment or Punishment, Rule 1; the Health Professionals Association's declarations, including The World Medical Association Declaration of Edinburgh on Prison Conditions and Spread of Tuberculosis and other Communicable Diseases, Preamble; and the International Council of Nurses Position Statement on Nurses' Role in the Care of Detainees and Prisoners.

10 Bernice Elger, 'Towards Equivalent Health Care for Prisoners: European Soft Law and Public Health Policy in Geneva' 29 *Journal of Public Health Policy* (2008), at 192–206.

11 Etat de Genève. Arrêté du Conseil de l'Etat, (entré en vigueur le 27.09.2000). Documents des HUG. Santé et soins en milieu carcéral. Référence Aml/2.4.4 publié le 12.04.2005.

12 Council of Europe. Committee of Ministers, 'Recommendation No. R(98) 7 of the Committee of Ministers to Member States Concerning the Ethical and Organizational Aspects of Health Care in Prison' 6(3) *European Journal of Health Law* (1999), at 267–278.

13 Dagmar Haller-Hester, Bernice Elger, Slim Slama, Hans Wolff, 'Prison Health Services: Opening an Access to the Community Healthcare Network' 3(126) *Revue Médicale Suisse* (2007), at 2171–2174.

14 Swissinfo, 'New Prison doesn't ease Pressure on Swiss Jail' (2008), available at http://www.

swissinfo.ch/eng/swissinfo.html?siteSect=43& sid=9198143.

15 Council of Europe, Committee of Ministers, *supra* note 11.

16 Council of Europe. Committee of Ministers, 'Recommendation No. R(2006) 2 of the Committee of Ministers to Member States on the European Prison Rules' (2006), available at https://wcd.coe. int/ViewDoc.jsp?id=955747.

17 Council of Europe, Committee of Ministers, 'European Prison Rules: Recommendation No. R(87)3' and updated version of 2006 (Rec (2006)2, available at https://wcd.coe.int/ViewDoc.jsp?id=703309 &BackColorInternet=9999CC&BackColorIntranet =FFBB55&BackColorLogged=FFAC75.

18 Gérard Niveau, 'Relevance and Limits of the Principle of "Equivalence of Care" in Prison Medicine' 33 *Journal of Medical Ethics* (2007), at 610–613.

19 André Duhamel and al., 'Social and Health Status of Arrivals in a French Prison: A Consecutive Case Study from 1989 to 1995' 49(3) *Revue d'Epidémiologie et de Santé Publique* (2001), at 229–238.

20 Jean-Marc Feron et al., 'Substantial Use of Primary Health Care by Prisoners: Epidemiological Description and Possible Explanations' 59 *Journal of Epidemiology and Community Health* (2005) at 651–655; Tom Marshall, Sue Simpson, Andrew Stevens, 'Use of Health Services by Prison Inmates: Comparisons with the Community' 55 *Journal of Epidemiology and Community Health* (2001), at 364–365.

21 Nancy Stoller, 'Space, Place and Movement as Aspects of Health Care in Three Women's Prisons' 56 *Social Science & Medicine* (2003), at 2263–2275.

22 Stoller, *supra* note 20, at 2265.

23 Luke Birmingham, Debbie Mason, and Donald Grubin, 'Prevalence of Mental Disorder in Remand Prisoners: Consecutive Case Study' 313 *British Medical Journal* (1996), at 1521–1524; Graham Durcan, *From the Inside. Experiences of Prison Mental Health Care* (London: Sainsbury Centre for Mental Health, 2008) available at http://www.scmh.org.uk/pdfs/From_the_Inside. pdf; World Health Organization & International Committee of the Red Cross, 'Information Sheet

Mental Health and Prisons' (2005), available at http://www.who.int/mental_health/policy/mh_in_prison.pdf; Linda A. Teplin, Karen M. Abram, Gary M. McClelland, 'Prevalence of Psychiatric Disorders Among Incarcerated Women: Pretrial Jail Detainees' 53 *Archives of General Psychiatry* (1996) at 505–512.

24 Frank Urbaniok, Jérôme Endrass, Thomas Noll, Stefan Vetter, Astrid Rossegger, 'Posttraumatic Stress Disorder in a Swiss Offender Population' 137 *Swiss Medical Weekly* (2007), at 151–156.

25 Joseba Achotegui, 'Emigration in Hard Conditions: The Immigrant Syndrome with Chronic and Multiple Stress (Ulysses' Syndrome) 16(60) *Vertex* (2005), at 105–113, available http://www.unipd.it/programmi/coimbra/ACP%20TF/DOCS/J_Achotegui%20Sept%205th.doc.

26 Seena Fazel, John Danesh, 'Serious Mental Disorder in 23 000 Prisoners: A Systematic Review of 62 Surveys' 359 *The Lancet* (2001), at 545–50.

27 Hans Wolff, Hans Stalder, Manuella Epiney, Angela Walder, Olivier Irion, Alfredo Morabia, 'Health Care and Illegality: A Survey of Undocumented Pregnant Immigrants in Geneva' 60 *Social Science and Medicine* (2005), at 2149–2154; Hans Wolff, Marius Besson, Marylise Holst, Eliana Induni, Hans Stalder, 'Social Inequalities and Health: Experiences of a Mobile Health Care Unit in Geneva' 1(34) *Revue Médicale Suisse* (2005), at 2218–2222; Platform for International Cooperation on Undocumented Migrants *Access to Health Care for Undocumented Migrants in Europe* (Brussels: PICUM, 2007), available at http://www.picum.org/HOMEPAGE/Health%20care/REPORT%20Access%20to%20Health%20Care%20for%20Undocumented%20Migrants%20in%20Europe%20(17).pdf.

28 Roman Romero-Ortuno, 'Access to Health Care for Illegal Immigrants in the EU: Should We Be Concerned?' 11 *European Journal of Health Law* (2004), at 245–272.

29 Haller-Hester, *supra* note 12.

30 Tom Marshall, Sue Simpson, Andrew Stevens, 'Health Care Needs Assessment in Prisons: A Toolkit' 23 *Journal Public Health Medicine* (2001), at 198–204.

31 Thomas Lincoln, Sofia Kennedy, Robert Tuthill, Cheryl Roberts, Thomas J. Conklin, Theodore M. Hammett, 'Facilitators and Barriers to Continuing Healthcare After Jail: A Community-integrated Program' 29(1) *Journal of Ambulatory Care Management Ambulatory Care and Conflict* (2006), at 2–16; Robert B. Greifinger (ed.) *Public Health Behind Bars: From Prisons to Communities* (New York: Springer, 2007) at 508–535.

32 Jeremy Travis, 'But They All Come Back: Rethinking Prisoner Reentry' 7 *Sentencing and Corrections* (2000), at 1–11, available at: http://www.ncjrs.gov/pdffiles1/nij/181413.pdf.

33 Tom J. Conklin, Thomas Lincoln, Timothy P. Flanigan TP, 'A Public Health Model to Connect Correctional Health Care with Communities' 88(8) *American Journal of Public Health* (1998), at 1249–1250; Zulficar Gregory Restum, 'Commentary: Public Health Implications of Substandard Correctional Health Care' 95 *American Journal of Public Health* (2005), at 1689–1691.

34 Catherine Ritter, 'Approche des addictions en milieu carcéral' in Dominique Bertrand, Gérard Niveau, (eds.) *Médecine, Santé et Prison* (Chêne-Bourg : Editions Médecine & Hygiène, 2006).

35 Ingrid A. Binswanger, Marc F. Stern, Richard A. Deyo, Patrick J. Heagerty, Allen Cheadle, Joann G. Elmore, and Thomas D. Koepsell, 'Release From Prison – A High Risk of Death for Former Inmates' 356 *The New England Journal of Medicine* (2007) at 157–65.

36 Roy Walmsley, 'World Prison Population List', International Centre for Prison Studies, Kings College London, 7th edition (2007), available at http://www.kcl.ac.uk/depsta/law/research/icps/downloads/world-prison-pop-seventh.pdf.

37 Quotation taken from Professor Andrew Coyle's inaugural lecture 'On being a prisoner in the United Kingdom in the 21st century: Does the Wilberforce judgement still apply?' given at King's College London, on 22 March 2005. A transcript of this lecture is available at http://www.kcl.ac.uk/depsta/law/research/icps/downloads/wilberforce-judgement.doc.

38 Human Rights Watch, *Punishment and Prejudice:*

Racial Disparities in the War on Drugs (New York: Human Rights Watch, 2000). See also 'Race and Incarceration in the United States', Human Rights Watch Press Backgrounder, 27 February 2002, available at http://hrw.org/backgrounder/usa/race.

39 A. M. Van Kalmthout, F. B. A. M. Hofstee-van der Meulen, and F. Dünkel (eds.) *Foreigners in European Prisons* (Nijmegen: Wolf Legal Publishers, 2007). This book is the result of a European collaborative project, the EU Foreign Prisoners Project, co-funded by the European Commission. The results and recommendations of this initiative are available at http://www.foreignersinprison.eu.

40 Gary Hill, *The Treatment of Foreign Prisoners* (IS-PAC, 2004), available at the International Scientific and Professional Advisory Council of the United Nations Crime Prevention and Criminal Justice Programme website: http://ispac-italy.org.

41 Van Kalmthout, *supra* note 39, available at http://www.foreignersinprison.eu.

42 Van Kalmthout, *supra* note 39, available at ibid.

43 W. Gratz and A. Pilgram, 'Managing Prisons in an Increasingly Complex Environment: Meeting Public Demands and Expectations: Current Challenges Faced by Prisons Administrations', Proceedings of the 14th Conference of Directors of Prison Administration (CDAP), Vienna, 19–21 November 2007, available at http://www.coe.int/t/e/legal_affairs/legal_cooperation/prisons_and_alternatives/conferences/cdap%20(2007)%2006%20-%20e%20(Gratz%20&%20Pilgram).pdf.

44 Van Kalmthout, *supra* note 39.

45 Nick De Viggiani, 'Unhealthy Prisons: Exploring Structural Determinants of Prison Health' 29(1) *Sociology of Health & Illness* (2007), at 115–135.

"As Full Rehabilitation as Possible": Torture Survivors and the Right to Care

Douglas A. Johnson and Steven H. Miles

Torture is a tool states use to shape their cultures through fear, often by destroying leaders of opposition or civic renewal. Amnesty International reports that torture is still practiced or tolerated in at least 150 nations of the modern world, and over 60 invest in the technology and infrastructure to carry it out. Some people argue that torture is as old as humanity and will be ever present. But some things do change. The ancient Greeks believed that a slave's testimony in court could only be considered truthful if derived from torture; and torture was an integral part of the Roman legal tradition, later revived in Medieval Europe. No state today argues that it should use torture; when one decides to do so, the leadership insists either that they are not in control, or that the techniques are merely "enhanced interrogation" falling short of torture. Mostly, though, the perpetrators hide the acts and the victims, with varying degrees of effectiveness. But hiding too much can reduce the effectiveness of torture as a tool against the community; plausible deniability is apparently the best approach.

Contrary to popular belief, the primary aim of torture is not to secure information. Torture and human rights atrocities are tools that repressive states use to create fear and prevent the emergence of effective leadership in civil societies. Torture teaches citizens that they should disengage from public life. This warning spreads throughout a victim's network of family, friends, and influence. An African religious leader, when discussing the torture used against him, said the message was clear: "If they will do this to me, what will they do to my flock?" Another torture survivor said that the purpose of torture was "to sever the links of solidarity". Survivors often find that even their families are afraid to hear what happened to them; friendships end, and isolation builds as the frightened eyes of the community turn away. The terrifying nature of torture can stifle opposition, creating habits of aversion, including the thought that, if both we and the victim can forget about what happened, then we can move forward as if it did not happen. People in denial often harbour the delusion that what happened was not, in fact, so bad and that therefore it need not be addressed. Another delusion is that torture is so bad that nothing can be done for its survivors, so why try? Fear inhibits the public's reaction to torture. This may at least partly explain why, until the late 1970s, there was no systematic effort to provide treatment or rehabilitation.

The idea of rehabilitation for survivors caught on and spread relatively quickly, helping global actors increasingly understand that the deep physical and psychological damage of torture creates lasting harm to individuals and their communities. The widespread commission of atrocities by governments, guerrilla groups, and terrorist organizations has created countless victims; torture is a public health crisis. Its pervasive use calls for new energy and creativity to provide care to its victims.

Establishing the right to health for torture victims

A right to health care for survivors of torture is explicitly stated in the UN Convention Against Torture and Other Cruel, Inhuman or Degrading Treatment and Punishment (CAT) that came into force on 26 June 1987.[1] Article 14 states:

> "Each State Party shall ensure in its legal system that the victim of an act of torture obtains redress and has an enforceable right to fair and adequate compensation including the means for *as full rehabilitation as possible*. In the event of the death of the victim as a result of an act of torture, his dependents shall be entitled to compensation." (emphasis added)

Few international treaties provide such an explicit statement of the right to care. The CAT calls on states to make the "means for as full rehabilitation as possible" along with other forms of redress, an "enforceable right". The treatment and rights of torture victims are also addressed in other international instruments.[2]

The practical realization of torture survivors' established right to rehabilitation remains problematic. A right to health care or rehabilitation differs from an effective entitlement, the latter requiring a set of policies, funding, and treatment infrastructure which reliably delivers the needed care. This volume on the right to health contains many examples of how various social needs compete for finite resources, such as the needs for education, for health care, and for responding to disasters. Torture survivors have not fared well in this competition. States often want to hide and deny the harm they have created. Torture is taboo, a topic that is so shameful that it is concealed. Hobbled by shame, trauma, and lack of knowledge of what rehabilitation is possible, torture survivors are often poorly equipped to assert their needs. Many health care workers underestimate the value of treatment. Furthermore, access to entitlements for treatment usually varies according to whether the survivor is a citizen, an undocumented immigrant or refugee, or a person with a work, tourist, or student visa. We believe that all torture survivors have the right to health care addressing their specific needs and that health policy must promote the development of special entitlements to meet those specialized needs.

The plight of survivors began to change with the emergence of the international treatment movement for torture survivors, started in the early 1980s by the Rehabilitation and Research Centre for Torture Victims (RCT) in Copenhagen, Denmark. Today, nearly two hundred other specialized programmes for torture victims have shown that despair need not inhibit victims or societies from setting out on the path to healing; these institutions have promoted new efforts to develop effective access to care for survivors of torture. However, deep structural problems continue to impede progress from the right to treatment to a workable entitlement to treatment.

Nations have different abilities to provide the infrastructure and trained personnel for treating torture survivors. At the time of its transition from civil war, Sierra Leone had only one psychiatrist in the entire country. It could hardly have been considered best practice to wait for care until more psychiatrists became available. At one point, the Canadian health care system only reimbursed psychiatrists, and not psychologists, for care of torture survivors. Literature emerging in that context tended to equate psychiatric care with best practice. The scope of the entitlement to health care services for torture survivors cannot be universal in the same way that the civil right to be free from torture is universal and unconditional. Is "as full rehabilitation as possible" defined by available health care resources? Or is it defined by the needs of the survivors? It is clear that treatment must include coordinated medical, psychological, social, and vocational services. To what extent does the right and corresponding entitlement to rehabilitation expand as research teaches us more about what forms of multimodal treatment are most effective?

The CAT defines torture as an act of a government, though most human rights organizations recognize that torture also can be committed by those seeking to destroy or replace particular governments. The CAT does not limit solely to the perpetrators the duty to provide rehabilitation for torture survivors. It asserts that each jurisdiction should address who is responsible for creating and funding an entitlement programme to make treatment possible.

The purpose and intentional effects of torture themselves provide important reasons to assure an enforceable entitlement to health care for torture survivors. A survey of clients at the Center for Victims of Torture in Minneapolis, USA, shows that they tend to be more highly educated than the refugee population as a whole and that they have often been leaders in a wide range of organizations and movements.[3] That a poor country would channel scarce resources into the targeted destruction of its best educated persons demonstrates the perceived value of destroying these individuals and their networks. Though we tend to focus on torture's victims as individuals, it is through these individuals' pain and suffering that whole communities can be misshapen through fear. Thus, finding new ways to address the traumas of human rights atrocities directed at communities and societies is an essential component of any effective strategy designed to move a nation toward democracy. It is of global interest to see that torture survivors regain their capacity for leadership, whether they live in nations of exile where they can contribute to the success of others from their communities, or return to their native countries to contribute to building nascent democracies.

Torture's impact

Most people think of torture as a horrific cruel and painful physical assault. This is generally true; the forms and creativity of these physical attacks stun the imagination. The Human Rights Information and Documentation Systems International (HURIDOCS)[4] database of human rights violations tallies 73 forms of torture. Each technique engenders short-term and long-term consequences, sometimes unique. There are countless variations of ways to puncture, burn, break, stretch, hang, beat, asphyxiate, drown, or otherwise abuse a human being. Some techniques leave physical scars or signs; others, such as suffocation or waterboarding, may leave no physical scar at all but do leave long-term psychological suffering. Purely psychological forms of torture, such as subjecting victims to mock execution, sexual humiliation, or forcing them to watch the rape of a loved one, may have exactly the same psychological consequences as physical torture. The likelihood of profound and long-lasting psychological effects from torture is independent of the intensity, nature, or duration of the abuse, although such effects may be partly related to poorly understood psychological attributes of the victim. Torture may attack the body, but the ultimate target is the mind of the victim during, and after, imprisonment.

Although the CAT recognizes that torture can be purely psychological in character and bans "any act by which severe pain or suffering, whether physical or mental, is intentionally inflicted", many policy makers and citizens underestimate the profound and intentional damage psychological forms of torture can produce. The psychological consequences for the individual can be more disabling than residual physical disabilities. They include nightmares and inability to sleep or rest, depression, anxiety, panic attacks, thoughts and acts of suicide, cognitive impairments, memory loss, difficulty concentrating, depression, post traumatic stress disorder, inability to form intimate social relationships, and the propensity for explosive rage. Even after the memories of the pain of a physical assault have abated or disappeared altogether, torture survivors tell their therapists of intrusive memories of mock executions and watching or hearing the torture of others.[5]

Torture as a public health catastrophe

Torture is so broadly used that it constitutes a public health disaster. Ten to thirty thousand persons disappeared during Argentina's dirty war during the late 1970s and early 1980s. Human rights organizations estimate that five times that number were arrested and tortured, sometimes briefly and sometimes over extended periods. The Human Rights Foundation of Turkey estimates that over 1 million Turkish citizens were tortured during the 1980s.[6] Other smaller nations, such as Sierra Leone and Liberia, were racked by years of civil war, and are renowned for a level of physical and psychological cruelty that affected the lives of nearly every living resident. The public dismemberment of men, women, and children by guerrilla forces in Sierra Leone illustrates how torture is used to control large populations by creating deep levels of anxiety and fear. Torture generates massive numbers of refugees, sending the ripples of atrocities around the globe. Even Minnesota, a state of only 5 million in the central United States, is home to about 30 000 torture survivors from over the world.

Different nations: Different approaches

Torture survivors do best where there is a general entitlement to health care and where already high levels of health care are augmented by specialized rehabilitation centres. This is true in Canada, Australia, and nations in Western Europe. Copenhagen's Rehabilitation and Research Centre for Torture Victims (RCT) was initially funded by the Danish Foreign Ministry, as part of its foreign policy against torture. Eventually, the Danish Ministry of Health took over its funding; torture survivor programmes are now a specialized care network, similar to other centres dedicated to particular medical and social needs. This is also true in Norway, Sweden, and the Netherlands. Although some European centres receive supplemental funding in recognition of the severe and chronic needs of survivors and their families, few receive sufficient funding to train experts needed for the larger health care system. Several Canadian rehabilitation programmes have most client care costs paid by the national health care system, but there is very little support for their infrastructure and supplemental specialized services. Thus, even though torture survivors do have an entitlement to health care, it does not meet the CAT's vision of "as full rehabilitation as possible".

The United States provides funding to torture treatment centres through the Torture Victims Relief Act of 1998. This funding includes about USD 10 million for domestic programmes, USD 12 million for rehabilitation programmes outside the U.S., and USD 7 million through the UN Voluntary Fund for Victims of Torture. The effect of these contributions is diminished by the lack of universal health insurance in the United States as well as by rules limiting public health coverage for foreign nationals.

In Romania, the ICAR Foundation's Medical Rehabilitation Centre for Victims of Torture organized a political campaign to pressure the government to pay for prescription drugs for torture survivors.[7] The government initially argued that it was not responsible for the crimes of the dictatorship that came before it. In 2006, the Romanian President, Traian Basescu, recognized the state's responsibility towards the almost 100 000 survivors of gross human rights violations committed during the Communist regime (1945–1989) and made a public apology to the victims and their families. It remains to be seen how this recognition will be leveraged to provide rehabilitation for the many survivors who have not had access to such services.

India's National Human Rights Commission encourages the right to rehabilitation for torture survivors. Chaired by a former Supreme Court Justice, the National Human Rights Commission reviews human rights violations, such as torture, and recommends relief and a measure of justice through the local state governments. It has sometimes recommended fining the police authorities and the responsible police station to provide the funds needed for rehabilitation and other compensation for injuries. The hope is that this approach will help deter torture as well. Although this system does eventually fund some rehabilitation, it results in long delays while verdicts are achieved and compensation collected.

Truth commissions in South Africa, Guatemala, and El Salvador have recognized torture survivors' needs for compensation and rehabilitation. Often the new government argues that it does not have sufficient resources or is not responsible for the acts of a criminal government which preceded it. Again, health care professionals, acting as individuals or in small, specialized centres – in the best case with international moral and financial assistance – have provided treatment with very limited budgets.

In the first years after Chile's Pinochet dictatorship, the new government cautiously explored the extent of human rights abuses. In his inaugural address, President Patricio Aylwin recognized the families of the disappeared, and later appointed a Truth and Reconciliation Commission to investigate political assassinations and disappearances. Torture, however, was not investigated even though the government asked Chilean torture treatment centres to train community health centres across Chile to provide appropriate care. The under-funded health care system was particularly short of mental health treatment infrastructure. Survivors and their families were afraid to self-identify or seek care. The indictment and arrest of General Pinochet in 1998 changed Chilean attitudes about accountability for human rights abuses and national legislation established a right to health care for survivors. A new commission established standards and accepted applications from survivors who, once authenticated by the commission, were guaranteed access to health care for the rest of their lives.[8]

Peru is grappling with similar problems. Its Truth and Reconciliation Commission recommended compensating victims of government-sponsored abuses, as well as victims of a guerrilla group, the Shining Path. An institution was created to craft guidelines and to assist provincial and national governments in registering survivors of human rights abuses, so that resources for reparations and rehabilitation could be equitably distributed.

These various national examples illustrate the complexity of establishing workable entitlements for delivering treatment to torture survivors. In industrialized countries with relatively small groups of immigrants who have been tortured, the general medical needs of torture survivors could be met by the national health care system if appropriate training for specialized torture care were available. In such countries, modest public funding can supplement the specialized centres to improve the care of survivors. In countries emerging from torture, however, the ability to acknowledge or respond to torture survivors' needs can be markedly limited by the need for political stability and can lead to mollifying the powerful military and political cliques that carried out torture under a preceding regime. As the political culture matures, the need for survivor rehabilitation is more likely to be recognized, and the demands for treatment then become part of the discussion of accountability for abuses.

Each of these national scenarios and historical evolutions away from torture is plagued by fundamental confusion regarding torture survivors and their rehabilitation. How does one define a victim? How does one define a secondary victim, such as a child of disappeared parents who was raised by police? How do clinicians measure the damage or assess the progress of rehabilitation? How does a country secure the resources to make such rehabilitation possible? In resource-poor countries, how do governments or external donors evaluate the priority for torture treatment compared to meeting other societal needs?

Conclusions

The development of entitlements for treatment of torture survivors is at an early stage. We can learn from and improve upon the diverse, preliminary efforts. Although there will always be debate about what can and should be offered, research and clinical evidence are producing similar findings about the emotional, physical, and cognitive impacts. This suggests that continued experience will have wide applicability. Surely new forms of treatment and rehabilitation will emerge that will have broad applicability in many cultural settings. "As full rehabilitation as possible" does not mean that the treatment community should promise complete healing for all survivors. But neither does it mean that funding agencies should fund "as little rehabilitation as possible". We should expand our infrastructure to provide rehabilitation for each torture survivor, as we simultaneously expand our understanding of what the healing process can accomplish.

Sufficient expertise and funds have not yet been invested to deal fully with torture survivors' needs for rehabilitation. New ideas are needed, especially with regard to funding. Debate in the United States in the 1970s demonstrated there was bipartisan support for the idea that victims of violent crime should receive support and compensation, as well as have an opportunity to participate in the conviction and sentencing of perpetrators. The resulting victims' compensation programme was funded from fines against the perpetrators of corporate fraud. Each year, the Justice Department gives an award to prosecutors who secure the greatest contributions to the victims' compensation fund. Ideally, as in the example of the Indian police station fines, these kinds of mechanisms should reinforce the accountability of torturers. Funds seized from rogue states or terrorist organizations, or their banks, could support the rehabilitation of victims of state terrorism.

Contributions from the United Nations Voluntary Fund for Victims of Torture, the Torture Victims Relief Act, the European Union, and other national contributions remain insufficient to cover the needs of survivors – and to mend nations damaged by the systematic commission of human rights atrocities. The best use of these funds is to invest in the creation or support of organizations that can demonstrate effectiveness of care. This will work to broaden their influence on mainstream providers, through the generation of knowledge, intensive training, and building constituencies in a given country, so that states develop their health care systems to be responsive to intense traumas. Victims of torture are a lost resource of leadership, skills, and education. Where atrocities have been more widespread, the scale of repression has been used to shape societies with fear so they are more brittle and less able to respond creatively. Both of these types of losses create notable economic and political consequences and will inhibit the growth of democratic cultures. Local, national, and international interventions to help victims and their communities recover from intense traumas are in the self-interest of each level of society, all the more so where resources are scarce.

Torture is universally condemned and, paradoxically, widely practiced. Governments around the world spend more money abusing prisoners than rehabilitating them. More clinicians supervise torture than treat its survivors. Rehabilitation will always be an uncertain and incomplete response. And yet, rehabilitation, like torture, is not simply about the individual. The act of rehabilitation requires that victims, crimes, and criminals be named; it requires that euphemisms like "enhanced interrogation" and "torture-lite" be exposed as the Orwellian frauds they are. Rehabilitation is treatment – it is also about accountability. Torture destroys civil society. Rehabilitation heals victims and communities, and prepares them to re-enter public life.

1 The text of the Convention Against Torture and other Cruel, Inhuman or Degrading Treatment and Punishment (CAT) can be found at http://www2.ohchr.org/english/law/cat.htm.

2 Other international instruments and conventions are applicable to the rights of torture survivors to rehabilitation. These include: The Standard Minimum Rules for the Treatment of Prisoners (1977); Additional Protocols to the Geneva Conventions of 1949 (1979); the Body of Principles for the Protection of All Persons under Any Form of Detention or Imprisonment (1988); International Covenant on Economic, Social and Cultural Rights as elaborated in General Comment No. 14 (2000); the Rome Statute of the International Criminal Court (2002); the Basic Principles and Guidelines on the Right to a Remedy and Reparation for Victims of Gross Violations of International Human Rights Law and Serious Violations of International Humanitarian Law (2005); and the Convention on the Rights of Persons with Disabilities (2007).

3 See the website of the Center for Victims of Torture (www.cvt.org) for information about clients and access to information about care.

4 See the HURIDOCS website at http://www.huridocs.org/.

5 For a more elaborated discussion of the impact of torture and a review of emerging practices in programmes of care, see Dr. Jose Quiroga and Dr. James M. Jaranson, 'Politically-Motivated Torture and Its Survivors: A Desk Study Review

of the Literature', in 15(2–3) *Torture: Journal on Rehabilitation of Torture Victims and Prevention of Torture* (Copenhagen: International Rehabilitation Council for Torture Victims (IRCT), 2005). See also www.irct.org.

6   Levent Kutlu and Ümit Fiahin (eds.) 'Treatment and Rehabilitation Centres Report 2006', Human Rights Foundation of Turkey Publications: 50, August 2007, at 12.

7   For a description of the campaign, see http://www.newtactics.org/MakingtheStatePay.

8   For a more comprehensive telling of the story, see Elizabeth Lira, 'The Reparations Policy for Human Rights Violations in Chile' in Pablo de Greiff (ed.) *The Handbook of Reparations* (Oxford: Oxford University Press and the International Center for Transitional Justice, 2006), see in particular Chapter 2, at 55–101.

Who Cares? The Right to Health of Migrants

Vincent Chetail and Gilles Giacca

The rapid changes associated with globalization have exacerbated the growing discrepancy between the social reality of migration and its legal regulation, which is traditionally understood through the lenses of national interest and security. Political and legal debates on international migration are traditionally focused on issues such as border control, labour demands, and a general willingness to prevent irregular migration, involving huge financial outlay.[1] In such a context, human rights considerations, as well as economic and developmental issues, remain subordinate, if not marginal, subjects of concern. While migrants often make significant socio-economic contributions to the country in which they work, states have not generally been willing to recognize the vulnerability of this particular group to human rights abuses.

The right to health exemplifies the typical tension between the state's reluctance to advance the protection of the human rights of migrants and the increasing need to clarify and articulate a comprehensive migrant-related framework of protection in a globalized world.[2] Against this background the first part of this chapter briefly addresses the vulnerability of migrants and the implications for their health, including questions of access to public health services. From a normative perspective, the realization of social rights such as the right to health should be understood within the broader framework of international human rights law; this is the subject of the second part of the chapter. Finally, we examine the impact of specific conventions dealing with migration on health-related matters.

Migrants as a vulnerable group

In the international discourse on migration, measures to protect specific groups of persons who find themselves outside the territory of their country of origin are typically justified by reference to their vulnerability, which depends on a variety of social, economic and political factors. Numerous General Assembly resolutions acknowledge "the situation of vulnerability in which migrants frequently find themselves, owing, inter alia, to their absence from their states of origin and to the difficulties they encounter because of differences of language, custom and culture, as well as the economic and social difficulties and obstacles for the return to their states of origin of migrants who are non-documented or in an irregular situation."[3] Based on these considerations, the General Assembly reiterates "the need for all States to protect fully the universally recognized human rights of migrants, especially women and children, regardless of their legal status, and to provide humane treatment, in particular with regard to assistance and protection."[4]

The two successive UN Special Rapporteurs on the human rights of migrants highlighted that vulnerability of migrants derives not only from the prevalent cultural bias against foreigners (stereotypes, racism, xenophobia ...), but predominantly from the structural distribution of power within the nation state.[5] Vulnerability is related to the migrant's powerlessness, in the etymological sense of the word; that is to say, "lack of empowerment", which itself, "derives from the existence of a power structure which shows that in any given national society, some have more power than others."[6] The perceived or de jure distinctions between citizens and non-citizens pave the way for a "widespread – and mistaken – view that migrants are somehow not entitled to the full protection of human rights law, often because of the belief that only citizens are entitled to these rights."[7] Other aggravating factors, such as the recurrent economic crisis and the spectre of terrorist violence, have led to highly irrational fantasies that serve to create an environment fertile for violations of human rights.

While personal situations and experiences vary greatly from one migrant to another, there are several possible barriers to the effective and full realization of migrants' social, economic and cultural rights. It should be acknowledged that in spite of the traditional link between low socio-economic status and poor health, which touches both nationals and non-nationals, migrants may be further disadvantaged and discriminated against in relation to "health determinants" and to the accessibility to adequate health care services. Indeed, a large body of empirical evidence shows that socio-economic conditions affect migrants' physical, mental and social situation in the new country and they may experience more health problems than the "average" person.[8] Many different aspects, closely intertwined, can be relevant to a migrant's health, such as living and working conditions, education, housing, or individual lifestyles.

Moreover, migrant workers, both regular and irregular, are frequently concentrated in labour markets that are sometimes characterized as "the bargain-basement of globalization."[9] The great majority of migrants are employed – often on a temporary basis – in low-skilled and labour-intensive occupations, including the informal sector, where general labour standards are rarely respected. This workforce fuels economic growth by taking jobs that are normally shunned by nationals, and which are frequently oriented towards mining, textile, agriculture, construction, heavy manufacturing, sweatshops, and sex work. These are commonly referred to as the "three-D jobs": Dirty, degrading and dangerous. Not surprisingly, occupational health and labour-related risks and injuries are prominent in this context.[10]

Another fundamental aspect governing the realization of the right to health is related to access to health care services. Migratory or legal status, educational and income level, as well as poor language skills can, inter alia, severely obstruct access to health care. Undocumented migrants may be severely constrained in their enjoyment of human rights, which is manifested by a constant fear of being arrested and expelled.[11] This can have a tremendous impact on access to medical care, as these migrants largely fall outside the protection offered by the receiving country to its residents.

The human rights law framework of the right to health of migrants

Vulnerability of migrants contrasts with the very nature of human rights law, as it is based on the assumption that human rights apply to everyone, irrespective of nationality, because of the inherent dignity of every human being. According to human rights instruments, everyone within a state's jurisdiction is entitled to all the rights and freedoms without distinction of any kind, such as race, colour, sex, language, religion, political or other opinion, national or social origin, property, birth or other status.[12] Thus, the applicability of human rights to migrants has been explicitly endorsed by the General Assembly in the 1985 Declaration on the Human Rights of

Individuals Who are Not Nationals of the Country in Which they Live,[13] as well as in many subsequent resolutions devoted to the protection of migrants.[14]

Article 8(1)(c) of the 1985 Declaration specifically refers to "the right to health protection, medical care, social security, social services, education, rest and leisure, provided that they fulfil the requirements under the relevant regulations for participation and that undue strain is not placed on the resources of the State." Entitlement of non-citizens to enjoy their right to health is thus qualified by two major conditions based, respectively, on domestic law and on the resources of the host state.[15] Such far-reaching requirements may, though, be in conflict with the prohibition on racial discrimination enshrined in the International Convention on the Elimination of All Forms of Racial Discrimination (ICERD). Indeed, under Article 5(e) (iv) of ICERD, States Parties are required to guarantee the right of everyone, without distinction as to race, colour, or national or ethnic origin, to equality before the law, notably in the enjoyment of "the right to public health [and] medical care."

Aware of this potential disjuncture between the 1985 Declaration and the relevant conventional obligations of states, subsequent resolutions of the General Assembly *strongly condemn* all forms of racial discrimination and xenophobia with regard to access to ... health services and social services."[16] Equal access to health services has also been restated by the treaty body of the ICERD. The Committee underlined the obligation for states to "respect the right of non-citizens to an adequate standard of physical and mental health by, inter alia, refraining from denying or limiting their access to preventive, curative and palliative health services."[17]

From the perspective of the International Covenant on Economic, Social and Cultural Rights (ICESCR), equal treatment and non-discrimination are critical components in securing the right to health for all. The supervisory body of the ICESCR, the Committee on Economic, Social and Cultural Rights (CESCR) stated that "the principle of non-discrimination mentioned in Article 2(2) of the Covenant operates immediately and is neither subject to progressive implementation nor dependent on available resources."[18] CESCR reaffirmed the importance of this fundamental principle in relation to the full realization of the right to health, understood as imposing an "immediate obligation" of non-discrimination.[19] The scope of the principle of non-discrimination under Article 2(2) clearly encompasses non-citizens, for it refers to "national origin" as a prohibited ground of discrimination.[20]

According to CESCR's General Comment No. 14, "States are under the obligation to *respect* the right to health by, inter alia, refraining from denying or limiting equal access for all persons, including prisoners or detainees, minorities, asylum seekers and illegal immigrants, to preventive, curative and palliative health services ..." (para. 34). The applicability of the right to health to migrants irrespective of their legal status has been further spelled out in regional human rights systems. For instance, the Committee on Social Rights of the Council of Europe considered that "legislation or practice which denies entitlement to medical assistance to foreign nationals, within the territory of a State Party, even if they are there illegally, is contrary to the Charter".[21]

In practice, however, domestic legislation on access to health coverage for undocumented migrants varies considerably between countries, some being more restrictive than others. A number of states may provide preventive and primary health care only on a payment basis, including for urgent care; some may offer free health care in limited cases; and others provide the widest health coverage to undocumented migrants. In all of these contrasting positions, the availability of emergency care continues to be the rule.[22] However, particular caution should be observed when referring to emergency or urgent medical care, as it can cover a variety of situations.

The lowest common denominator appears to include at least access to medical care that can not be delayed without putting in danger the life or health of the migrant concerned. As a result, this may imply that early diagnosis and medical follow-up could be excluded. However, such inequalities in health care are evidently neither legally permissible, nor, from a general public health perspective, justified and reasonable. First, state health policies, legislation and other measures limiting access to health care to mere basic medical treatment would contravene the principle of non-discrimination as set out in Article 2 of the ICESCR. Second, the fact of not being subject to any type of primary medical care could create risks for migrants and to the host society of propagating contagious diseases. As a result, these inequalities in health care provisions could lead to excessive or inefficient use of health services and thereby increase the cost of emergency care.[23]

Another cause for concern is the duty imposed in certain states on civil servants working in health care services to report the presence of undocumented migrants to immigration officials.[24] Such a practice not only undermines the right to equal access to health care, but contravenes the independence and the obligation of confidentiality of the health profession.

The denial of health care has also been interpreted as conflicting with the prohibition of inhuman and degrading treatment in the context of expulsion of migrants. Indeed, human rights treaty bodies have extended the notion of inhuman and degrading treatment to socio-economic conditions in situations where a person is to be returned to a country where his or her illness cannot be treated. In a landmark expulsion case, the European Court of Human Rights held that "the abrupt withdrawal of medical treatment caused by the deportation of D. to St. Kitts would expose him to a real risk of dying under most distressing circumstances and would thus amount to inhuman treatment."[25] This purposive interpretation has been subsequently endorsed by the Committee against Torture[26] as well as the Human Rights Committee.[27] It substantially enlarges the scope of the customary principle of non-refoulement and, as a result, restricts the power of states in the enforcement of migration control.

The increasing role of health considerations in the context of expulsion highlights the interdependent and interrelated nature of human rights. The right to health is indivisibly linked to the inherent dignity of the human person and is indispensable for the fulfilment of other human rights. Following the same approach, the CESCR has included as an integral component of the right to health the underlying determinants of health, such as adequate supply of safe food, nutrition and housing, healthy occupational and environmental conditions. This is in line with the general clause of the Universal Declaration of Human Rights (UDHR) Article 25(1) which reads "[e]veryone has the right to a standard of living adequate for the health and well-being of himself and of his family, including food, clothing, housing and medical care and necessary social services ..."

The underlying preconditions of health prove crucial for low-skilled and seasonal or temporary migrant workers who are often concentrated in sectors with high levels of occupational health risks. In that context, realization of the right to health is closely linked to the right of everyone to "safe and healthy working conditions" as reflected in the ICESCR[28] and other regional treaties.[29] International Labour Organization (ILO) standards also provide, in a more specific and detailed manner, for the practical implementation at the national level of such a right. Examples of health-specific standards include the Occupational Safety and Health Convention and later Protocol as well the Occupational Health Services Convention, which applies to all workers irrespective of their nationality or migration status. In addition to these basic standards, there are several other aspects related to the right to just and favourable conditions of work that, with few exceptions, apply to all workers without distinction of any kind. They deal with a wide range of issues including, inter alia, limitation of working hours,[30] maternity[31] and holiday with pay.[32]

The plain applicability of fundamental labour standards to migrant workers has been stressed by the Inter-American Court of Human Rights in its landmark *Advisory Opinion on Juridical Condition and Rights of the Undocumented Migrants*. The Court held that the principle of non-discrimination should be considered irrespective of migrant status. When an employment relationship is established between a migrant and an employer, the migrant acquires as a worker a series of economic and social rights which must be recognized independently of his or her migratory status, as these rights derive directly from the labour relationship.[33] For the Court, these rights notably consist of the prohibition of forced labour, freedom of association and the rights to organize and join a trade union, and the right to adequate working conditions, including safety and health.[34]

The migration conventions and the right to health

The general human rights law framework is crucial for reinforcing and complementing the more specific treaty regimes devoted to refugees and migrant workers. With regard to the first traditional category of migrants protected by international law, the 1951 Convention Relating to the Status of Refugees and its 1967 Protocol[35] provide them with economic and social rights which are, in many respects, equivalent to those accorded to the receiving country's own citizens.

Once asylum is granted, refugees are entitled to social and medical assistance. Under the headings of "public relief", Article 23 states that "[t]he Contracting States shall accord to refugees lawfully staying in their territory the same treatment with respect to public relief and assistance as is accorded to their nationals." Although this article does not explicitly mention health care, public relief and assistance have been interpreted as including access to health services.[36] Moreover, according to Article 24(1)(b), states "shall accord to refugees lawfully staying in their territories the same treatment as is accorded to nationals in respect of ... [s]ocial security", which covers employment injury, occupational diseases, maternity, sickness, disability, old age, death, and unemployment as they appear in social security schemes.

However, this protective regime does not contain any specific provisions for asylum-seekers and other migrants in need of international protection. In such a normative context, general human rights law instruments play a critical role for bridging the protection gap of the Refugee Convention. The Special Rapporteur on the Right to Health acknowledged in his report on his mission to Sweden that: "The right to health is to be enjoyed by all without discrimination. It is especially important for vulnerable individuals and groups. Asylum seekers and undocumented people are among the most vulnerable in Sweden. They are precisely the sort of vulnerable group that international human rights law is designed to protect."[37] This highlights in turn the primary importance of human rights law as a complementary source of international refugee law, especially with regard to health-related issues.

With regard to migrant workers, the right to health is relatively well acknowledged by the specific instruments adopted under the auspices of the ILO and the UN. These conventions suffer, however, from two substantial drawbacks. They are not ratified by a majority of states and their provisions on the right to health of undocumented migrant workers remain disputable from a human rights law perspective. This is notably the case of the two following ILO treaties: The Migration for Employment Convention of 1949 (C97) and the Convention Concerning Migrations in Abusive Conditions and the Promotion of Equality of Opportunity and Treatment of Migrant Workers of 1975 (C143).

This latest Convention (C143) and Recommendation No. 151 – which supplements the C97 provisions – represent the first multilateral efforts to deal with irregular migration and acknowledge the obligation of states to "respect the basic human rights of all migrant workers."[38] Despite this general acknowledgment, the right to health is further developed through its recommendation solely with regard to those lawfully present in the host country. Migrants should enjoy effective equality of opportunity and treatment with nationals in respect of conditions of life, including housing and the benefits of social services and educational and health facilities.[39] Whatever their normative content with regard to the right to health, the practical impact of both Conventions (C97 and C143) is rather limited for they have not attracted a large number of ratifications. Receiving countries have been particularly reticent.[40]

The same observation can be made with regard to the 1990 International Convention on the Protection of the Rights of All Migrant Workers and Members of their Families (ICMW). As an instrument, it is notable more for the poor level of adherence it has attracted than for the substantive legal protection it affords this group. Not surprisingly, the Convention is structured along the division between "regular" and "irregular" migrants. In Part III (Articles 8 to 35), fundamental rights are afforded to all migrant workers and members of their families without regard to the (ir)regularity of their stay, while those contained in Part IV (Articles 36 to 56) are restricted to those migrant workers and their families in a regular situation.

In light of the broad understanding of fundamental social rights enshrined in the ICESCR, this difference in treatment might be problematic as it generates grounds for disappointment, and indeed dissatisfaction: Although Article 28 of the ICMW guarantees the right to emergency medical treatment to all migrant workers and members of their families,[41] only regular migrants are granted the fully fledged right to health (Article 43). As a result of the consensus principle that "watered down" most ICMW provisions, the scope of the right to health in the ICMW is clearly narrower than the corresponding provision afforded to all persons in the ICESCR as encompassing a holistic notion of health care. This potential conflict of norms may however be resolved through Article 81(1) of the ICMW which ensures that migrant workers remain under the protection of more favourable rights or freedoms granted by virtue of domestic law or any other international treaty.

Conclusion

At the time of the commemoration of the 60th anniversary of the Universal Declaration of Human Rights, it is worth reiterating the universality and inclusiveness of human rights. The struggle for equality of treatment of all human beings is a constitutive feature of the UDHR. The inclusive and holistic approach of the right to health implies a paradigm shift in governments' and people's collective perception of migrants. As long as the migrant is perceived as an individual who can be exploited at will, subject to discrimination, racism and other forms of intolerance, existing rules governing their rights will not be effective. Even though human rights law does not contain all the solutions, its framework can be considered a universal and appropriate standard for dealing with various aspects of the migration phenomena, and ensuring a minimum of consistency in protection. It recalls in turn that migrants' rights are human rights.

1   The 25 richest countries are spending approximately USD 25–30 billion a year on immigration enforcement and asylum processing mechanisms: P. Martin, 'Bordering on Control: Combating Irregular Migration in North America and Europe', IOM Migration Research Series No. 13, at 6.

2   See more generally on this issue V. Chetail (ed.), *Globalization, Migration and Human Rights: International Law under Review* (Brussels: Bruylant, 2007); A. Aleinikoff and V. Chetail (eds.), *Migration and International Legal Norms* (The Hague: T.M.C. Asser Press, 2003).

3   See for instance the General Assembly resolution on Protection of migrants, resolution A/RES/54/166 (2000) at para. 5.

4   Ibid.

5   See UN Doc. E/CN.4/2000/82 (2000), 15–16.

6   Working paper prepared by Jorge A. Bustamante, Chairman/Rapporteur of the Working Group of intergovernmental experts on the human rights of migrants, UN Doc. E/CN.4/AC.46/1998/5 (1998).

7   F. De Varennes, 'Strangers in Foreign Lands – Diversity, Vulnerability and the Rights of Migrants', 2003 UNESCO-MOST Working Paper 9, Paris, at 9.

8   A. Amato-Gauci and A. Ammon (eds.), *The First European Communicable Disease Epidemiological Report* (Stockholm: European Centre for Disease Prevention and Control, 2007), 270–271; M. Carballo and Mourtala Mboup, *International Migration and Health* (Geneva: Global Commission on International Migration, 2005). See also S. Da Lomba, 'Fundamental Social Rights for Irregular Migrants: The Right to Health Care in France and England', in B. Bogusz, R. Cholewinski (eds.), *Irregular Migration and Human Rights: Theoretical, European and International Perspectives* (Leiden: Martinus Nijhoff Publishers, 2004), at 366.

9   ILO, *Towards a Fair Deal for Migrant Workers in a Global Economy* (Geneva: ILO, 2004).

10 A number of studies have confirmed that occupational injuries appear to be approximately two times higher amongst migrant workers in Europe: P. Bollini, 'No Real Progress Towards Equity: Health of Migrants and Ethnic Minorities on the Eve of the Year 2000' 41(6) *Social Science and Medicine* (1995), at 819–828.

11 D. W. MacPherson and B.D. Gushulak, Irregular Migration and Health, Global Migration Perspectives (Geneva: Global Commission on International Migration, 2004).

12 See Articles 2 and 7 of the Universal Declaration of Human Rights (UDHR); Articles. 2(1), 3, 26 and 27 of the International Covenant on Civil and Political Rights (ICCPR); and Articles 2(2) and 3 of the International Covenant on Economic, Social and Cultural Rights (ICESCR).

13 Resolution A/RES/47/144 of 13 December 1985.

14 General Assembly Resolutions on the Protection of Migrants: A/RES/55/92 (2000), A/RES/56/170 (2001), A/RES/57/218 (2002), A/RES/58/190 (2003), A/RES/59/194 (2004), A/RES/60/169 (2005), A/RES/61/165 (2006), and A/RES/62/156 (2007).

15 These qualifications are however not applicable to "the right to safe and healthy working conditions" restated in Article 8(1)(a) of the Declaration.

16 See, for instance, 'Protection of migrants', A/RES/54/166 (2000), para. 2.

17 Committee on the Elimination of All Forms of Racial Discrimination (CERD), General Recommendation No. 30: Discrimination Against Non Citizens, para. 36.

18 Committee on Economic, Social and Cultural Rights (CESCR), General Comment No. 18 on the Right to Work, UN Doc. E/C.12/GC/18 (2005), para. 33. See also General Comment No. 3 on the nature of States Parties' obligations, UN Doc. E/1991/23 (1990), para. 1; General Comment No. 9 on the domestic application of the Covenant, UN Doc. E/C.12/1998/24 (1998), para. 9.

19 CESCR, General Comment No. 14 on the right to the highest attainable standard of health, 11 August 2000, UN Doc. E/C.12/2000/4, at para. 30.

20 The only exception is given by Article 2(3) which reads: "Developing countries, with due regard to human rights and their national economy, may determine to what extent they would guarantee the economic rights recognized in the present

Covenant to non-nationals." This provision can, however, be applied only by developing countries for the purpose of their economic development and it relates exclusively to "economic rights". It thus does not concern social rights, such as the right to health, which remain plainly applicable to both nationals and non-nationals.

21 CESCR, *International Federation of Human Rights Leagues (FIDH) v. France*, Complaint No. 14/2003, 3 November 2004, para. 32.

22 Platform for International Cooperation on Undocumented Migrants (PICUM), *Access to Health Care for Undocumented Migrants in Europe* (Brussels: PICUM, 2007), at 8.

23 Council of Europe, Parliamentary Assembly, 'Health conditions of migrants and refugees in Europe', Doc. 8650, Strasbourg, 2000.

24 Médecins du Monde, *European Survey on Undocumented Migrants' Access to Health Care* (Paris: MDM: European Observatory on Access to Health Care, 2007) 14.

25 European Court of Human Rights (ECHR), *D v. United Kingdom*, Judgment of 2 May 1997, (1997) 24 EHRR 423, paras. 53–54.

26 Committee Against Torture (CAT), *G.R.B. v. Sweden*, CAT/C/20/D/83/1997, 15 May 1998, para. 6.7.

27 Human Rights Committee (HRC), *C. v. Australia*, CCPR/C/76/D/990/1999, 28 October 2002, para. 6.

28 ICESCR, Article 7(b)

29 San Salvador Protocol to the American Convention on Human Rights, Article 7(e) and (f); Revised European Social Charter, Part I (3) and Part II, Article 3.

30 Hours of Work (Industry) Convention (C1), 1919, Article 2.

31 Maternity Protection Convention (C183), 2000, Article 1.

32 Holidays with Pay Convention (Revised) (C132), 1970, Article 2.

33 Inter-American Commission on Human Rights (IACHR), Advisory Opinion OC-18/03 of September 17, 2003, Juridical Condition and Rights of the Undocumented Migrants, paras. 133–134.

34 Ibid., paras. 157–159.

35 As of 2008, there are 146 states parties to the Refugee Convention or its 1967 Protocol.

36 Paul Weis, *The Refugee Convention, 1951: The Travaux Preparatoires Analysed, with a Commentary* (Cambridge: Cambridge University Press, 1995), 174. See also at the regional level Article 29(1) of the European Union (EU) Directive of 29 April 2004 on minimum standards for the qualification and status of third country nationals or stateless persons as refugees or as persons who otherwise need international protection and the content of the protection granted, Council Directive 2004/83/EC of 29 April 2004 (Official Journal L 304, 30/09/2004 P. 0012–0023).

37 Report on Mission to Sweden, A/HRC/4/28/Add.2, 2007, para. 73.

38 See also 'Toward a fair deal for migrant workers in the global economy', Report VI, International Labour Conference, 92nd session, 2004, ILO, Geneva, para. 229, 82.

39 Migrant Workers Recommendation (R151), 1975, Article 2(I).

40 C97 and C143 have been ratified by 45 and 19 states respectively. Only nine Western receiving states have ratified one or both instruments, but none of them did so after 1981, indicating a lack of interest in the past 25 years.

41 "Migrant workers and members of their families shall have the right to receive any medical care that is urgently required for the preservation of their life or the avoidance of irreparable harm to their health on the basis of equality of treatment with nationals of the state concerned. Such emergency medical care shall not be refused them by reason of any irregularity with regard to stay or employment."

Sexual Orientation, Gender Identity and the Right to Health

Claire Mahon

Lesbian, gay, bisexual, transgender and intersex persons and violations of their right to the highest attainable standard of health

The problems posed by heteronormativity

Most societies are structured around two binary genders, male and female, and only one "normal" sexual orientation, heterosexual. Medical practitioners, health care workers, policy-makers, and educators often fail to talk about, or even consider, those who fall outside of this norm, particularly those who are lesbian, gay, bisexual, transgender, or intersex (LGBTI). When they do appear on the radar, the predominant concern is too often how LGBTI people "correct" the physical or psychological "problems" that make them this way. Little or no thought is given to how the right to health of these individuals is being violated, or could be better protected. This invisibility, and associated isolation and marginalization, can have tragic consequences for the health and well-being of many members of LGBTI communities.

LGBTI people have long been the victims of violations of the right to health. They have been subjected to direct violations, whereby their physical or mental health is compromised because of their actual or perceived sexual orientation[1] or gender identity[2]. Lesbians, gays, bisexuals and transgender persons have been attacked,[3] arrested,[4] tortured,[5] killed,[6] sentenced to death,[7] committed to medical or psychiatric institutions and treated with "aversion therapy" including electroshock therapy or forced rape.[8] Intersex individuals, especially those with visibly atypical anatomy, have been subjected to surgery against their will, for example to "correct" their "ambiguous genitalia".[9] LGBTI persons have also been indirectly victimized, as they are denied access to the full enjoyment of their right to the highest attainable standard of health, through failures to recognize and consider this diverse group as healthcare recipients with specific needs. Further, their status as LGBTI persons means that other human rights are frequently violated, which impact upon their right to health. For example, LGBTI persons often suffer violations of the right to privacy, the right to education, the right to family life, even housing and employment rights, particularly when they are discriminated against on the grounds of their sexual orientation or gender identity,[10] and these violations aggravate their vulnerability to violations of the right to health.

This situation is an unacceptable affront to human dignity, particularly given the startling statistics that have been well known for many years: LGBTI people, especially LGBTI youth, are highly susceptible to poor health and health risks.[11] Male teenagers who identify as gay are 2–3 times more likely than their peers to attempt suicide (although some studies put this figure as high as 6–30 times more likely[12]), and suicide attempts amongst LGBTI youth in general are reportedly 3–7 times higher than for heterosexual youth.[13] For these young people, family or social pressure to conform to the heterosexual norm makes them highly susceptible to mental health problems and places their personal safety at risk.

The rate of suicide and suicide attempts amongst LGBTI adults is also higher than in the heterosexual community, although this is not the only health concern: studies have shown that "sexual minorities" have a higher rate of other mental health problems including depression, bipolar disorder, panic attacks, as well as substance abuse including tobacco, alcohol and drug addictions and other "unhealthy behaviours" such as high-risk/unsafe sex, and higher infection rates for HIV/AIDS and other sexually transmitted diseases.[14] For example, it has been shown lesbian woman are more likely to smoke, abuse alcohol, weigh more, and suffer stress, than heterosexual women, placing them in a higher risk category for heart disease, stroke, cervical and other forms of cancer.[15] As lesbians usually have fewer pregnancies and live births than their heterosexual counterparts, their greater hormone exposure again increases their risk of breast, uterine and ovarian cancer.

The health and well-being of LGBTI people is in danger, yet little action seems to be taken to address this situation.

Violations of the right to the highest attainable standard of health

The United Nations Special Rapporteur on the right to the highest attainable standard of physical and mental health explained in his 2004 report:

> "The legal prohibition of same-sex relations in many countries, in conjunction with a widespread lack of support or protection for sexual minorities against violence and discrimination, impedes the enjoyment of sexual and reproductive health by many people with lesbian, gay, bisexual, or transgender identities or conduct."[16]

It is not only sexual and reproductive health that is impeded – all forms of physical and mental health can be affected by discriminatory policies and practices, and the homophobia or heterosexism of society in general and medical practitioners in particular.

Homophobia: A health hazard

LGBTI student activists have described some of the problems they see resulting from heterosexism:[17]

> "Once the heterosexist assumption is made, many gay men feel the necessity to maintain it. If you can't talk to your doctor about who you have sex with, you won't get the information you need ..."[18]

> "One health challenge is that providers don't necessarily know the sexual orientation of their patients. This can prevent them from asking certain questions, probing for certain risk behaviours, or looking for indications of a particular illness – which does a disservice to their patients ..."[19]

> "There's another potential barrier to health care ... regarding 'coming out': Is your provider friendly? How do you know that what you say to them will be private? What are the implications of whether or not you have privacy? ... It's a greater risk for youth because if you come out to your doctors, are they going to tell your parents or the people you're living with? With teens coming out at a younger age, the risk of homelessness has skyrocketed

for adolescents whose parents aren't ready for their coming out even if the person is young. That's a major health concern right there."[20]

Sharing your sexual orientation or gender identity with others, by "coming out", is important for positive mental health. A society that discourages coming out, discourages recognition of each individual's worth and dignity. It also fosters a culture where, from an early age, LGBTI people are unlikely to be able to properly access the full range of health services and health information that should be available to them, because traditional views about sexuality create obstacles to the provision of health services.[21] Researchers have found that in health care situations LGBTI patients can suffer "ostracism, invasive questioning, rough physical handling, derogatory comments, breaches of confidentiality, shock, embarrassment, unfriendliness, pity, condescension, and fear".[22] They "respond to this mistreatment by delaying medical care or risking potential misdiagnosis by hiding their sexual orientation."[23] Homophobia, ignorance and fear are not just impediments to accessing healthcare, but also to research,[24] further perpetuating the cycle of mistreatment.

Homophobic societies also inhibit education and advocacy about safe sex and other health matters. In places where homosexual activities are criminalized, HIV/AIDS education and other forms of preventive health care that should be tailored to LGBTI communities are suppressed. For example, non-governmental organizations (NGOs) such as Human Rights Watch have reported that the crackdown on lesbians and gays in Uganda, prompted by "state homophobia", is "undermining Uganda's efforts to combat the spread of HIV/AIDS".[25] Amnesty International reports that the arrest, detention, and compulsory testing of men suspected of having HIV in Egypt "not only violates the most basic rights of people living with HIV ... [i]t also threatens public health, by making it dangerous for anyone to seek information about HIV prevention or treatment."[26] Marginalizing LGBTI people undermines public health initiatives, leaving this significant sector of the community underserved and often afraid to seek treatment, even if they could, due to stigmatization or criminalization.[27] Other prejudices, such as those associated with HIV/AIDS, may reinforce and exacerbate discrimination on the grounds of sexual orientation or gender identity, or vice versa, making it less likely that those in need access health services, even if such services are available.[28]

Failure to take into account LGBTI persons in health policy setting

Another way in which the right to health of LGBTI people can be violated is through a failure to adequately take into account their specific needs, and tailor health care systems, including training for health care practitioners, to be more sensitive to the concerns of the LGBTI community. Gays and lesbians are "overlooked and underserved" when it comes to their unique health care needs.[29] Transgender persons face many obstacles in accessing "gender-appropriate services".[30] Health policy makers simply fail to prioritize this particular group of consumers of health services, along with other LGBTI people.

While national health systems are often poorly designed to serve the needs of "sexual minorities", likewise international health care programming is not effectively targeting these groups in need. In 2007 the International Gay and Lesbian Human Rights Commission (IGLHRC) published a study that analysed how the international funding community, governments, and NGOs, are failing LGBTI people because HIV/AIDS programming is not addressing same-sex practicing people, and only leads to further denying LGBTI patients' access to effective HIV prevention, counselling and testing, treatment, and care.[31] "Moving the mountain" is how the group have described the epic struggle to get HIV programmers and policymakers to address how anti-gay discrimination fuels the HIV/AIDS crisis in Africa and elsewhere.[32]

Indeed it could be said that the failure to protect health rights for LGBTI people is as much a failure of human rights practitioners and the human rights system, as it is a failure of health practitioners and health systems, because "[h]uman rights law has developed ... while keeping the issues of sexuality firmly in the closet".[33] Even as human rights law has developed, it has continued to marginalize and it has failed to adequately integrate the rights of LGBTI people.[34]

Further, it is not just health policies which are failing LGBTI individuals: Good health starts with good health education, and school curricula often fail to address LGBTI health education needs. In many countries, educational materials that address sexual orientation and gender identity issues, or even acknowledge the existence of LGBTI concerns, are banned from schools. For example, in some state education systems in the USA, sex education is focused on abstinence-only messages, which risks ignoring the needs of LGBTI youth and failing to protect their health education requirements, not just in the USA but also further afield.[35] In many countries around the world the hetero-norm is reinforced through withholding education about sexual and gender diversity,[36] and risking the health of young LGBTI people in the process.[37]

Protecting LGTBI persons and their right to health
Protection offered by international human rights law

As has been explained in several other chapters in this book, the right to the highest attainable standard of health (often referred to simply as "the right to health"), is protected under international human rights law through article 25 of the Universal Declaration of Human Rights (UDHR), article 12 of the International Covenant on Economic, Social and Cultural Rights (ICESCR), and multiple other international and regional treaties and conventions.[38] It is important to remember that all of these international legal protections apply to people of all sexual orientations and gender identities – the right to health contained in the UDHR and ICESCR is not only relevant for straight men or women.[39] It is after all, "the right of *everyone* to the highest attainable standard of physical and mental health",[40] not just the right of heterosexual males and females. The Committee on Economic, Social and Cultural Rights (CESCR) explained in its General Comment No. 14 on the right to the highest attainable standard of health, that discrimination on any basis, including on the basis of sex and sexual orientation, is contrary to Article 2(2) (non-discrimination) and Article 3 (equal rights of men and women) of ICESCR.[41] This is consistent with the case law of the Human Rights Committee, which decided in the matter of *Toonen v. Australia*, that the prohibition against discrimination on the basis of "sex" should be taken to include sexual orientation.[42] The European Court of Human Rights has also confirmed that discrimination in treatment due to a person's sexual orientation is the "embodi[ment of] a predisposed bias on the part of a heterosexual majority against a homosexual minority, [and] these negative attitudes cannot of themselves be considered by the Court to amount to sufficient justification for the differential treatment any more than similar negative attitudes towards those of a different race, origin or colour."[43]

The European Court of Human Rights has long upheld that LGBTI persons should not be subjected to human rights violations stemming from their sexual orientation. In a variety of cases, the Court has addressed issues that are highly relevant to the enjoyment of the right to the highest attainable standard of health for LGBTI persons, although this has usually been achieved through applying the right to privacy. For example, in the cases of *Goodwin v. United Kingdom*[44] and *I. v. United Kingdom*,[45] the Court ruled that the United Kingdom (UK) Government's refusal to recognize the post-operative genders of two transsexual women was discriminatory and a violation of their right to privacy and right to a family. This is relevant for the right to health, as upholding a right to privacy in relation to their past and present gender identity, and the ability to change their legal identities to protect this privacy, helps to ensure that these women are less likely to be subjected to unlawful discrimination, harassment, and psychological harm.

Protecting a person's freedom to be recognized as the gender they wish to identify as is, however, just one aspect: Protecting one's freedom to change genders, including through the use of medical procedures, is another aspect which is relevant for protecting the right to health, and very important for considering what the content of the right to health means for transgender persons. As the Court described in a case about a female-to-male gender reassignment patient unable to complete his transformation:

> "His continuing inability to complete gender-reassignment surgery left him with a permanent feeling of personal inadequacy and an inability to accept his body, leading to great anguish and frustration. Furthermore, due to the lack of recognition of his perceived, albeit pre-operative, identity, the applicant constantly faced anxiety, fear, embarrassment and humiliation in his daily life. He has had to submit to severe hostility and taunts in the light of the general public's strong opposition, rooted in traditional Catholicism, to gender disorders. Consequently, he has had to follow an almost underground life-style, avoiding situations in which he might have to disclose his original identity, particularly when having to provide his personal code. This has left him in a permanent state of depression with suicidal tendencies."

Freedom to define one's own gender identity, the Court has said, is "one of the most basic essentials of self-determination."[46] This belief was enumerated in a recent case from 2003, where the Court ruled that Germany had failed to respect this freedom (part of the right to privacy) when its civil courts refused a woman's appeal against her health insurance company and its rejection of her claim for reimbursement of the costs of her sex-reassignment surgery.[47] This could be seen as part of a positive obligation to facilitate the self-determination of gender identity, including through the provision (and funding) of relevant health care procedures. Indeed, the Court recently ruled in September 2007 that it was necessary for a state, in this instance Lithuania, to make changes to their civil code in order to protect the right to full gender-reassignment surgery, and allocate budgetary measures to facilitate the fulfilment of this right.[48]

At the international level, there also exists an understanding that positive obligations are part of the right to health. The Committee on Economic, Social and Cultural Rights, in General Comment No. 14, describes the content of the right to health as including:

> "... both freedoms and entitlements. The freedoms include the right to control one's health and body, including sexual and reproductive freedom, and the right to be free from interference, such as the right to be free from ... non-consensual medical treatment ... By contrast, the entitlements include the right to a system of health protection which provides equality of opportunity for people to enjoy the highest attainable level of health."[49]

This interpretation of the right to health, along with the prohibition on discrimination on the grounds of sex or sexual orientation, has been used by LGBTI advocates to advance a more comprehensive understanding of the legal protection of the right to health regardless of sexual orientation or gender identity.[50]

The Yogyakarta principles 17 and 18 on the right to the highest attainable standard of health and protection from medical abuses

In relation specifically to protecting the right to health for LGBTI persons, a relatively new international legal instrument has been established to identify the relevant obligations under international human rights law. The Yogyakarta Principles on the Application of Human Rights Law in Relation to Sexual Orientation and Gender Identity (the Yogyakarta Principles) were launched on 26 March 2007.[51] They comprehensively examine the situation of protection of all human rights for all persons, regardless of sexual orientation or gender identity: Principles 17 and 18 in particular address the right to the highest attainable standard of health, and protection from medical abuses. As set out in their preamble, the Yogyakarta Principles are based on the premise that:

> "... international human rights law affirms that all persons, regardless of sexual orientation or gender identity, are entitled to the full enjoyment of all human rights, [and] that the application of existing human rights entitlements should take account of the specific situations and experiences of people of diverse sexual orientations and gender identities."[52]

Principle 17 of the Yogyakarta Principles states: "Everyone has the right to the highest attainable standard of physical and mental health, without discrimination on the basis of sexual orientation or gender identity. Sexual and reproductive health is a fundamental aspect of this right." This Principle goes on to detail nine aspects of state obligations related to this right, including: the duty to take legislative and other measures to ensure the right to health and access to healthcare; the treatment of medical records with confidentiality; the design and development of healthcare resources and programmes to improve the health status of LGBTI people and address discrimination and prejudice; the need for informed and empowered decisions regarding medical treatment and care; non-discrimination and respect for the diversity of sexual orientations and gender identities in sexual health, education, prevention, care and treatment, including recognition of next of kin; facilitating access to gender reassignment treatments; and adopting policy-making and education and training programmes for healthcare workers to improve treatment for LGBTI people.

Principle 18, which addresses the need for LGBTI persons to be protected from medical abuses, states:

> "No person may be forced to undergo any form of medical or psychological treatment, procedure, testing, or be confined to a medical facility, based on sexual orientation or gender identity. Notwithstanding any classifications to the contrary, a person's sexual orientation and gender identity are not, in and of themselves, medical conditions and are not to be treated, cured or suppressed."

Again, this is broken down into a set of five obligations for states, including: Taking the necessary legislative and other measures to ensure protection against harmful medical practices, including the irreversible alteration of a child's body through attempts to impose a gender identity; establishing child protection mechanisms to reduce risk of medical abuse; ensuring LGBTI people are not used to unethically or involuntarily test medical procedures or conduct research, and reversing funding programmes that would enable such abuses; and ensuring medical and psychological treatment does not treat sexual orientation and gender identity as a pathology.

These provisions in the Yogyakarta Principles provide some guidance as to how international human rights law can be applied in the specific context of respecting, protecting and promoting the right to health for LGBTI persons.

Prospects for the future

The solution to the myriad of health and human rights problems faced by LGBTI people is not to be found merely through the adoption of health systems strategies, but also through human rights strategies directed towards ending discrimination: "There is a pressing need for homosexual orientation to be understood as a benign human variation,"[53] not just by the medical profession, but by the general community. State-sponsored and/or state-sanctioned homophobia is the pathology, and the cure for this must include better training for medical practitioners regarding the needs of the LGBTI community and other same-sex practicing people. Governments must act on their responsibility to respect, protect and fulfil the highest attainable standard of physical and mental health by devising and implementing policies which are not just LGBTI-friendly, but which are specifically directed towards enhancing the health of the LGBTI community and addressing their unique health service requirements. Particular attention needs to be paid to LGBTI youth and the culture shift necessary in society as a whole to ensure that their health needs are protected: "If we cannot change some of the environment in which [LGBTI] youths come to maturity ... alienation, isolation, and victimization will continue their lethal work."[54] Creating a society that is more accepting of diversity, including diversity in gender and sexual practices, is a task for both health professionals and human rights advocates.

1   This chapter draws on the definition of "sexual orientation" used in the Yogyakarta Principles: "'Sexual orientation' ... refer[s] to each person's capacity for profound emotional, affectional and sexual attraction to, and intimate and sexual relations with, individuals of a different gender or the same gender or more than one gender": *The Yogyakarta Principles on the Application of International Human Rights Law in relation to Sexual Orientation and Gender Identity* (The Yogyakarta Principles) (2006), available at http://www.yogyakartaprinciples.org/.

2   This chapter draws on the definition of "gender identity" used in the Yogyakarta Principles: "'Gender identity' ... refer[s] to each person's deeply felt internal and individual experience of gender, which may or may not correspond with the sex assigned at birth, including the personal sense of the body (which may involve, if freely chosen, modification of bodily appearance or function by medical, surgical or other means) and other expressions of gender, including dress, speech and mannerisms": *The Yogyakarta Principles, supra* note 1.

3   See, e.g., Concluding Observations of the Committee Against Torture regarding Venezuela, 23 December 2002, UN Doc. CAT/C/CR/29/2 at para. 10(d).

4   Nigel S. Rodley, *Report of the Special Rapporteur on the question of torture and other cruel, inhuman or degrading treatment or punishment*, 12 January 1995, UN Doc. E/CN.4/1995/34.

5   See, e.g., Concluding Observations of the Committee Against Torture regarding Argentina, 10 December 2004, UN Doc. CAT/C/CR/33/1 at para. 6(g); Concluding Observations of the Committee Against Torture regarding Egypt, 23 December 2002, UN Doc. CAT/C/CR/29/4 at para. 5(e).

6   Francis M. Deng, *Report of the Representative of the Secretary-General on Internally Displaced Persons: Mission to Colombia*, 3 October 1994, UN Doc. E/CN.4/1995/50/Add.1; and Nigel S. Rodley and Bacre Waly Ndiaye, *Joint Report of the Special Rapporteur on the question of torture and other cruel,* *inhuman or degrading treatment or punishment and the Special Rapporteur on Extrajudicial, Summary or Arbitrary Executions: Mission to Colombia*, October 1994, UN Doc. E/CN.4/1995/111.

7   Maurice Copithorne, *Report of the Special Representative on the situation of human rights in the Islamic Republic of Iran*, 21 March 1996, UN Doc. E/CN.4/1996/59.

8   See, e.g., Paul Hunt, *Report of the Special Rapporteur on the right of everyone to the enjoyment of the highest attainable standard of physical and mental health*, 16 February 2004, UN Doc. E/CN.4/2004/49 at para. 38; Nigel S. Rodley, *Report of the Special Rapporteur on the question of torture and other cruel, inhuman or degrading treatment or punishment*, 3 July 2001, UN Doc. A/56/156; Theo van Boven, *Report of the Special Rapporteur on the question of torture and other cruel, inhuman or degrading treatment or punishment*, 23 December 2003, UN Doc. E/CN.4/2004/56; International Commission of Jurists, *Sexual Orientation and Gender Identity in Human Rights Law: References to Jurisprudence and Doctrine of the United Nations Human Rights System* (Geneva: ICJ, 2007); Amnesty International, 'Crimes of Hate, Conspiracy of Silence: Torture and Ill-Treatment Based on Sexual Identity', AI Index ACT 40/016/2001, August 2001; Amnesty International, *Breaking the Silence: Human Rights Violations Based on Sexual Orientation*, (London: Amnesty International Publications, 1994); Human Rights Watch, 'Hated to Death: Homophobia, Violence and Jamaica's HIV/AIDS Epidemic', November 2004, available at http://hrw.org/reports/2004/jamaica1104/jamaica1104.pdf; Human Rights Watch and The International Gay and Lesbian Human Rights Commission, 'More Than A Name: State-Sponsored Homophobia and its Consequences in Southern Africa', 1 January 2003, available at http://www.hrw.org/reports/pdfs/g/general/safriglhrc0303.pdf.

9   Michael O'Flaherty and John Fisher, 'Sexual Orientation, Gender Identity and International Human Rights Law: Contextualizing the Yogyakarta Principles' 8(2) *Human Rights Law Review* (2008) 207–248, at 213; Intersex Society

of North America, 'Frequently Asked Questions', available at http://www.isna.org/faq/; Esther Morris, 'The self I will never know' 364 *New Internationalist* (2004) available at http://newint.org/features/2004/02/01/self/.

10 Amnesty International (1994), *supra* note 8.

11 See, inter alia, Kroll and Warneke, *The Dynamics of Sexual Orientation and Adolescent Suicide: A Comprehensive Review and Development Perspective* (Calgary: University of Calgary, 1995).

12 Ross White, 'Growing Up as a Gay Young Person in Ireland – So What's the Story?' in Rainbow Project, 'Carers are Ignoring Gay Teens' *Irish News*, 5 June 1988, as referred to in Northern Ireland Human Rights Commission, *Enhancing the Rights of Lesbian, Gay and Bisexual People in Northern Ireland*, report published August 2001, available at www.nihrc.org.

13 See, e.g., Stephen T. Russell and Kara Joyner, 'Adolescent Sexual Orientation and Suicide Risk: Evidence From a National Study', 91 *American Journal of Public Health* (2001) 1276; Elvia R. Arriola, 'The Penalties for Puppy Love: Institutionalized Violence Against Lesbian, Gay, Bisexual and Transgendered Youth', 1 *Journal of Gender, Race and Justice* (1998) 429, at 439–47; Jay Paul et al., 'Suicide Attempts Among Gay and Bisexual Men: Lifetime Prevalence and Antecedents' 92 *American Journal of Public Health* (2002) 1338; Michael D. Boucai, 'Legal Remedy for Homophobia: Finding a Cure in the International Right to Health' 6 *Georgia Journal of Gender and Law* 21 (2005).

14 Boucai, ibid.

15 University of Washington Women's Health, 'Lesbian Health: Getting the care you deserve', available at http://depts.washington.edu/uwcoe/healthtopics/lesbianhealth.html.

16 Hunt, *supra* note 8, at para. 38.

17 Heterosexism refers to the presumption that everyone is heterosexual and that opposite-sex attractions and relationships are the norm.

18 Danni (interview subject), 'Sexual Orientation and Other Sexual Minorities', in *Healthy Maine 2010: Opportunity For All*, available at http://www.maine.gov/dhhs/boh/files/hm2010/oppforall/b10sexor.pdf, at 62.

19 Rick Galena (interview subject), ibid., at 63.

20 Penthea Burns (interview subject), ibid., at 62.

21 Hunt, *supra* note 8, at para. 14.

22 Patricia E. Stevens and Joanne M. Hall, as quoted in Nadine Gartner, 'Articulating Lesbian Human Rights: The Creation of a Convention on the Elimination of All Forms of Discrimination Against Lesbians' 14 *UCLA Women's Law Journal* (2005) 61, at 82–3. See further, Boucai, *supra* note 13, at 32.

23 Gartner, ibid., at 83.

24 Laura Dean et al., 'Lesbian, Gay, Bisexual and Transgender Health: Findings and Concerns' 4 *Journal of the Gay and Lesbian Medical Association* (2000) 101. See also, Boucai, *supra* note 12.

25 Human Rights Watch, 'Uganda: State Homophobia Threatens Health and Human Rights', press release, 23 August 2007, available at http://hrw.org/english/docs/2007/08/22/uganda16729.htm.

26 Amnesty International, 'Egypt: Spreading Crackdown on HIV Endangers Public Health', press release, 19 February 2008.

27 James Wilets, 'Using International Law to Vindicate the Civil Rights of Gays and Lesbians in United States Courts' 27 *Columbia Human Rights Law Review* (1995) 33, 34; Boucai, *supra* note 13.

28 Hunt, *supra* note 8, at para. 35.

29 Gartner, *supra* note 20.

30 O'Flaherty and Fisher, *supra* note 9, at 211.

31 International Gay and Lesbian Human Rights Commission (IGLHRC), *Off the Map: How HIV/AIDS Programming is Failing Same-Sex Practicing People in Africa* (New York: IGLHRC, 2007).

32 IGLHRC, 'Moving the Mountain: Getting HIV Programmers and Policymakers to Pay Attention to the Needs of Men Who Have Sex with Men in Kenya', Press Release, 8 March 2007; IGLHRC, 'IGLHRC's New Study Reveals How Anti-Gay Discrimination Fuels HIV/AIDS Crisis in Africa', Press Release, 9 July 2007.

33 Wayne Morgan, 'Queering International Human Rights' in Carl Stychin and Did Herman (eds.)

Law and Sexuality: The Global Arena (Minneapolis: University of Minnesota Press, 2001), at 208, 209.

34 For example, Nadine Gartner writes of how the Convention on the Elimination of All Forms of Discrimination Against Women (CEDAW) "fails to adequate represent lesbians ... [t]he woman who emerges from CEDAW is heterosexual, married, with children, and primarily focused on her home": Gartner, *supra* note 22.

35 Hazel Glenn Beh and Milton Diamond, 'The Failure of Abstinence-Only Education: Minors Have a Right to Honest Talk about Sex' 15 *Columbia Journal of Gender and Law* (2006), at 12; and IGLHRC, 'What Happened to Safer Sex? How the US Abstinence-Only and Global Gag Rule Policies Affect Sexual Minorities', available at www.iglhrc.org.

36 Kelli Kristine Armstrong, 'The Silent Minority Within a Minority: Focusing on the Needs of Gay Youth in our Public Schools', 24 *Golden Gate University Law Review* (1994), at 67.

37 Carlo A. Pedrioli, 'Lifting the Pall of Orthodoxy: The Need for Hearing a Multitude of Tongues in and Beyond the Sexual Education curricula at Public High Schools', 13 *UCLA Women's Law Journal* (2005), at 209, at 211–2.

38 Including, inter alia, the Convention on the Rights of the Child (Article 24); the International Convention on the Elimination of All Forms of Racial Discrimination (Article 24); the International Convention on the Elimination of all Forms of Discrimination Against Women (Article 11); the Convention on the Rights of Persons with Disabilities (Article 25); the African Charter on Human and Peoples' Rights (Article 16); the African Charter on the Rights and Welfare of the Child (Article 14); the Protocol to the African Charter on Human and Peoples' Rights on the Rights of Women in Africa; the Additional Protocol to the American Convention on Human Rights in the Area of Economic, Social and Cultural Rights (the Protocol of San Salvador) (Article 10); the Arab Charter on Human Rights (Article 39); and the European Social Charter (common Article 11).

39 See further, International Commission of Jurists (ICJ), *Sexual Orientation and Gender Identity: A Practitioner's Guide* (Geneva: ICJ, 2008), in particular 'Chapter 8: Right to Health'; and Eric Heinze, *Sexual Orientation – A Human Right: An Essay on International Human Rights Law* (Dordrecht: Martinus Nijhoff Publishers, 2005).

40 Article 12(1), ICESCR, *emphasis added.*

41 Committee on Economic, Social and Cultural Rights (CESCR), *General Comment No. 14 on the right to the highest attainable standard of health,* 11 August 2000, UN Doc. E/C.12/2000/4.

42 *Toonen v. Australia,* Human Rights Committee, Views on Communication 488/1992 (1994), UN Doc. CCPR/C/50/D/488/1992.

43 *S.L. v. Austria* (2003) 37 EHRR 39, at para. 44. These cases concerned the differing age of consent for homosexuals and heterosexuals.

44 *Goodwin v. United Kingdom* (2002) 35 EHRR 18.

45 *I. v. United Kingdom* (2003) 36 EHRR 53.

46 *Van Kück v. Germany* (2003) 37 EHRR 51, 2003-VII 1.

47 Ibid.

48 *L. v. Lithuania,* Application No. 27527/03, Judgment of 11 September 2007.

49 CESCR, *General Comment No. 14,* at para. 8.

50 Douglas Sanders, 'Getting Lesbian and Gay Issues on the International Human Rights Agenda', 18 *Human Rights Quarterly* (1996), at 67–106; Center for Constitutional Rights, *Promoting Lesbian and Gay Rights through International Human Rights Law* (New York: Center for Constitutional Rights); James D. Wilets, 'International Human Rights Law and Sexual Orientation' 18(1) *Hastings International and Comparative Law Review* (1994) 1–120; James D. Wilets, 'Using International Law to Vindicate the Civil Rights of Gays and Lesbians in United States Courts' 27(1) *Columbia Human Rights Law Review* (1995) 33–56; Laurence R. Helfer and Alice M. Miller, 'Sexual Orientation and Human Rights: Toward a United States and Transnational Jurisprudence' 9 *Harvard Human Rights Journal* (1996), at 61–103. See further the work of the International Lesbian and Gay Association (ILGA), available at http://www.ilga.org.

51 *The Yogyakarta Principles* were signed by 29 international human rights experts, after a draft process and workshop organized by the International Commission of Jurists and the International Service for Human Rights.

52 *Yogyakarta Principles*, preambular paragraph 6.

53 Boucai, *supra* note 13, at 41.

54 Ibid., at 29, quoting Paul, *supra* note 13, at 1343.

Mental Health as a Human Right

Lance Gable and Lawrence O. Gostin

Introduction

The goal of achieving good mental health remains an important global concern, although one that is often overlooked and undermined by policymakers and politicians. Persons living with mental disabilities often face substantial obstacles to improving their mental health and participating fully in their communities and societies. They have been subjected to discrimination, stigmatization, and other indignities, including involuntary confinement without fair process, inability to access needed care and treatment, and the erection of social and economic barriers that limit their opportunities.

The impact of these persistent human rights violations exacerbates the burden of mental disabilities throughout the population and may preclude persons with mental and intellectual disabilities from successfully seeking and obtaining mental health services. While these problems have received widespread recognition by international agencies and governments, human rights abuses continue to occur with frustrating regularity around the world. Paul Hunt, the former United Nations Special Rapporteur on the Right to Health, has described mental health as "among the most grossly neglected elements of the right to health."[1]

This chapter will articulate a robust conception of a human right to mental health, and illustrate the need to conceive of the right to mental health in a broader way within a human rights framework. Our conception of a right to mental health embraces a complex and interrelated relationship between mental health and physical health, and between the right to mental health and other human rights. Mental health comprises an integral component of overall health and well-being. Likewise, the right to health, as it exists in international human rights instruments, necessarily and clearly encompasses both physical and mental health. Just as it is difficult to address the right to health without contemplating other related human rights, mental and physical health cannot be considered separately in the context of human rights – a minimum level of both mental and physical health are necessary to ensure the ability to enjoy and benefit from other human rights.[2] Thus, efforts to recognize and uphold a human right to health must incorporate strategies to protect, respect, and fulfil mental health as well as physical health. Establishing and upholding affirmative mental health rights can fundamentally advance the dignity and welfare of persons with mental disabilities, and, simultaneously, advance the recognition and development of the right to health generally.

The global burden of mental disabilities

Mental disabilities occur around the world with great frequency. The World Health Organization (WHO) estimates that approximately 450 million people worldwide have mental, neurological, and behavioural health conditions.[3] These conditions range from depression (more than 150 million people at any time) to schizophrenia (approximately 25 million people) to substance abuse (90 million people).[4] The coexistence of mental health problems with other characteristics of vulnerability often renders persons with mental and intellectual disabilities especially vulnerable to human rights abuses and consequently less able to advocate for their human rights. Mental disabilities occur more frequently in poor populations,[5] and often disproportionately affect women, children, and other disempowered groups.[6]

At the national level, data indicate that mental health services routinely receive inadequate funding from public and private sources.[7] Insufficient resources often are coupled with an absence of enforceable legal protections for persons with mental and intellectual disabilities. Economic, social, and cultural rights, such as the right to health, are frequently ignored in national public policy discourse, because these rights can be costly to secure, and may only address concerns salient to small – and politically powerless – groups within a society.[8] Approximately 62% of countries do not have mental health legislation, or have legislation more than ten years old.[9] Older legislation typically does not incorporate human rights protections. Consequentially, persons with mental disabilities may lack valuable legal protection rooted in human rights, or protection may be under-enforced, even where available under law.[10]

The three myths of mental disabilities

Three pernicious myths about persons with mental and intellectual disabilities continue to impede efforts to eliminate discrimination, diminish stigma, and foster political support for mental health services.[11] These myths have fuelled misperceptions about persons with mental disabilities and perpetuated enduring negative stereotypes. As a result, these myths have become pervasive and influential on the public discourse surrounding mental disability and the right to mental health.

The myth of incompetency relies on the false assumption that persons with mental disabilities cannot competently make decisions or grant consent. In actuality, mental disabilities vary substantially, and a continuum of competency exists. While some mentally disabled people lack competency, others have full competency or merely limited incapacity. Policies that presume automatic or perpetual incompetency for mentally disabled individuals, or fail to assess separately a person's competency with regard to specific services, decisions, or functions, violate human rights. A person's right to mental health clearly may be undermined if he or she is inappropriately denied the ability to make health-related decisions.

A second destructive myth is the common misconception that persons with mental disabilities generally pose a threat to others. Research on this issue demonstrates that persons with mental disabilities have no greater propensity to commit violent acts than persons who do not have a mental disability.[12] The key variable in predicting dangerousness is co-morbidity with alcohol and drug dependency. Moreover, most violent acts are committed by people who do not have a mental disability.[13] Nevertheless, the media often give disproportionate attention to the rare cases when a mentally disabled person commits a violent crime.[14] Even a single high-profile incident of this nature can fuel public outrage and stigma against all persons with mental disabilities, and additionally may provide the impetus to enact more punitive mental health laws. Recent changes to mental health legislation in the United Kingdom reflect this tendency. In reaction to a highly-publicized violent crime, Parliament enacted the Mental Health Act of 2007,[15] which embraces the aforementioned stereotypes about dangerousness and enhances government powers of preventive confinement at the expense of treatment and patients' rights.[16] Such approaches threaten to eviscerate the right to mental health by enacting punitive measures instead of treatment.

The third myth invokes the misconception that the deinstitutionalization movement resolved the most important human rights issues facing persons with mental and intellectual disabilities. After effective psychotropic medications were discovered and made available in the 1960s, thousands of people with severe mental disabilities became able to receive treatment in the community, and were released from institutional settings. These medications held great promise to benefit patients with more effective treatments and greater freedom. Additionally, governments strongly supported deinstitutionalization for its economic benefits. Costly psychiatric institutions could be shuttered and resources directed elsewhere.[17]

The promising benefits of deinstitutionalization did not accrue as planned. First, while the medications effectively alleviated symptoms of schizophrenia and other serious conditions, they also had significant side effects when used in high dosages over long periods. Many people taking these medications, for example, developed tardive dyskinesia, a debilitating neurological condition, which causes uncontrollable tics and shaking.[18] Second, efforts to implement community care and treatment were undercut by ineffective planning and meagre economic support.[19] Effective treatment with pharmaceuticals in the community requires a robust infrastructure to ensure that medications and other support services are available and affordable. Many countries did not create community mental health systems to support persons who had been deinstitutionalized. In jurisdictions that have established community services, these services often remain chronically under-funded, fragmented, and punitive.[20]

The sad consequence of these policy choices has been an explosion in the number of mentally disabled people who have become homeless without any access to health services. Equally troubling is the steady transmigration of mentally disabled people from psychiatric institutions to other institutions – jails, prisons, remand centres, and nursing homes – where they do not receive appropriate treatment, if any.[21] In many countries around the world prisons have become the de facto mental health systems, leaving this population isolated, forgotten, and deprived of their human rights.

The evolution of a human right to mental health

The connection between human rights and health has gained increasing salience in international human rights law as norms and infrastructure have expanded across many jurisdictional levels, international to domestic.[22] In many ways, the linkage between health and human rights represents the culmination of the collective efforts of the human rights movement and the disability rights movement, two of the great international social movements of the last sixty years.[23] Yet, the recognition of an affirmative right to mental health has evolved comparatively slowly and gradually within international human rights law. Even within the disability rights movement, mental and intellectual disabilities were historically marginalized while the focus remained on physical disabilities. Additionally, most efforts targeting human rights violations related to persons with mental disabilities addressed infringements on civil and political rights: Issues involving liberty, dignity, and to a lesser extent, equality.[24] Relevant jurisprudence in regional human rights courts, and at the national level, has focused on issues related to involuntary confinement of persons with mental disabilities, including ensuring scientific criteria and fair procedures for admission and release,[25] appropriate review processes,[26] and adequate conditions of confinement and treatment.[27] Only more recently have initiatives sought to take the additional step of formulating a right to mental health that acts also as an entitlement to the conditions necessary for good mental health.

Nevertheless, the right to mental health is firmly grounded in numerous international documents going back sixty years. The Constitution of the World Health Organization, drafted in 1946 and adopted in 1948, recognizes that "[h]ealth is a state of complete physical, mental, and social well-being and not merely the absence of disease or infirmity."[28] The Universal Declaration of Human Rights, adopted in 1948, acknowledges the right to health as a component of "a standard of living adequate for the health and well-being of [a person and that person's] family, including ... medical care and necessary social services, and the right to security in the event of ...

sickness."[29] The 1966 International Covenant on Economic, Social, and Cultural Rights (ICESCR) adopts a broad concept of health as a human right, declaring "the right of everyone to the ... highest attainable standard of physical and mental health."[30] The Principles for the Protection of Persons with Mental Illness (MI) Principles, drafted by the United Nations in 1991, afford a right to the "best available mental health care."[31]

Other international and regional instruments have incorporated variations of the right to health into their respective texts. Both the European Social Charter and the Protocol of San Salvador in the Inter-American Human Rights System describe expansive conceptions of a right to health that encompass rehabilitation and social resettlement of people with mental or physical disabilities,[32] and "[s]atisfaction of the health needs of the highest risk groups."[33] The African Charter on Human and Peoples' Rights contains "the right to enjoy the best attainable state of physical and mental health", requiring the State to "take the necessary measures to protect the health of their people and to ensure that they receive medical attention when they are sick."[34] An increasing number of recently drafted national constitutions and legislation, for example in Brazil and South Africa, also establish a right to health.[35] These various versions of a right to health follow a clear trajectory: More recent definitions of the right to health are more likely to include detailed description of the contents of the right, and many of these definitions explicitly invoke a right to mental health as a component of the right to health more generally.

Several contemporary initiatives have further elucidated the right to health and by extension the right to mental health. In 2001, the United Nations Committee on Economic, Social and Cultural Rights issued General Comment No. 14 on the Right to Health.[36] General Comment No. 14 provides an authoritative examination of the scope and meaning of the right to health that adopts a broad normative interpretation of the right. Accordingly, the right encompasses public health, health care, and the underlying determinants necessary for healthy living, including safe homes and workplaces, adequate access to nutritious food and uncontaminated drinking water, healthy environmental conditions, and sufficient sanitation. The right to health also contains both "freedoms and entitlements". The freedoms are protections essentially drawn from the context of civil and political rights: The right to have control over one's health and body, the right to sexual and reproductive freedom, and freedom from interference, which includes the right to be free from torture and medical treatment or experimentation without consent. The entitlements, by comparison, include an affirmative "right to a system of health protection which provides equality of opportunity for people to enjoy the highest attainable level of health."[37]

The United Nations Human Rights Commission subsequently appointed a Special Rapporteur with a mandate to focus on the right to health.[38] The Rapporteur's first report in 2003 identified three primary objectives: Promote the right to health as a fundamental human right; clarify its contours; and identify good practices for the implementation of the right.[39] In 2005, the Rapporteur (Professor Paul Hunt) published a report examining the right to health in the context of mental and intellectual disabilities, which provides a detailed, thoughtful assessment of the significance of mental health as a component of the right to health.[40] The Report recognizes that the scope of the right to mental health goes beyond entitlements to mental health services and the availability of underlying determinants of mental health. The right also encompasses freedoms encapsulated in other human rights, such as prohibitions against discrimination, involuntary detention without due process, and non-consensual medical treatment.[41]

The recently completed Convention on the Rights of Persons with Disabilities (CRPD) also affirms a right to the highest attainable standard of health,[42] access to habilitation and rehabilitation services,[43] and inclusion in the community for persons with physical and mental disabilities.[44] The CRPD articulates a detailed right to health, including ensuring "access for persons with disabilities to health services" without discrimination, providing for early intervention and identification "to minimize and prevent further disabilities," and facilitating community-based health services.[45] Moreover, the Convention requires substantive participation by persons with disabilities in the implementation of the enumerated rights.[46]

Finally, several notable cases have expanded the jurisprudential recognition of the right to health and to conditions necessary to maintain health. The Inter-American Commission of Human Rights has been particularly progressive in this regard. In *Victor Rosario Congo v. Ecuador,* the Commission found a violation of the right to humane treatment when a mentally disabled person was denied health services in a state-run facility.[47] A key aspect of this decision was the willingness of the Commission, not only to apply human rights standards from the American Convention on Human Rights, but also to refer to, and incorporate, norms from other sources, including the MI Principles and decisions of the European Court of

Human Rights.[48] In a later case, the Inter-American Court of Human Rights went further and found violations of the right to health in *Damiao Ximenes v. Brazil* based upon standards found in the American Convention, the Protocol of San Salvador,[49] and a number of other international declarations and interpretive guidance sources.[50] A few national courts have begun to uphold the right to health as well. Courts in both Argentina[51] and South Africa[52] have required their national governments to provide access to specific medical treatments in order to fulfill the right to health.

The right to mental health as an affirmative right

Prior scholarship has assessed the "ideology of entitlement" – the idea that international human rights law affords a right to mental health.[53] Framing mental health as a human right, rather than a mere moral claim, suggests that states possess binding obligations to respect, defend, and promote that entitlement.[54] Considerable disagreement persists, however, on the issue of whether "mental health" is a meaningful, identifiable, operational, and enforceable right, or whether it is merely aspirational or rhetorical. A right to mental health that is too broadly defined lacks clear content and is less likely to have a meaningful effect.[55] For example, if health is, in the World Health Organization's words, truly "a state of complete physical, mental and social well-being", then no one can ever achieve it.[56] Even if this definition were construed as a relative, as opposed to an absolute standard, it remains difficult to implement, and is unlikely to be justiciable. Thus, the concept of entitlement is more vague and variable than concepts of liberty and dignity, because it involves the right of access to core mental health services. Yet all articulations of the right to health concede that the "entitlement" components of the right are subject to the economic realities in the country to support such entitlements, and consequently to "progressive realization".[57]

The expansive and ambitious definitions of the right to health developed by General Comment No. 14, the Special Rapporteur's Mental Health Report, the CRPD, and the developing right to health jurisprudence set a precedent that, if followed, could substantially benefit the lives of persons with mental and intellectual disabilities. Persons with mental disabilities and their advocates could utilize these standards to insist that governments deliver on their obligations related to the right to mental health, including the provision of community-based preventive mental health services, treatment facilities, and rehabilitation services. A broad right to health would require governments to assure that mental health services and the determinants of good mental health were available, accessible, acceptable, and of appropriate quality, pursuant to the norms established in the General Comment. Further, the establishment of a broad right to health increases the likelihood that national and local governments will augment the mental health services available to the public, undertake public education initiatives about mental and intellectual disabilities to reduce stigma, and implement other preventive and population-based mental health services.

General Comment No. 14 and the Special Rapporteur's Mental Health Report also highlight the linkages between the right to health and other human rights. Normatively, this correlation of rights grants the right to health equal standing with other rights. Practically, it expands the options for mental health promotion through human rights. Many of the activities that violate the right to health may also be seen as violations of other human rights. For instance violations of the prohibition on inhuman and degrading treatment where a mentally ill person is detained in squalid, inhumane conditions and does not receive appropriate treatment, are, in addition to violations of the right to health, due to the potential for significant physical and mental deterioration or even death.[58]

Another conceptual way to consider the interconnected relationship between the right to mental health and other human rights is to view protection of other human rights as themselves underlying determinants of mental health. Strong and consistent protections for liberty, equality, and dignity are not only beneficial for their own sake: These conditions are likely to reduce stress, anxiety, discrimination, and depression. The availability of robust social services and community engagement even beyond the health sector can also foster good mental health. These synergistic results suggest that upholding human rights can positively impact mental health in numerous ways.[59]

The right to mental health, together with other human rights, supports modern trends in mental health policy and practice such as community integration initiatives for persons with mental disabilities and the newer concept of public mental health. Community integration seeks to provide persons with mental disabilities effective treatment in a community setting and to maximize opportunities for social integration. However, to avoid the problems that have undermined past efforts to implement community care, governments must ensure that community mental health services are well-funded and supported.

Efforts to implement the right to mental health should also incorporate both individual and population-based approaches to mental health. An individualized concept of mental health emphasizes the conditions most relevant to the mental health status of a particular individual. If the government implements policies and practices that are harmful to the mental health of individuals or withholds services necessary to maintain the mental health of individuals, it may violate the right to mental health. Public mental health, on the other hand, approaches issues of mental health from a population-based perspective. Under this approach, the state must not only provide care and rehabilitation services, but also must assure the existence of multiple conditions in which people can be mentally healthy. Public mental health imposes a duty on the state, within the limits of its available resources, to assure the conditions necessary for people to attain and maintain mental health, including by providing decent economic conditions, education and health information, opportunities for meaningful employment, social and welfare services, primary and secondary mental health care, community mental health services, and hospital-based treatment and services. Governments can also positively affect mental health by improving underlying societal conditions, for example by implementing policies that favour humane working conditions, time and space for recreation and relaxation, and assistance with stress-causing circumstances such as child rearing and debt.

Conclusion

The persistent violations of human rights that continue to affect persons with mental disabilities will only be reduced through diligent efforts to recognize and remedy these violations at all levels. Legal initiatives should comprise a core aspect of theses efforts. Countries should ratify international and regional human rights treaties that include the right to health and pass legislation implementing an affirmative right to mental health. Courts at all levels of jurisdiction should enforce this right consistently and expansively. Countries should also take practical measures to disarm societal barriers that hinder full social participation of persons with mental disabilities; eliminate stigma and discrimination; encourage understanding, cooperation, and participation; uphold dignity and equality; and provide mental health services in settings that are less restrictive and more humane.

Many of these initiatives will require significant political and economic support and a concerted effort to prioritize the right to mental health despite resource limitations. The widespread adoption of policies and practices consistent with the right to mental health can help address the enduring inequity and injustice faced by this population. Moreover, this effort can provide the impetus at long last to eliminate the insidious myths that surround mental disabilities.

1   Paul Hunt, *Report of the Special Rapporteur on the right of everyone to the enjoyment of the highest attainable standard of physical and mental health*, 11 February 2005, UN Doc. E/CN.4/2005/51.

2   L. O. Gostin, 'Beyond Moral Claims: A Human Rights Approach in Mental Health' 10 *Cambridge Q. Healthcare Ethics* (2001), at 264.

3   World Health Organization (WHO), *Investing in Mental Health* (Geneva: WHO, 2003), at 8.

4   Ibid.

5   Ibid., at 25.

6   Ibid., at 84–87.

7   World Health Organization, *Mental Health Atlas 2005* (Geneva: WHO, 2005).

8   P. Harvey, 'Human Rights and Economic Policy Discourse: Taking Economic and Social Rights Seriously' 33 *Columbia Human Rights Law Review* (2002), at 363.

9   WHO, *Mental Health Atlas 2005* (Geneva: WHO, 2005), at 15.

10 L. O. Gostin and L. Gable, 'The Human Rights of Persons with Mental Disabilities: A Global Perspective on the Application of Human Rights Principles to Mental Health' 63(1) *Maryland Law Review* (2004) 20–121, at 44.

11 L. Gable and L. O. Gostin, 'Global Mental Health: Changing Norms, Constant Rights' 1 *Georgetown Journal of International Affairs* (2008), at 83–92.

12 MacArthur Violence Risk Assessment Study, Executive Summary, April 1999, available at http://www.macarthur.virginia.edu/risk.html.

13 Seena Fazel and Martin Grann, 'The Population

Impact of Severe Mental Illness on Violent Crime' 163 *American Journal of Psychiatry* (2006), at 1397–1403.

14 M. Smith, 'Role of the Popular Media in Mental Illness' 349 *The Lancet* (1997).

15 UK Mental Health Act of 2007, available at http://www.opsi.gov.uk/acts/acts2007/pdf/ukpga_2007 0012_en.pdf.

16 Lawrence O. Gostin, 'From a Civil Libertarian to a Sanitarian' 34 *Journal of Law and Society* (2007), at 594–616.

17 Richard G. Frank and Sherry A. Glied, *Better But Not Well: Mental Health Policy in the United States Since 1950* (Baltimore: The Johns Hopkins University Press, 2006).

18 L. Gable and L. O. Gostin, 'Global Mental Health: Changing Norms, Constant Rights' 1 *Georgetown Journal of International Affairs* (2008), 83–92 at 85.

19 Robert A. Burt, 'Promises to Keep, Miles to Go: Mental Health Law Since 1972' in L. E. Frost and R. J. Bonnie (eds.) *The Evolution of Mental Health Law* (Washington, D. C.: American Psychology Association, 2001), 11–30; David L. Bazelon, 'Institutionalization, Deinstitutionalization and the Adversary Process' 75(5) *Columbia Law Review* (1975), at 897–912.

20 'The Unseen: Mental Illness's Global Toll' 311 *Science* (2006), at 458–461.

21 G. N. Grob, 'Mental Health Policy in America: Myths and Realities' 11(3) *Health Affairs* (1992) 7–22; Gerhard Langle, Birgit Egerter, Friederike Albrecht et al., 'Prevalence of Mental Illness among Homeless Men in the Community: Approach to a Full Census in a Southern German University Town' 40 *Soc Psychiatry Psychiatr Epidemiol* (2005), at 382–390.

22 L. Gable, 'The Proliferation of Human Rights in Global Health Governance' 35(4) *Journal of Law, Medicine & Ethics* (2007) 534–544, at 539.

23 SS. Herr, L. O. Gostin, H. H. Koh (eds.), *Persons with Intellectual Disabilities: Different But Equal* (Oxford: Oxford University Press, 2003).

24 R. J. Bonnie, 'Three Strands of Mental Health Law: Developmental Mileposts' in L. E. Frost and R. J. Bonnie (eds.), *The Evolution of Mental Health Law* (Washington, D. C.: American Psychological Association, 2001), at 31–54.

25 *Winterwerp v. The Netherlands*, 33 European Court of Human Rights (1979) Series A, at 23.

26 *X v. United Kingdom*, 46 European Court of Human Rights (1981) Series A, at 23.

27 Victor Rosario Congo, Case 11.427, Inter-American Commission on Human Rights 63/99 (1999) para. 66, available at http://www1.umn.edu/humanrts/cases/1998/ecuador63-99.html.

28 Constitution of the World Health Organization, signed 22 June 1946, available at http://www.who.int/governance/eb/constitution/en/.

29 Universal Declaration of Human Rights (1948), Article 25.

30 International Covenant on Economic, Social and Cultural Rights (1966).

31 'Principles for the protection of persons with mental illness and the improvement of mental health care', General Assembly resolution A/RES/46/119, available at http://www.unhchr.ch/html/menu3/b/68.htm.

32 European Social Charter (1961), Articles 11 and 15, available at http://conventions.coe.int/Treaty/en/Treaties/Html/035.htm.

33 Additional Protocol to the American Convention on Human Rights in the Area of Economic, Social and Cultural Rights (1988) (Protocol of San Salvador), Article 10(2)(f) and Articles 10(2)(a)–(e), available at http://www.cidh.org/Basicos/English/basic5.Prot.Sn%20Salv.htm.

34 African Charter on Human and Peoples' Rights (1981), Article 16.

35 L. Gable, 'The Proliferation of Human Rights in Global Health Governance' 35 *Journal of Law, Medicine & Ethics* (2007) 534–544, at 538.

36 Committee on Economic, Social and Cultural Rights, *General Comment No. 14 on the right to the highest attainable standard of health*, 11 August 2000, UN Doc. E/C.12/2000/4.

37 Ibid.

38 Paul Hunt, *Report of the Special Rapporteur on the right of everyone to the enjoyment of the highest at-*

tainable standard of physical and mental health, 13 Februrary 2003, UN Doc. E/CN.4/2003/58.

39 Paul Hunt, 'The UN Special Rapporteur on the Right to Health: Key Objectives, Themes, and Interventions' 7 *Health and Human Rights* (2003), at 1–26.

40 Paul Hunt, *Report of the Special Rapporteur on the right of everyone to the enjoyment of the highest attainable standard of physical and mental health,* 11 February 2005, UN Doc. E/CN.4/2005/51.

41 Ibid., para. 33–34.

42 Convention on the Rights of Persons with Disabilities (2006), Article 25.

43 Ibid., Article 26.

44 Ibid., Article 19.

45 Ibid., Article 25.

46 Ibid., Article 34.

47 *Victor Rosario Congo, Case 11.427,* Inter-American Commission on Human Rights, Case No. 63/99 (1999), at para. 66.

48 L. Gable et al., 'Mental Health and Due Process in the Americas: Protecting the Human Rights of Persons Involuntarily Admitted to and Detained in Psychiatric Institutions' 18(4/5) *Pan American Journal of Public Health* (2005), at 366–373.

49 Additional Protocol to the American Convention on Human Rights in the Area of Economic, Social and Cultural Rights (1988) (Protocol of San Salvador).

50 *Damaio Ximenes v. Brazil,* Inter-American Court of Human Rights, Judgment of 4 July 2006.

51 *Mariela Viceconte v. Argentina Ministry of Health and Social Welfare,* Case No 31.777/96 (1998).

52 *Minister of Health v. Treatment Action Campaign,* Constitutional Court of South Africa, 10 BCLR (2002), at 1033.

53 L. O. Gostin, 'The Ideology of Entitlement: The Application of Contemporary Legal Approaches to Psychiatry' in P. Bean (ed.), *Mental Illness: Changes and Trends* (1983), at 27–54.

54 L. O. Gostin, 'Beyond Moral Claims: A Human Rights Approach in Mental Health' 10 *Cambridge Quarterly on Healthcare Ethics* (2001), at 271.

55 L. O. Gostin, 'The Human Right to Health: A Right to the "Highest Attainable Standard of Health"'31 *Hastings Center Report* (2001), at 29.

56 World Health Organization, 'Declaration of Alma-Ata', adopted 6–12 September 1978, available at http://www.who.int/hpr/NPH/docs/declaration_almaata.pdf.

57 CESCR, *General Comment No. 14 on the right to the highest attainable standard of health,* UN Doc. E/C.12/2000/4 (2000).

58 See *Keenan v. United Kingdom,* App. No. 27229/95, 33 Eur. H. R. Rep. 913, 964 (2001).

59 Jonathan M. Mann et al., 'Health and Human Rights' in 1(1) *Health and Human Rights* (1994), at 6.

05

KEY HEALTH CHALLENGES

A Human Rights-Based Approach to Non-Communicable Diseases

Helena Nygren-Krug*

Scope, magnitude and risk factors

In recent years, the global public health community has increasingly been calling for intensified action to prevent and control non-communicable diseases (NCDs).[1] NCDs represent 60% of all deaths globally, with 80% of deaths due to non-communicable diseases occurring in low- and middle-income countries, and approximately 16 million deaths involving people less than 70 years of age.[2] Total deaths from NCDs are projected to increase by a further 17% over the next 10 years.[3] NCDs, principally cardiovascular diseases, diabetes, cancers, and chronic respiratory diseases, caused an estimated 35 million deaths in 2005.[4] These NCDs, often considered "lifestyle epidemics", have a number of common modifiable risk factors – tobacco use, unhealthy diet and physical inactivity and the harmful use of alcohol. These risk factors are mainly behavioural and are on the rise everywhere due to the "nutrition transition" with diets rich in saturated fats and poorer in complex carbohydrates and dietary fibre, fruit and vegetables; the growth of urban lifestyles involving less physical exertion; and the promotion and rising consumption of tobacco and alcohol.[5] While some of these risk factors, such as tobacco consumption, have received attention in recent years, others have been much neglected. Obesity, for example, is one of today's most blatantly visible – yet most neglected – public health problems.[6]

A human rights approach to non-communicable diseases

The most recent World Health Assembly adopted a draft action plan to prevent and control non-communicable diseases (NCDs), recognizing that the global burden continues to grow.[7] This plan sets out three strategic directives as follows:

1.   Map the epidemics and analyze their social, economic, behavioural and political determinants as the basis for providing guidance on effective interventions;
2.   Reduce the level of exposure of individuals and populations to the common modifiable risk factors and their determinants while strengthening the capacity of individuals and the population to make healthier choices and follow lifestyle patterns that foster good health;
3.   And strengthen health care for people with NCDs.[8]

Human rights are relevant to each of these strategic directives. Overall, integrating a human rights-based approach to the efforts to address NCDs means that the realization of health-related human rights[9] becomes the overall goal of these efforts and that human rights principles[10] guide all actions towards this goal. Moreover, a human rights-based approach supports action to build the capacity of rights-holders to claim their rights, and duty-bearers to meet their obligations.[11] There are two main rationales for using a human rights approach to address NCDs. The intrinsic rationale, acknowledging that a human rights-based approach is the right thing to do, morally or legally; and the instrumental rationale, recognizing that a human rights-based approach leads to better and more sustainable human development outcomes.[12]

The human right to health is the right to the enjoyment of a variety of facilities, goods, services and conditions necessary for the realization of the highest attainable standard of health.[13] It provides a universal normative framework to design and assess health-care and health determinants in relation to NCDs. Other human rights that guide and support action to address NCDs include equality and non-discrimination and the rights to information, education and participation.

Specific human rights instruments have been adopted over the years that have articulated rights in relation to specific groups of populations that have been exposed disproportionately to human rights violations, including the enjoyment of the right to health. Indigenous peoples; persons with disabilities; migrant workers; prisoners; ethnic, religious and linguistic minorities; women; children; are examples of population groups addressed in specific human rights instruments. Addressing the health of these population groups effectively requires an approach, which begins from their perspective, keeping in mind their needs and situations and with their full participation.

In addition to normative and analytical guidance, the human rights framework contains a number of international, regional and national mechanisms that can support monitoring and accountability in relation to action to address NCDs.

Analyzing and addressing NCDs

A human rights-based approach provides not only a conceptual framework but also a practical methodology for analyzing and addressing the determinants of NCDs.[14] It involves various steps of analysis, starting with a causal one, to identify the immediate, underlying and root causes of NCDs. This helps to go beyond the behavioural risk factors, such as smoking and overeating, to consider underlying and root causes, such as the enjoyment of a range of health-related human rights such as freedom from discrimination and the rights to safe and healthy working conditions, nutritious food, information and education. Secondly, a pattern (also called role/obligation) analysis aims at identifying who are the rights-holders and duty-bearers and their corresponding entitlements and obligations. This step in the analysis maps the various stakeholders involved in promoting or undermining actions to address NCDs. Under international human rights law, the government is the prime duty-bearer; it is under an obligation to promote and protect human rights across all sectors. Within government, in the context of NCDs, specific duty-bearers identified will range across sectors such as agriculture, finance and taxation, education, recreation and sports, media and communication, transportation, and urban planning. However, beyond the government, a range of other duty-bearers can be identified that have specific responsibilities. These may range from family members to multinational corporations and donors. In the area of NCDs, moreover, the private sector plays a significant role, including the tobacco, food, sugar, and alcohol industries. This does not, however, absolve the obligations of the government, which must protect human rights by regulating the private sector so that it acts in conformity with human rights.[15]

Some identified stakeholders may be both duty-bearer and rights-holder. For example, a teacher is a duty bearer vis-à-vis children who should be educated on healthy eating habits, but is also a rights-holder in relation to local and national authorities that should give him or her the authority and resources to carry out health-promotion activities in schools.[16]

In a human rights-based approach to programming, human rights principles guide all stages of the analysis, including the principles of equality and the right to participation. The latter means that those groups identified as most affected should be involved in decisions about possible interventions. The human rights-based approach is concerned with the population groups most exposed to human rights violations: This stems from the focus on equality and non-discrimination in human rights discourse.[17] Focusing the analysis on individuals and groups experiencing a disproportionate burden of exclusion, marginalization and discrimination will help unveil further underlying and root causes of NCDs. As such, the identity of the rights-holder(s) becomes an important and central feature in analyzing why the right to health is not being enjoyed. Addressing NCDs from a human rights perspective thus requires collecting disaggregated data on the prevalence of NCDs, to identify which population groups are most affected. Where there is no systematic collection of disaggregated data, efforts should nevertheless be made to identify the most vulnerable and/or marginalized population groups through research and interviews with those knowledgeable about the national and local context. Such an analysis usually reveals that some populations groups suffer consistently poorer health than others in the same country. For example, across countries, available mortality and morbidity data provide scientific evidence of significant inequalities in the health status of indigenous populations.[18] Smoking, alcoholic and substance abuse are serious health and social problems, along with cardiovascular diseases, diabetes and cancer.[19] Many of these illnesses are associated with lifestyle changes resulting from land displacement and acculturation, which constitute underlying and root causes of NCDs in indigenous communities. In this context, the UN Committee on Economic, Social and Cultural Rights has recognized that development-related activities that lead to the displacement of indigenous peoples against their will from their traditional territories and environment, denying them their sources of nutrition and breaking their symbiotic relationship with their lands, has a deleterious effect on their health.[20] To improve indigenous health, therefore, a holistic approach is required, considering the range of underlying, structural and root causes, and with full participation of the indigenous communities affected.

The third, and final, step in a human rights analysis is the capacity gap analysis, to reveal why rights are not realized, paying particular attention to why duty-bearers are not living up to their human rights obligations or responsibilities. This involves considering questions such as the authority, motivation, commitment, ability to communicate and leadership of duty-bearers, as well as their access to, and control over, resources. This analysis will reveal where interventions will be most effective and how they can be designed so as to enhance the capacities of rights-holders to claim their rights and duty-bearers to meet their obligations. The involvement of rights-holders in all stages of a rights-based analysis is not only a question of safeguarding the right to participation, but also has instrumental value, ensuring that interventions are culturally appropriate and sustainable. Anchored in human rights law, interventions should span across government actors and other stakeholders and generate change at different levels synergistically, from the local and community level to the national and international levels. At all these levels, a priority focus for a human rights-based response is how to enhance accountability of the duty-bearers so that they live up to, and deliver on, their obligations and responsibilities.

Holding the duty-bearers to account

A human rights analysis of NCDs reveals those required to take action and what human rights obligations and responsibilities they have assumed. Accountability is one of the most important features of human rights and requires effective monitoring. To facilitate the monitoring of State Parties' performance in realizing the various rights enshrined in the core UN human rights treaties, the human rights treaty bodies have been engaged in identifying appropriate indicators. Indicators proposed for the monitoring of the right to health include some particularly relevant to monitoring the commitment of governments to address NCDs. Such indicators include: Death rates associated with and prevalence of NCDs (an "outcome indicator"); the proportion of school-going children educated on health and nutrition issues (a "process indicator") and, finally, the timeframe and coverage of national policy on child health and nutrition (a "structural indicator").[21]

Human rights law focuses on state obligations and thus mechanisms at international, regional and national levels focus on monitoring government performance. Since the 1990s, however, there has been an ongoing debate regarding the roles and responsibilities of the private sector in promoting and violating human rights. This debate has focused predominantly on labour standards, with a plethora of initiatives unfolding, mainly in the form of self-regulation and voluntary codes of conduct. In recent years, moreover, attempts are being made at clarifying duties and roles of the private sector specifically in relation to the right to health.[22] Meanwhile, work in public health is increasingly engaging the private sector to attract resources, attention and increase outreach and impact of public health interventions. This poses inherent risks, particularly when there are tremendous commercial interests involved and there is no common framework to address human rights and businesses. The Special Representative of the Secretary-General on the issue of human rights and transnational corporations and other business enterprises, John Ruggie, has sought to address the lack of a framework by proposing three foundational principles: Protect, respect and access to remedy.[23] The first element aims to underscore the role of the state as the steward and prime-duty bearer. Governments need to mainstream the business and human rights agenda across all sectors and ensure adequate domestic policy coherence in order to ensure policy coherence at the international level.[24] The second principle – the principle to respect – is directed at companies themselves, recognizing a corporate responsibility to "do no harm". This poses particular challenges in the context of NCDs and tobacco in particular. How can the tobacco industry operate in a way consistent with human rights? Can a tobacco company respect the right to life – the most fundamental of all human rights – or is there a contradiction given that the substance that it produces, tobacco, kills a third to a half of all those who use it?[25] Application of this principle in practice challenges the very raison-d'être of some businesses. The third and final principle in the framework proposed is that of effective remedy.

It is the first principle – to protect – that has evolved most substantively in international law given that states are the principal actors in this field. As far back as in the 70s, high profile non-governmental organizations' (NGO) campaigns sought to protect and promote breast-feeding for babies and prevent the inappropriate marketing of breast milk substitutes.[26] Supported by UNICEF and the WHO, these campaigns led governments in the World Health Assembly to adopt the International Code of Marketing of Breast-Milk Substitutes (1981) which constitutes a set of recommendations to regulate the marketing of breast-milk substitutes, feeding bottles and teats.[27] Breastfeeding has long-term benefits associated with NCDs. Adults who were breastfed as babies often have lower blood pressure and lower cholesterol, as well as lower rates of overweight, obesity and type-2 diabetes.[28] Although most of the countries that have adopted the Code have put in place some implementing measures, frequently by enforceable legislation, voluntary means are also being used. Despite this now long-standing code, however, manufacturers of infant formula milks are still accused of using manipulative marketing techniques that have an adverse affect on breastfeeding rates around the work.[29] According to Save the Children, an international treaty on Baby Milk marketing is required, based on the WHO code but with much stronger state obligations and institutional oversight.[30] Others argue that the Code has become a flexible, clear and authoritative reference and contains more detailed standards than could have been expected in a binding convention.

Accountability is closely linked to the need for legal standards that bind duty bearers to take action. General Comment No. 14 notes that "(t)he realization of the right to health may be pursued through numerous, complementary approaches, such as the formulation of health policies, or the implementation of health programmes developed by the World Health Organization (WHO), or the adoption of specific legal instruments ..."[31] As such, the General Comment assumes that WHO focuses on policies, guidelines and other non-binding instruments to address health challenges, rather than legally binding instruments. Indeed, despite extensive powers to establish health-related standards and adopt treaties under its constitution, WHO has not been notably active in using such instruments to address public health challenges.

The first treaty negotiated under the auspices of WHO was the WHO Framework Convention on Tobacco Control (FCTC).[32] Mergers and trade liberalization, and the resulting globalization of the tobacco epidemic, generated support for the development of global legal norms for tobacco control.[33] Moreover, clear evidence demonstrated that tobacco kills. With strong leadership from the WHO secretariat, the WHO FCTC was developed and adopted. It helps governments to live up to their right-to-health obligations. The UN Committee on Economic, Social and Cultural Rights has specifically identified "the failure to discourage production, marketing and consumption of tobacco" as a violation of the obligation to protect the right to health in General Comment No. 14.[34] This follows from the failure of a state to take all necessary measures to safeguard persons within their jurisdiction from infringements of the right to health by third parties, and includes such omissions as the failure to regulate the activities of individuals, groups or corporations to prevent them from violating the right to health of others.[35] From a human rights perspective, regulation is often a necessity, particularly when it comes to protecting vulnerable groups. To protect young people, for example, WHO has urged governments to ban all tobacco advertising, promotion and sponsorship, in light of recent studies that prove that the more young people are exposed to tobacco advertising, the more likely they are to start smoking.[36]

Arguments are being put forward for the development of international legal standards in select areas of diet and nutrition, as a strategy for ensuring that the health of future generations does not become dependent on corporate charity and voluntary commitments.[37] However, in the area of diet and nutrition, a voluntaristic approach has so far dominated. In 2004, the member states of the FAO agreed upon the Voluntary Guidelines on the Right to Food, which encourage states "to take steps, in particular through education, information and labeling regulations, to prevent over-consumption and unbalanced diets that may lead to malnutrition, obesity and degenerative diseases."[38] The same year, 2004, the World Health Assembly adopted a Global Strategy on Diet, Physical Activity and Health to address non-communicable diseases. Ironically, the paragraph in the resolution that adopted the Strategy, containing the strongest language, is the one which urges member states to avoid trade-restrictive or trade-distorting impact of public policies adopted in the context of implementation of the Strategy.[39] In reviewing food labels and their impact on free trade, the WTO extensively relies on a decision of the Codex Alimentariaus Commission.[40] A WTO Dispute Resolution Panel has distinguished between foods that pose a danger to the life or health of the consumer, and foods that were nutritionally disadvantageous due to the quality or quantity of their nutrients, but without necessarily presenting a danger to the health of the consumer.[41] The implications of this distinction are that health warnings about nutritional quality of food are likely to be treated under the Agreement on Technical Barriers to Trade ("TBT Agreement").[42] The TBT Agreement states that "technical regulations shall not be more trade-restrictive than necessary to fulfill a legitimate objective, taking account of the risks non-fulfillment would create. Such legitimate objectives are, inter alia: ... protection of human health or safety".[43] To address NCDs, arguments have been made for global standards in relation to labelling of product constituents, fair warning of health risks, and health claims to enable consumers to make informed and healthy food choices.[44] Such standards would support the realization of the right to information as well as the empowerment of rights-holders to demand healthier choices and hold duty-bearers more accountable.

Empowering the rights-holders

Under international human rights law, the government is under the obligation to protect the right to health and thus must regulate non-state actors – companies and other stakeholders – to act in a way consistent with this right. This raises the question as to how far the state can regulate, particularly in relation to the enjoyment of other human rights. The aforementioned Special Representative refers to the UN human rights treaty monitoring bodies for guidance on how far the duty to protect human rights applies.[45] In general terms, the Human Rights Committee has underscored that the protection of the right to life requires that states adopt positive measures to increase life expectancy.[46] But how far do individuals have a free choice to overeat, smoke or consume alcohol in a way harmful to their own health? In the case of tobacco, the courts have been willing to limit the interpretation of the right to privacy to safeguard public health. In this context, the British courts held that preventing a person from smoking did not generally involve such adverse effect upon his physical or moral integrity as would amount to an interference with the right to respect for private or home life within the meaning of Article 8 of the European Convention on Human Rights.[47] However, denying a job or dismissing qualified persons solely on the basis of their obesity or because they are off-duty smokers would amount to discrimination and constitute an undue intrusion in their private life.[48] An important test in reviewing the balance between the right to privacy and measures taken to safeguard public health are the Siracusa Principles.[49] These can protect individuals against punitive, discriminatory and disproportionate measures taken by governments to ostensibly protect the public's health. Unfortunately, however, many societal measures adopt punitive approaches to NCDs on the assumption that those affected are solely responsible for their predicament. Some argue, and some health insurance companies maintain, that people who overeat and become obese should not burden society by having others pay for their health care costs. Indeed, the tobacco industry managed to avoid compensating any of its victims for the first 40 years of litigation not only by persistently refusing to admit that smoking caused any disease, but also by convincing judges and juries that the smoker was entirely at fault for "choosing" to smoke in the face of known risks as well as government mandated health warnings included on cigarette packs since 1966.[50] These arguments fail to consider the underlying and root causes of ill-health, which are as important to determining someone's level of health as the immediate causes. These underlying causes go beyond the immediate risk factors and implicate a broad range of duty-bearers that may play a role in influencing a person's health throughout his or her life-cycle, ranging from local communities, private companies and international actors. The government needs to act as the steward to ensure that society as a whole acts coherently and in a way that is health enhancing. International human rights instruments thus focus on the state as the prime duty-bearer, and these treaties may contain explicit duties to encourage individual responsibility for health. For example, the original European Social Charter (1961) and its revised form (1996) sets out the obligation of the state to ensure that the population is adequately informed and educated about health matters in order to encourage individual responsibility in health matters.[51]

Greater awareness among the general public of health-related human rights is generating increased demand for transparency and accountability from duty-bearers, particularly governments, to take action for better health. Significantly, under international human rights law, rights-holders are able to hold duty-bearers to account. In recent years, there has been an upsurge in litigation in the area of health rights in general. Increasingly, people are demanding access to medicines, treatments and care before the courts. However, in relation to NCDs, which are often chronic, courts have been reluctant to review decisions taken by political organs and medical authorities as to how to allocate budgets and decide on priorities. For example, in 1997, the Constitutional Court of South Africa held that a hospital that had refused renal dialysis treatment to a patient suffering from terminal illness had not violated the constitutional right not to be "refused emergency medical treatment" as the treatment did not amount to an "emergency" in the sense of a sudden catastrophe, but rather an "ongoing state of affairs".[52] However, the increased recognition of health rights and some successful claims being brought before the courts, are empowering claim-holders to secure treatment even without going to the courts. For example, in 2006, a woman with breast cancer shamed Somerset Primary Care Trust in the United Kingdom into providing a drug, Herceptin, after threatening to take her case to the European Court of Human Rights.[53]

Conclusion

Analysing and addressing NCDs from a human rights perspective brings to the forefront the most challenging and pressing issues in public health, such as how to ensure a more intersectoral and coherent response to address upstream determinants of health; how far the private sector can be held responsible and accountable; the nature and scope of state obligations under international law; the extent of the role of the state in protecting public health versus allowing individual freedom and choice; and how to empower people affected by ill-health to demand action from powerful actors to promote and protect health.

Human rights provide an internationally recognized legal framework under which governments have concrete obligations relevant to NCDs. However, these obligations should be further articulated to better address the challenges posed by NCDs, not only in relation to specific applicable human rights norms such as the rights to life, health, food and education, but also in relation to the human rights responsibilities of the private sector. Although some industries are engaged in an ongoing and constructive dialogue on how to address NCDs,[54] they, along with many governments that benefit from their profits, are generally adverse to international legal standards, particularly in areas dominated by powerful commercial interests. In the absence of specific, internationally binding standards to address NCDs, beyond the WHO FCTC, human rights norms should be further and better articulated to incorporate the risk factors and underlying determinants of NCDs. This would ensure that the accountability mechanisms dedicated to human rights monitoring at the international, regional and national levels pay greater attention to NCDs.

Moreover, the emerging "health rights movement" should forge stronger alliances with the public health community. The health rights movement brings with it the skills of the international human rights movement including advocacy, litigation, social mobilization and societal transformation skills. The public health community has the authoritative tools of epidemiology, which are revealing causal links not only between smoking and death, but also between unhealthy diets and a range of chronic diseases, including cardiovascular diseases, cancer, diabetes and other conditions linked to obesity. Together, the human rights and public health communities can generate stronger leadership from governments and international organizations to address NCDs through a human rights-based approach.

* The author is a staff member of the World Health Organization (WHO). The author alone is responsible for the views expressed in this publication and they do not necessarily represent the decisions, policy or views of the World Health Organization. The author would like to thank Sabina Hassanali, WHO Health and Human Rights intern, for background research on this paper.

1 Although WHO does not have an official definition of what is meant by non-communicable diseases, diseases within this category are generally those diseases which are not caused by infectious agents (excluding diseases of pregnancy and gynaecological diseases).

2 See Sixty-First World Health Assembly, 'Prevention and Control of Non-communicable Diseases: Implementation of the Global Strategy', Resolution A61/8, 18 April 2008.

3 Ibid.

4 Ibid.

5 Ibid.

6 WHO, 'Controlling the Global Obesity Epidemic', available at http://www.who.int/nutrition/topics/obesity/en/index.html.

7 See World Health Assembly Resolution, *supra* note 2.

8 Ibid.

9 Health-related human rights include the rights to health, information, food, education, equality and non-discrimination.

10 Key human rights principles that guide all actions which are rights-based are: Universality and inalienability; indivisibility; interdependence and interrelatedness; equality and non-discrimination; participation and inclusion; and accountability and the rule of law. See UN Common Understanding on a Human Rights-Based Approach to Development Cooperation 2003, available at http://www.undg.org/?P=221.

11 Ibid.

12 Office of the High Commissioner for Human Rights (OHCHR), 'Question 17: What Value Does A Human Rights-Based Approach Add To Development?' in *Frequently Asked Questions on a Human Rights-Based Approach to Development Cooperation* (Geneva: OHCHR, 2006), at 16.

13 Committee on Economic, Social and Cultural Rights (CESCR), *General Comment No. 14 on the*

right to the highest attainable standard of health, 11 August 2000, UN Doc. E/C.12/2000/4, para. 9.

14 UN Common Learning Package on a Human Rights-Based Approach, available at http://www.undg.org/index.cfm?P=531.

15 See 'Question 10' in *25 Questions and Answers on Health and Human Rights,* at 15, available at http://www.who.int/hhr/NEW37871OMSOK.pdf.

16 For more detailed analysis of how to operationalize a human rights-based approach to programming, see Urban Jonsson, 'Human Rights Approach to Development Programming' (UNICEF, 2003).

17 According to General Comment No. 14 discrimination is prohibited "on the grounds of race, colour, sex, language, religion, political or other opinion, national or social origin, property, birth, physical or mental disability, health status (including HIV/AIDS), sexual orientation and civil, political, social or other status".

18 See *The Lancet,* volume 367, 17 June 2006, available at www.thelancet.com.

19 WHO, *The Health of Indigenous Peoples,* WHO publication No. WHO/SDE/HSD/99.1, available at http://whqlibdoc.who.int/hq/1999/WHO_SDE_HSD_99.1.pdf.

20 Paragraph 27 of General Comment No. 14 specifically discusses health as it relates to indigenous peoples.

21 See 'List Of Illustrative Indicators On The Right To Enjoyment Of The Highest Attainable Standard Of Physical And Mental Health', UN Doc. HRI/MC/2008/3, at 25.

22 See for example, Draft Guidelines for Pharmaceutical Companies, open for consultations until 15 May 2008, available at http://www2.ohchr.org/english/issues/health/right/.

23 John Ruggie, Report of the Special Representative of the Secretary-General on the issue of human rights and transnational corporations and other business enterprises, 7 April 2008, UN Doc. A/HRC/8/5.

24 John Ruggie, 'Next Steps in Business and Human Rights', speech at Chatham House, London, 22 May 2008, available at http://www.reports-and-materials.org/Ruggie-speech-Chatham-House-22-May-2008.pdf.

25 WHO, World Health Statistics 2008: *Reducing Deaths from Tobacco* (Geneva: WHO, 2008), at 18.

26 International Council of Human Rights Policy (ICHRP), *Beyond Voluntarism: Human Rights and the Developing International Legal Obligations of Companies* (Versoix: ICHRP, 2002), available at http://www.ichrp.org/files/reports/7/107_report_en.pdf.

27 World Health Assembly Resolution 34.22, 21 May 1981, available at http://www.ibfan.org/english/resource/who/whares3422.html.

28 See WHO, '10 Facts on Breast-Feeding: Long-Term Benefits for Children', available at http://www.who.int/features/factfiles/breastfeeding/en/index.html.

29 Save the Children, 'Case Study 7: "Baby milk" Marketing' in Jennifer A. Zerk, *Corporate Abuse in 2007: A Discussion Paper on What Changes in the Law Need to Happen* (London: The Corporate Responsibility (COHE) Coalition, 2007), available at http://www.corporate-responsibility.org/module_images/corporateabuse_discussionpaper.pdf.

30 This would harmonize corporate obligations, requiring disclosure by companies of policies regarding marketing, research, lobbying and promotional activities, and provide for effective enforcement at the state level.

31 *General Comment No. 14, supra* note 13, para. 1.

32 See http://www.who.int/fctc/en/index.html.

33 Roger S. Magnusson, 'Short Report: Non-Communicable Diseases and Global Health Governance: Enhancing Global Processes to Improve Health Development' 3(2) *Globalization and Health* (2007), at 6, available at http://www.globalizationandhealth.com/content/3/1/2.

34 *General Comment No. 14, supra* note 13, para. 1.

35 Ibid.

36 'WHO Wants Total Ban on Tobacco Advertising', News Release, 30 May 2008, http://www.who.int/mediacentre/news/releases/2008/pr17/en/index.html.

37 Magnusson, *supra* note 33.

38 Guideline 10, Voluntary Guidelines to Support the Progressive Realization of The Right to Adequate

Food in the Context of National Food Security, Adopted by the 127th Session of the FAO Council, November 2004, available at http://www.fao.org/docrep/meeting/009/y9825e/y9825e00.htm.

39 Global Strategy on Diet, Physical Activity and Health, adopted by the Fifty-Seventh World Health Assembly, 22 May 2004, WHO Doc. No. WHA57.17, Operative paragraph 4(7).

40 The Codex Alimentarius is available at http://www.codexalimentarius.net.

41 *EC-Biotech Products Case* (European Communities-Measures Affecting the Approval and Marketing of Biotech Products), WT/DS291, WT/DS292, WT/DS293, www.wto.org.

42 http://www.wto.org/english/docs_e/legal_e/17-tbt.pdf.

43 Article 2.2 of the TBT Agreement.

44 Magnusson, *supra* note 33, at 11.

45 Ruggie, *supra* note 23, para. 18.

46 Human Rights Committee, *General Comment No. 6 on the right to life,* 30 April 1982, UN Doc. HRI/GEN/1/Rev.1, at para. 5.

47 See further, 'Smoking is Not a Right Protected by Law' in *The Times,* 28 May 2008, available at http://business.timesonline.co.uk/tol/business/law/reports/article4015677.ece, discussing the case of *Regina (G) v Nottingham Healthcare NHS Trust; Regina (N) v Secretary of State for Health; Regina (B) v Nottingham Healthcare NHS Trust,* Queen's Bench Divisional Court.

48 ILO, 'Declaration on Fundamental Principles and Rights at Work', ILO Fact Sheet series, available at www.ilo.org/public/english/region/eurpro/budapest/download/pressrelease/european_fact_sheet_eng.pdf.

49 See WHO, 'Question 13' in *25 Questions and Answers on Health and Human Rights,* WHO Health and Human Rights Publication Series, Issue No. 1, July 2002, at 18.

50 Richard A Daynard, Clive Bates, Neil Francey, 'Tobacco Litigation Worldwide', 320 *British Medical Journal* (2000), at 111–113.

51 European Social Charter, Article 11 on the right to protection of health, and Revised European Social Charter (which reads that among appropriate measures to be taken by the contracting parties is the provision of "advisory and educational facilities for the promotion of health and the encouragement of individual responsibility in matters of health").

52 *Soobramoney v Minister of Health (KwaZulu Natal)* CCT32/97 (1997) ZACC 17; 1998 (1) SA 765 (CC).

53 See further http://www.independent.co.uk/lifestyle/health-and-wellbeing/health-news/breast-cancer-drug-hailed-as-stunning-breakthrough-511695.html.

54 See e.g. 'WHO Talks Held With Members Of The Alcohol Industry', http://www.who.int/substance_abuse/openconsultalcind/en/.

The HIV/AIDS Epidemic and Human Rights Responses

Mary Crewe

"The real world is endlessly fertile in its yield of sobering, wrenching, clarifying contexts for thinking about the idea of human rights".[1]

The HIV and AIDS epidemics yield sobering, wrenching and clarifying contexts for thinking about human rights and pose one of the most fascinating and challenging problems of our times. Despite the pain and suffering, the epidemic offers new and compelling ways to look at how individuals, communities, societies and states can and should respond to such challenges.

Throughout the history of the epidemic we have witnessed, in many parts of the world, acts of cruelty and horror[2] but also acts of support and protection.[3] In the political domain there have been attempts, through legislation, to ensure that people living with HIV and AIDS suffer no discrimination or violation of their rights. At the same time there have been official acts of discrimination and violations of human rights. This tension remains between the work to get the human rights of all people living with HIV and AIDS secured and protected and the work of politicians to have HIV and AIDS as part of legislation that will restrict rights and freedoms, and is highlighted by the move of some African governments to criminalize "wilful" transmission of HIV and to put in place laws that target people living with HIV and AIDS.[4]

At the UN World Conference Against Racism in Durban in 2001, Mary Robinson declared HIV/AIDS poses the greatest challenge to human rights we have had to face.

Human rights speak in broad terms about the fundamental entitlement of all human beings to live in dignity and in conditions of social justice.[5] The approach of human rights provides a foundation from which to mount a set of demands premised on the intrinsic worth of the person whose rights are being threatened or denied. As Connors argues, claims based on human rights require no justification, with claimants inherently entitled to human rights.[6] Usually, an approach based on human rights promises the engagement of the state in a way that is internationally recognized and acknowledged; their denial or violation immediately raises the question, both at the national and international levels, of the legal responsibility of the state.

Is it possible that the emphasis on human rights in relation to HIV and AIDS has influenced the larger world of public health and the access of people to proper health care and support? It has been argued[7] that this awareness of a fundamental connection between HIV and human rights has slowly but increasingly led to a new and deeper collaboration between public health officials and human rights advocates.

Initial responses to the HIV epidemic focused the blame on others: Foreigners, sex workers, gay men, injecting drug users, uneducated people, rich men, sinners, and women. Countries started to exclude foreigners with HIV, to test sex workers and to make HIV a notifiable disease.[8]

This early response to HIV was consistent with the history of disease and ways to deal with perceived threats to the general population. Wars and panics as well as epidemics have all served at one time or another in history to justify significant incursions on the rights of individuals or groups.

Between 1918 and 1920, due to fears of sexually transmitted infections (STIs) and the health of soldiers and sailors conscripted to fight in World War I, the Government of the United States promoted and paid for the detention of over 18 000 women suspected of prostitution.[9] Earlier, when cholera struck New York City in 1832, officials rounded up alcoholics, especially poor Irishmen; and in the polio epidemic of 1916 health officials conducted house-to-house searches and forcibly removed and quarantined children thought to have polio. In short, it was common to violate the civil rights of the ill to protect the healthy – to abuse some to protect others.[10]

Although early responses to HIV and AIDS were based on discrimination and the application of standard public health measures such as isolation, mandatory testing, and quarantine, as the epidemic unfolded it became clear that the most effective way to address the issue was through a protection of rights rather than allowing for any restriction of freedoms and movements, and from this developed the very strong movement that linked HIV and AIDS to human rights and the attainments and protection of such rights. HIV is no respecter of gender, nationality, sexual orientation, occupation, skin colour or age.[11] Rather HIV is about the risks that each of us takes and our personal ability to make choices about those risks – and some of us have far more choice than others. But it was with regard to risk and choice that many of the punitive decisions about HIV and AIDS were taken.

This point was emphasized by Jonathan Mann in 1997:[12] In HIV/AIDS, it has become clear that the traditional public health approach, combining information and education with specific health services (counselling, HIV testing, needle exchange, condom distribution) is necessary and helpful, yet clearly insufficient for HIV prevention. Vulnerability to the epidemic has now been associated with the extent of realization of human rights. For as the HIV epidemic matures and evolves within each community and country, it focuses inexorably on those groups who – before HIV/AIDS arrived – were already discriminated against, marginalized, and stigmatized within each society. Now that a lack of respect for human rights has been identified as a societal level risk factor for HIV/AIDS vulnerability, HIV prevention efforts are starting to go beyond traditional educational and service-based efforts – to address the rights issues which will be a precondition for greater progress against the epidemic.

In this way, the human rights emphasis on HIV started to strengthen work on access to health care, the position of women in society, the rights of young people to good health care and education, the rights of orphans and other young people left homeless and the rights of the elderly as they grapple with the needs of their grandchildren left in their care.

Despite this, some caution is needed. In various publications from UN agencies and from the international donor community, there are introductory paragraphs that emphasize that the work discussed is considered within a human rights framework. However, what that framework is or how it influences policy, legislation or behaviour is often quite unclear. It is as if by the mere statement of intent the right actions will follow. Some kind of nod is made in the direction of rights but measures that are discriminatory continue. This would be particularly the case, for example, in discourse about the rights of women and access to health care. The real challenge is to the power of patriarchy, the increasing feminization of poverty, and the disproportionate burden of infection that women have to face. Stating that work about women and health needs to be in a human rights framework would be supported by most states – but seldom is there a real interrogation of what this would actually mean for state policy, action and social change.

Human rights discourse is placed within the existing status quo and has the intention of trying to make the status quo more acceptable. It is important that the human rights approach should be about challenging the status quo on all levels – no longer asking status quo questions which give status quo answers – but finding ways to ask oppositional questions which will give oppositional answers and ways to a radically transformed society.

That is what HIV and AIDS offers – a dramatic way to challenge the status quo and the prevailing patterns of discrimination and prejudice. AIDS gave us ways to challenge the status quo on issues of sex and sexuality – highlighting the needs and exploitation of those people who have sexual identities and practices outside of the mainstream. It gave us a new language to talk about intravenous drug users and the ways in which they were addressed within the status quo. We could think about sex work differently, about the position of women and young people, and it allowed for creative new ways to address how men have been marginalized in traditional public health discourse and AIDS prevention and care programmes.

Challenging the status quo is extremely complex and difficult and it is all too easy to dismiss these concerns as being outside of existing social norms and values. But it is precisely this dynamic that created the space for human rights lobbyists and activists to make the links and then the demands for greater attention to the abuse of the rights of people living with HIV and AIDS, for attention to the rights of women, attention to access to health care and treatments, and to emphasize the importance of the right to good nutrition, housing, employment and security as fundamental to an HIV and AIDS response.

While this remains fundamental to HIV and AIDS work, it is also the case that, deep within the epidemic, HIV and AIDS hold the possibility for expanded control and legislation to try to limit or prevent transmission. So while the human rights approach is acknowledged, there are also worrying signs that some governments are increasingly trying to use the law to criminalize infection, to enforce mandatory testing and disclosure, and to set back many of the human rights gains that have been made over the past two decades. And they are doing this precisely to try and buttress the status quo against the social challenges and political action that addressing rights at all levels would entail.

Combined, the HIV/AIDS epidemic and the failure to realize and protect the human rights of both the infected and the affected represents a human tragedy and betrayal of huge proportions. Yet by using the existing conventions and protocols and by exposing how prevailing gender relations and other patterns of structural inequality are implicated in its spread, the AIDS epidemic offers the possibility of real change – change in terms of human rights being realized and along with that the real possibility to turn the AIDS epidemic around. AIDS highlights all the areas in which all of our vulnerability is increased through the failure to respect rights. In addressing AIDS, it is also possible to ensure the full protection of rights.

HIV and AIDS came into a world in which commitment to human rights was already established in the Universal Declaration and through various treaties already signed and ratified by most states. They came into a post-colonial world where the rights and dignity of previously oppressed and marginalized groups was recognized and protected and they came into a world in which equality between races, gender and nations was high on the agenda.[13]

Unlike other contagious diseases for which harsh public health interventions remained applicable, AIDS was supposedly treated in an exceptional manner. Nevertheless it was possible to try to restrict individuals' rights on behalf of overall epidemiological security. AIDS went beyond a public health issue, beyond being a contagious disease, and in the attempts to curtail the epidemic's rise – in the guise of public health – the most enduring political dilemma was how to reconcile individuals' claim to autonomy and liberty with the community's concern with safety. How does the polity treat the patient who is both citizen and a carrier of disease? How are individual rights and the public good pursued simultaneously?[14]

AIDS then caused a deeper analysis of instincts and attitudes lying just below the surface of expressed ideology. What AIDS forced people to confront in very real terms were their own prejudices – prejudices which before they had been able to mask. AIDS stripped bare those who were and are homophobic; those who judge sex workers and people of alternative sexual lives; of young people and how they behave and exposed in very stark forms the extent of our prejudice; our intolerance and the depth of our social hypocrisy and dishonesty. And so it was possible not to intervene as the attacks started on the gay people, IV drug users and sex workers and very soon the attacks and the distaste were not addressed to those groups but rather to the virus itself – to the extent that anyone living with the virus moved in a slow but persistent side stream of society.

Should we, the question seemed to be, focus on the lives saved by traditional public health interventions albeit if these violate rights or focus on the rights that have been violated? Tactics adopted 150 years ago with cholera, leprosy and tuberculosis created a template for the responses to AIDS. Old mentalities and old ways of doing things remained remarkably consistent. Decisions about how to treat AIDS, and the subsequent violations of rights and dignity, were taken in accord with a deep public health ideology set in place during the last century and health is the last site where many people doubtful of the value of and sceptical of the need for human rights reside.[15] This view has been echoed by amongst others Kevin de Cock who suggested:

> "We think that the emphasis on human rights in HIV/AIDS prevention has reduced the importance of public health and social justice, which offer a framework for prevention efforts in Africa that might be more relevant to people's daily lives and more likely be effective."[16]

How then do we shift away from the idea that a restriction of freedoms is part of the universal good when dealing with public health crisis?[17] How do we put rights first and public health second and how do we break the stranglehold of those who believe that in a time of crisis rights can be set aside and placed on the back burner?

How is it possible that in the world in which people are developing AIDS prevention and intervention programmes, various positions, for which there is very little evidence or which could clearly violate human rights, come to be taken as authoritative, and therefore to some degree socially determinant, statements about the nature of the world and the ways to address the epidemic?

According to Foucault, discourses develop and gain their determinative power as a consequence of interaction between four elements:[18]

___ "Objects" – the things they are about
___ Modes of enunciation – the way these things are spoken of
___ Concepts – the intellectual constructs we need to speak about them
___ Strategies – the ways in which these constructs are developed

In the field of HIV and AIDS and human rights, there are many examples of where a decision has been reached where the outcome may serve one purpose, but in execution may lead to an abuse of human rights. This analysis can apply to the ways in which routine/opt out or mandatory testing has been debated. The concept of mandatory testing was debated and discussed by people with authority and power – doctors operating from a deeply public health model, steeped in the public heath history of individual rights for the general good. So skilfully did they employ their constructs that it was almost impossible for the non-medic – the community person, the human rights activist, or the AIDS worker, to challenge this – they lacked the required social authority. The strategy then became the provider-initiated test which became the routine offer, and then the mandatory test with the subsequent potential abuse and violation of rights.

Overwhelmingly the voice of testing was the medical voice, the voice of public health authority, and there seemed little ground for the non-medic – the lawyer, the judge, the teacher or the priest – to move. Through WHO, the 3x5 programme[19] started and we learned that in the developing world, people required less counselling, that the numbers tested mattered, and those who were opposed to testing in this way were negatively portrayed.

Multiple social, political and economic rights were potentially rolled aside in this emphasis on testing. Reports describe increased domestic violence, losing jobs, family support and family homes.[20] There is now mainstreamed into public health a programme and policy counter-intuitive to the understanding of the epidemic and disrespectful of people's rights, privacy and dignity.

No one denies that treatments and treatment access are a basic and fundamental human right which should be freely and openly available to all people. When people raise concerns and questions about testing and treatment, they are not questioning the right to treatments or that people should freely choose to have them; rather they are questioning what comes with it – the very real potential for a reduction in human rights, a reduction in counselling and confidentiality, and a reduction of nuanced prevention as everything gets subsumed into voluntary counselling and testing and routine offers of a test.

A huge burden lies on treatment to succeed in ways where other ideas have failed. The urgency of the need to save lives in the face of this epidemic, and the hope that treatment would succeed where prevention seems to have failed have led to a situation where treatments are assumed to take on all kinds of symbolic powers beyond their actual capacity to address the virus in the body.

But in Foucault's terms, testing has become a mainstreamed public and policy response leading to all kinds of rights violations that are not being challenged. Although the programme was at pains to link treatments to prevention, this instrumentalist approach seemed to close the door on research about sexuality, power, patriarchy and rights. Open and ongoing debates about sex, sexuality and modern sexual behaviour have been largely pushed to the margins.

There are similar concerns about male circumcision.[21] Trials seemed to show that circumcision lowered the level of risk for infection in men. Experts were called in to give the social and scientific language. The strategy is to roll out male circumcision at least in the developing world with scant regard for individual choice or autonomy. Indeed examples from Kenya[22] already tell us of discrimination against non-circumcized men and pressures on men presenting with a negative test result to be circumcized.

Little attention has been paid to the sexual rights of men in this regard. What of cultural, sexual and traditional rights? How will these be ensured and protected? What of the right to refuse the procedure? What about the rights of mothers in terms of decisions about their infant sons' health? Men will still have to use condoms and what about the rights of circumcized men who become infected after all. What about the sexual experiences of women? What voice do women have in this decision?

Through the WHO and UNAIDS, circumcision is to be a mainstreamed health intervention which offers no real insights into social and cultural rights and practices. So-called protection of rights is disingenuously claimed in the right of patients to choose. None but the most naive are in any doubt about how patients actually have very few rights in the face of medical authority.

There are many other examples of how, through a mainstreamed public health intervention, individual, social and community rights have been pushed aside, ignored or quite clearly abused. And most worrying of all is how this mainstreaming of an abuse of rights has been tolerated. All too often we debate the right and not the transgressor.

When confronted with these kinds of interventions we need to apply the Foucault analysis:

___ What is the object?
___ How is the intervention being articulated?
___ Whose is the voice that is talking and why is it legitimate?
___ What is the strategy?

And we need to add a fifth and most crucial point of analysis: What is the right of the individual that is being transgressed or abused and how would we move to protect it and challenge such interventions?

As South Africa's history under Apartheid showed, it is very easy to abuse rights, to deny them and take them away on the basis of a perceived public good at the time – and once rights are taken away it is very difficult to restore them.

1   William J. Perry, *The Idea of Human Rights: Four Ideas* (Oxford: Oxford University Press, 2000) 4.

2   For example, the murder of Gugu Dhlamini and other women in South Africa because of their HIV status, to people living with HIV and AIDS being rejected by their families, suffering from violence, losing jobs and housing, and young children facing exploitation and violence.

3   Many people living with HIV are lovingly and effectively cared for by family and volunteers; many young people have been taken in and cared for by other families and community members.

4   Examples of this from Africa include: From Angola, *Law 8/04 on HIV and AIDS* (2004); from Kenya, *HIV and AIDS Prevention and CONTROL Act 14 of 2006* and the *Sexual Offences Act 3 of 2006;*

from Lesotho, the *Sexual Offences Act of 2003*; and other examples from Madagascar, South Africa, Swaziland, Tanzania, Uganda and Zimbabwe. See also the concerns raised in the Open Civil Letter to the participants of the Capacity building workshop on human rights and gender in the HIV legal framework (held in Dakar 16–18 April 2008) concerning how some of the provisions in the N'Djamena "model law" violate international human rights law and the Office of the High Commissioner for Human Rights (OHCHR) Guidelines on HIV/AIDS and Human Rights.

5   Jane Connors, 'Mainstreaming Gender Within the International Framework' in A. Stewart (ed.) *Gender Law and Social Justice* (London: Blackstone Press, 2000) at 19.

6   Ibid.

7   S. Gruskin, K. Tomasevski and A. Hendriks, 'Human Rights and Responses to HIV/AIDS' in Jonathan Mann and David Tarantola (eds.), *AIDS in the World II* (Oxford: Oxford University Press, 1996) at 326.

8   A. Welbourn, 'Gender, Sex and HIV: How to Address Issues that No One Wants to Hear About' in A. Cornwall and A. Welbourn (eds.), *Realizing Rights* (London: Zed Books, 2002) at 99, 101.

9   T. Stoddard and W. Reiman, 'AIDS and the Rights of the Individual: Toward a More Sophisticated Understanding of Discrimination' in D. Nelkin et al. *A Disease of Society: Cultural and Institutional Responses to AIDS* (Oxford: Oxford University Press, 1992) at 241.

10 See P. Baldwin, *Disease and Democracy: The Industrialized World Faces AIDS* (California: University of California Press, 2005) at 1.

11 Welbourn, *supra* note 8.

12 Jonathan Mann, 'Public Health and Human Rights' 27(3) *Hastings Centre Report* (1997).

13 It should not have been possible for the levels of discrimination around HIV to have developed over what is essentially another physical characteristic like race or gender.

14 Baldwin, *supra* note 10.

15 Ibid.

16 Ibid.

17 This is not to suggest that its an either/or scenario – either individual rights or public health – but rather to question the ways in which public health has been able, through its history and social standing, to violate human rights and defend this position.

18 See this discussion in A. Woodiwiss, *Making Human Rights Work Globally* (London: Glasshouse, 2003) at 19.

19 The 3x5 programme was the undertaking to get three million people in the developing world onto ARV treatments by the year 2005. This target was not met.

20 Many of these are anecdotal but many are well documented and some have been dealt with through non-governmental organizations such as the AIDS Law Project.

21 See the work of, for instance, Peter Aggleton and Gary Dowsett and others and the UNAIDS position papers.

22 See 'Uncircumcized pupils sent home', BBC News, 12 February 2007, available at http://news.bbc.co.uk/2/hi/africa/6355447.stm; 'Circumcision row divides Kenya town', BBC News, 16 February 2007, available at http://news.bbc.co.uk/2/hi/africa/6367807.stm. See also see the effects of persecution of men in Eastern Europe in the recent ethnic struggles depending on their being circumcized or not.

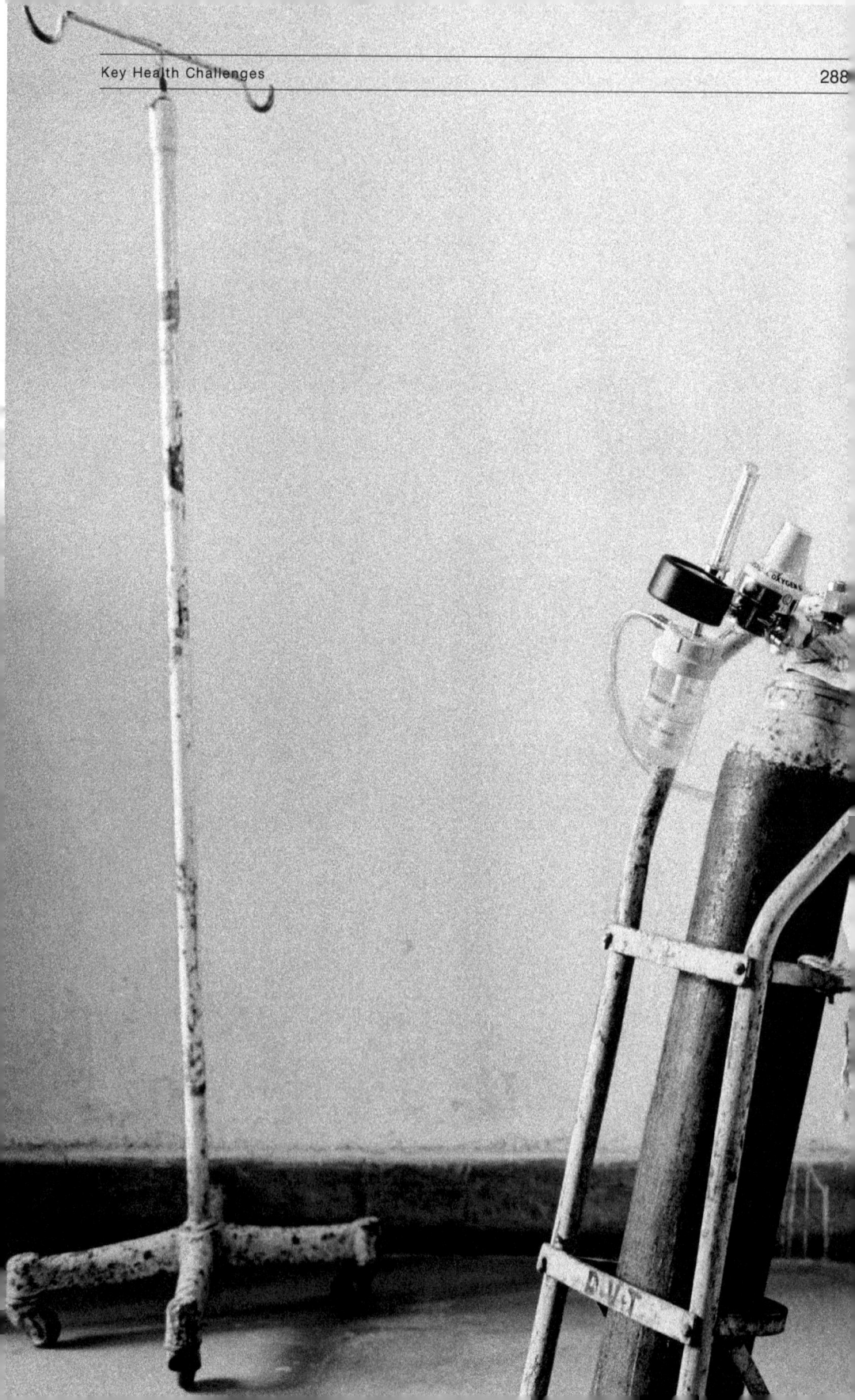

Drug-Resistant Tuberculosis

Tido von Schön-Angerer*

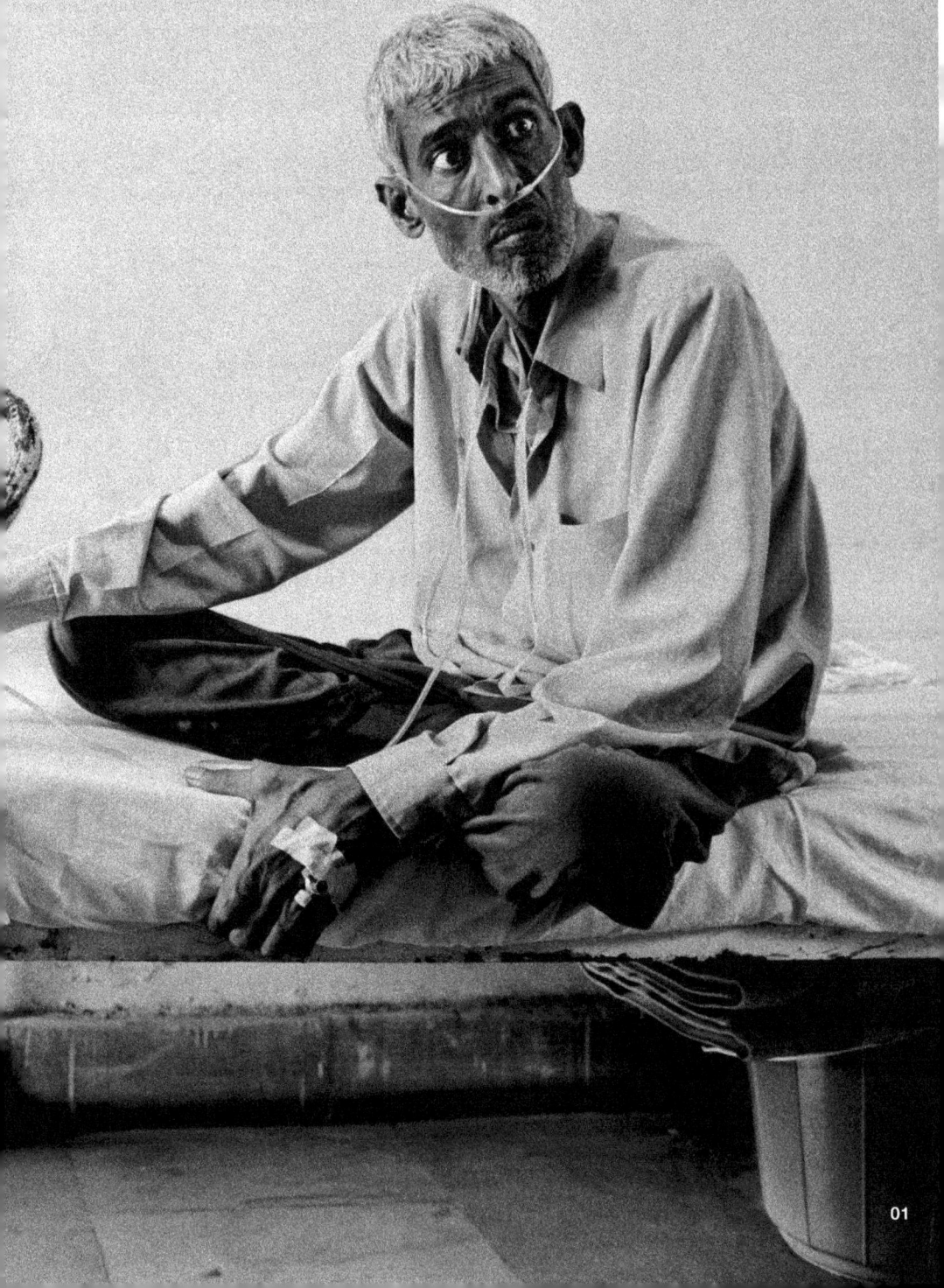

01
Lala Ram Sarup Institute of Tuberculosis and Allied
Diseases in New Delhi, India. A man with
advanced TB receives oxygen in the intensive care ward.
(Photograph by James Nachtwey / VII)

"They said I must cough the sputum and I said I have no sputum. I asked them to do an X-ray but they said they couldn't do it because I was pregnant. I told them that I wanted to sign the form so that I could have an X-ray. I was getting worse, getting thin and very weak. The X-ray showed I had TB. Now I was very, very worried because I had TB, HIV and I was pregnant. This was August 2005.

I started the TB treatment in September and in December I had to deliver my baby. I looked at the calendar and I thought: I am not going to make it, I will die before.

I made it and my baby was born on 2nd December 2005. But my TB treatment was not working. The doctor made a test and in February told me I had MDR-TB. I was so shocked because it was my first time to hear about this MDR. I knew nothing about it."

Busisiwe Beko, Khayelitsha, South Africa, MDR-TB counsellor

These few words immediately highlight the major problems associated with tuberculosis (TB) care. Ordinary, or drug-susceptible TB, is a major killer, affecting nearly 9.2 million per year and killing about 1.7 million.[1] A disease that is already difficult to diagnose and treat has now become very common among people living with HIV, for whom diagnosis and cure options are even more complex and limited. At the same time, multidrug-resistant TB (MDR-TB) and even extensively drug-resistant strains (XDR-TB)[2], already widespread in Eastern Europe and parts of Asia – are also increasing in Africa, in particular South Africa, where HIV rates are very high.

Busisiwe was lucky because she belongs to the minority of people living with HIV where the multidrug-resistant tuberculosis infection was diagnosed in time and who survived the lengthy and complex treatment of limited effectiveness.

The TB epidemic in Africa is being fuelled by HIV – tuberculosis is now the most common cause of death for HIV infected persons in Africa. The combination of HIV and MDR-TB is particularly deadly as TB progresses much more rapidly in the presence of HIV/AIDS and MDR-TB is very difficult to treat with the currently available medications. The overlapping of the HIV and MDR-TB epidemics in some populations today threatens the control of both of these two epidemics. The spread of XDR-TB, which has been reported in at least 49 countries, further exacerbates the situation, as treatment options are then severely restricted.

Globally, there are some 490 000 new patients with active MDR-TB every year and about ten times as many MDR-TB infections. Less than 2% of patients with active MDR-TB receive appropriate treatment.[3] Treating MDR-TB is extremely onerous – for the patient, and for health services. The difficulties associated with diagnosis and treatment, and the level of resources required to overcome these, pose a serious challenge to progressively ensuring access to effective MDR-TB treatment for all.

First, sophisticated laboratories with specialized staff are needed to detect drug resistance. Many developing countries do not yet have this capacity at all – others only have it in university hospitals or research laboratories. Most patients therefore go undiagnosed and will die. In fact, even "regular" TB disease is often not diagnosed as the most available test, sputum microscopy, only detects 40–60% of cases.

Second, treatment of MDR-TB is highly impractical, with treatment duration between 18 to 24 months, with up to ten different drugs, including six months or longer of daily painful injections. In addition, long hospitalizations, away from home and work, place an enormous psychological and economic burden on the patient and the family. The challenge for the health service to providing such highly sophisticated care is equally high. The best standard of care is for treatment to be individualized according to the individual patient's drug resistance pattern, further adding to the complexity.

In addition, the effectiveness of the available drugs to treat MDR-TB is limited. 5 to 20% of HIV-uninfected patients, and up to 66% of HIV-infected patients, die during treatment.[4] In a Médecins Sans Frontières (Doctors Without Borders, or MSF) project in Uzbekistan, in a context with few

HIV infections, treatment is successful in only 64% of patients, and this is despite the investment of very significant support and resources.[5] These outcomes are similar to those observed elsewhere. Worse, MSF witnesses the emergence of XDR-TB, even when best practice MDR-TB treatment is given, in up to 13% of patients.[6] In other words, XDR-TB is actively created by the poorly efficacious drugs used for MDR-TB treatment.

To add to the burden, many of the drugs are also highly toxic, comparable to the toxicity experienced with anticancer treatment. Often individual drugs have to be stopped because of severe side effects. The number of patients stopping treatment altogether is very high among MDR-TB patients – 14% in the MSF project in Uzbekistan.

Finally the cost is an issue. Even considering negotiated price reductions, MDR-TB treatment costs between USD 2000–8000 per patient, and over USD 15 000 for XDR-TB.[7]

The delayed response to the MDR-TB epidemic

In 1993, WHO declared TB a global emergency and launched the DOTS (Direct Observed Therapy Short Course) strategy to advance TB control by promoting a simple set of interventions. At the time however, WHO made no programmatic recommendations for drug-resistant TB, which was left to individual initiatives of national programmes. Instead, the UN health body promoted treatment of drug-sensitive cases as a way to prevent and reduce drug-resistant TB.[8] MDR-TB was not regarded yet as a public health problem, and it was argued that drug-susceptibility testing, and second-line drugs, were not cost-effective, and that intense clinical management was impossible because of lack of infrastructure.[9]

It took considerable effort by a number of groups, including Partners in Health/Harvard Medical School, the United States (US) Center for Disease Control, and MSF, to overcome this situation of active neglect in the name of public health priority settings. One of the key advocates, Dr. Paul Farmer, identifies a number of myths that had to be overturned for this policy change to occur:[10]

1. **"MDR-TB is untreatable."** It was demonstrated that MDR can be treated in resource-poor settings with results comparable to Western settings. Farmer and his colleagues demonstrated in Peru that even ambulatory, community-based therapy is possible[11].

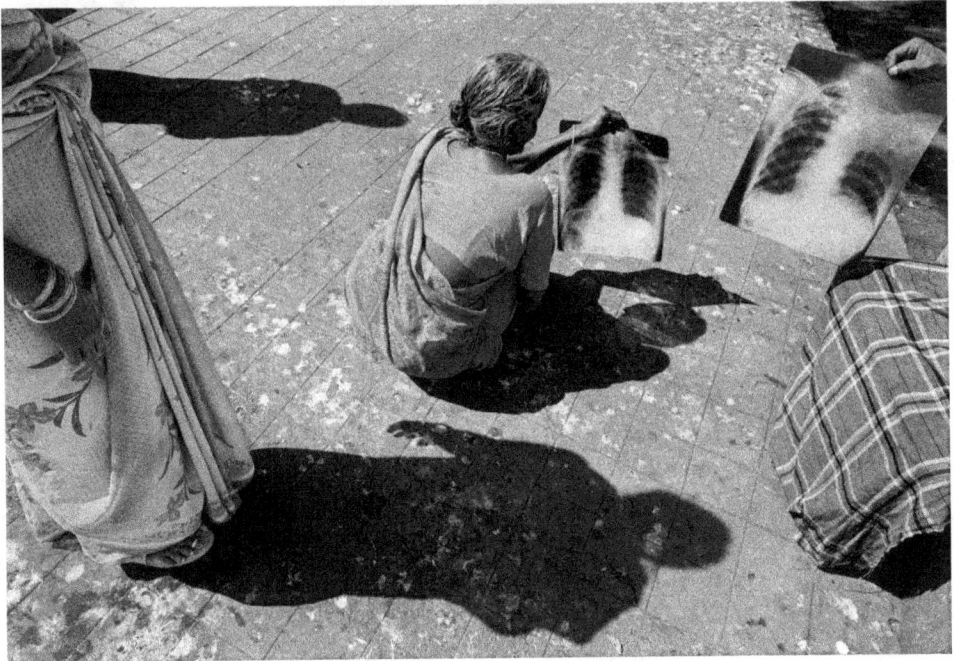

02

Tambaran Tuberculosis Hospital, Chennai, India. People
who came to the hospital to be examined for
TB wait with their x-rays for a medical consultation.
(Photograph by James Nachtwey / VII)

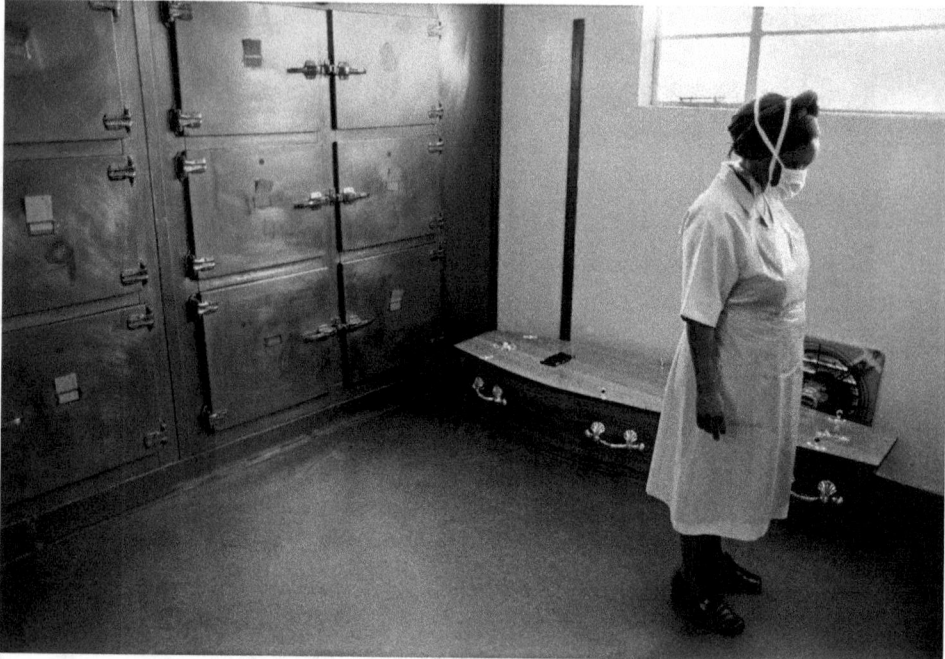

03

Church of Scotland Hospital, Tugela Ferry, Kwazulu Natal,
South Africa. A nurse who just helped bring
a deceased MDR-TB patient to the hospital morgue.
(Photograph by James Nachtwey / VII)

2.   **"MDR-TB is too expensive to treat in poor countries; it diverts attention and resources from treating drug-susceptible disease."** It was successfully argued that the discussion should not be a "zero sum" approach of how to spread limited resources available for TB control, but that more financial resources are needed.

3.   **"Treating drug-susceptible tuberculosis is the best way to address epidemics of drug-resistant disease."** That MDR-TB continued to spread even in countries that were running successful DOTS programmes for regular TB served to defeat this argument. In fact, giving repeated courses of standard treatment to drug-resistant patients further amplified resistance.[12]

4.   **"Patient non-compliance is the chief cause of MDR-TB."** Much blame continues to be placed on programmes and patients for causing drug resistance. While poorly functioning TB programmes certainly contribute to the development of drug-resistance, this is quite clearly not the only factor. A six month standard treatment, involving multiple drugs with many side effects, is inherently difficult to implement in low-resource settings. Also a bad international treatment policy for patients where TB relapses or where treatment fails (so-called category 2) substantially contributed to resistance development. In addition, people with HIV generally suffer multiple TB episodes over time – such repeated treatments provide fertile ground for the development of resistance. Too often there is a culture of blaming non-compliant patients. Farmer rightly points to the "structural violence", i.e. the institutional inequities of power and wealth, that puts so many constraints on the lives of poor people, so much so, that, in many instances, the limitations placed on their ability to adhere to treatment are largely beyond their control.

These international discussions triggered a number of important changes.

First, the programmatic response to MDR-TB was developed by WHO and partners through its "DOTS-plus" strategy.

Second, several organizations, including MSF (in part through its recently established Campaign for Access to Essential Medicines), negotiated price reductions with the producers of second-line drugs. These reduced prices are now available to programmes approved by the WHO-housed Green Light Committee (GLC). Prices are still not low enough, but MSF experience suggests further price reductions will only be possible once global demand increases as MDR-TB treatment is scaled up.

Lastly, funding streams available to MDR-TB have increased substantially through, among others, the creation of the Global Fund to fight AIDS, Tuberculosis and Malaria.

Dr. Mario Raviglione, Director of the Stop TB Department at WHO, acknowledges the importance of an implicit rights perspective in changing the approach to MDR-TB by the international medical community in the late 1990s: "The era of a renewed, human rights-based approach to medicine and public health had just begun, and the advent of the principle of access to care for all favourably influenced those discussions."[13]

Following these advances, MDR-TB treatment has expanded over the last decade to over 50 GLC-approved programmes in resource-limited settings, set to treat more than 30 000 patients. While significant efforts were necessary to get this far, this is clearly nowhere near enough. The question today is why are we not any further advanced in providing MDR-TB treatment, when only 2% of those who need it are accessing appropriate care?

Ambitious international targets will remain unachievable with current tools

The "Global Plan to Stop TB 2006–2015" foresees a dramatic scale-up of MDR-TB treatment as part of a routine component of TB control, with the aim, in the 2007 revised plan, to treat 1.6 million MDR-TB patients by 2015.[14]

Current scale-up is far too slow to achieve this goal. We are already behind schedule: Even the 30 000 patients reached through GLC-supported programmes represent fewer than half of the 66 000 people that were foreseen to be treated in 2007. In addition, the Global Plan does not even aim to treat all new patients with MDR-TB (with more than 1 million already existing and 490 000 new patients each year many more will need treatment).

The main obstacle to scaling up is the long, complex, toxic and often inadequate treatment and poor diagnostic test. The goals of treatment scale up are simply unrealistic with current tools. This situation dramatically highlights how countries can only achieve the highest attainable standard of health for their population once efficient tools to detect, prevent or treat disease are developed and made available.[15]

Of course, until better tools are available there is no other option than to scale up treatment with what we have at our disposal today. This burden falls almost entirely on national level programmes. While international policy change has been crucial, it is not sufficient to mobilize actions at country level. Technical expertise is still scarce and there is an important need for training. The lack of human resources has already been identified as a major bottleneck to expanding antiretroviral treatment coverage for HIV in many African countries,[16] and limited human resources can therefore not simply be redirected to fighting another international health priority. Given the high degree of overlap within the HIV and TB epidemics, the political and programmatic momentum for HIV programmes must be harnessed as much as possible, so that strategies against MDR-TB are also developed.

Considering the severity of the MDR-TB epidemic, one has to wonder whether WHO should not be more proactive. The founding members of the WHO agreed that "The enjoyment of the highest attainable standard of health is one of the fundamental rights of every human being without distinction of race, religion, political belief, economic or social condition" (WHO Constitution adopted 19 June – 22 July 1946 and entered into force on 7 April 1948). The attainment by all peoples of the highest possible level of health is the objective of the WHO (Article 1, WHO Constitution). From this mandate follows a series of functions the WHO shall carry out in order to fulfil the mandate. A minimalist position is that WHO cannot do much without the request of its member states.

Indeed, currently WHO treads carefully, refraining from any direct country critique regarding TB treatment other than through regular global reports that point to the disparity between individual countries in disease burden and TB control efforts. However WHO's own Constitution and the recently revised International Health Regulations, and the Global Strategy and Plan of Action on Public Health, Innovation and Intellectual Property adopted by the WHA in 2008 give the WHO more policy space than the organization is currently willing to take up. While assisting governments in strengthening health services indeed can only be done upon request from the country, many other activities do not need such a trigger. For example the WHO constitution lists the following functions that may be relevant for TB treatment: To stimulate and advance work to eradicate epidemic and other diseases, to promote co-operation among scientific and professional groups which contribute to the advancement of health, promote and conduct research study, report and make recommendations, standard setting with respect to food, biological, pharmaceutical and similar products. All of these functions allow the WHO to be forceful and outspoken if it wishes to do so.

But perhaps an interesting mechanism to enhance the response to the TB epidemic by both the WHO and its member countries is WHO's mandate to propose conventions, agreements and regulations that are binding on the member states. This instrument was used for the first time in response to the globalization of the tobacco epidemic when in 2003 the World Health Assembly adopted the WHO Framework Convention on Tobacco Control in 2003 (World Health Assembly resolution 56.1).

Like tobacco control, MDR-TB requires an international response. It is hard to see how progress can be made without much stronger leadership from the WHO and international collaboration. Also WHO's limited ability to push for progress in MDR-TB treatment and TB control in countries that are not on track to control the MDR-TB epidemic, such as some Eastern European states, needs to be strengthened. An international agreement on TB with a specific focus on control and treatment of MDR-TB would certainly help to strengthen WHO's role and increase attention to the MDR-TB problem at national level.

The key actions to improve access to care for MDR-TB will also need to take place at the national level. It remains to be seen if court rulings on issues of MDR-TB care will play a role in countries such as South Africa or India where courts have had an important role in directing health reform. In South Africa, for example, the Constitutional Court ruled in favour of an action brought by the Treatment Action Campaign (TAC) for provision of nevirapine to prevent mother-to-child transmission of HIV.[17] An analysis of 71 legal cases regarding access to medicines in which the enforcement of the right to health was sought shows that in 59 of the cases plaintiffs were successful. In 14 cases the judgment was extended to all individuals in similar circumstances. While the majority of the cases concerned access to HIV/AIDS care, others concerned cancers, neurological disease, transplant surgery and chronic diseases such as diabetes. This study shows the important role the courts can play in case the health authorities fail to provide what people are entitled to.[18]

Experience with the HIV epidemic suggests that the involvement of civil society will be crucial to increase access to MDR-TB treatment, similar to its role as a catalyst for stimulating access to treatment for anti-retrovirals. Despite the efforts of a dedicated few, civil society mobilization for TB remains, for the moment, limited.

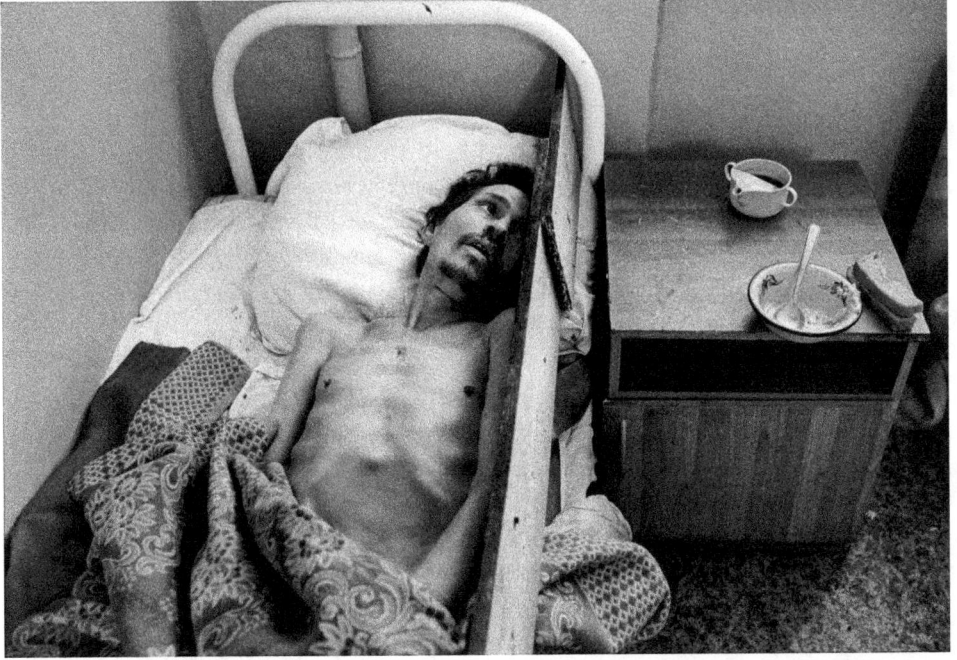

04

04
A patient with advanced tuberculosis at the Tomsk
Regional Clinical Tuberculosis Hospital, Building #3.
(Photograph by James Nachtwey / VII)

Paying the price for decades of neglecting research and development

Development of drug resistance is a well known problem for all kinds of antibiotics. It was indeed predictable that TB mycobacteria would develop resistance against current drugs, and that resistance would start spreading.

The three main strategies to address the problem of drug resistance are to prevent, for as long as possible, the development of resistance through rational drug use, to treat resistant cases appropriately when they occur and to start developing new generation antibiotics well ahead of time before resistance becomes widespread.[19]

Clearly, in the case of TB, this second aspect has been sorely neglected. Until recently, research and development (R&D) for drugs, diagnostics and vaccines for TB and other neglected diseases were at a standstill due to lack of commercial interest.[20] The drugs used in the current first-line therapy were all discovered and developed in the 1950s and 1960s.[21]

The cost in human lives due to a rapidly spreading MDR-TB epidemic is the price we are paying for decades of neglect of R&D. This price is arguably much higher than if R&D investments had been made in time: In addition to the unnecessary loss of human lives, society today has to pay the price, both of the high cost of providing MDR-TB treatment, and the R&D cost.

Pharmaceutical companies received criticism – and rightly so – for their lack of investment into R&D for neglected diseases. But there are obvious limits to investment into non-profitable diseases by for-profit companies. Arguably, with today's system for medical R&D, little else should have been expected. In fact, the lack of R&D is the direct result of our predominant reliance on a patent and profit-driven system for drug development. There is therefore a clear need for a greater role of the public sector to set priorities for health-needs-driven R&D. We also need to establish alternative incentive mechanisms for innovation, in particular ones that do not lead to high drug prices, and that de-link the costs of R&D from the price of health products.[22]

TB research and development has only recently been revived with the creation of three not-for-profit product development partnerships: The TB Alliance (for drugs), Aeras (for vaccines) and FIND (for diagnostics). There are also some renewed activities by a few drug companies, notably Tibotec and Otsuka.

But these developments remain fragile. The three partnerships receive most of their funding through the Bill and Melinda Gates Foundation, while government funding remains limited. Crucially, financing of the more costly clinical development stages is not yet secured. Companies have agreed to disclose their investment into TB drug R&D. This is a good step, but eight companies collectively invest only close to USD 50 million a year. This is a fraction of the amount needed.[23] Overall the drug pipeline remains weak and is unlikely to deliver the urgently needed breakthroughs.[24] The likelihood of introducing a new first-line treatment with at least two new drugs by 2015 is under 1%.[25]

The strategies adopted could also be questioned. The goal of the TB Alliance, which is associated with about half of the drugs currently in the pipeline, is to develop a new first-line treatment for TB that is shorter, active against drug-resistant TB, and can be taken together with HIV drugs. While there is wide agreement on the importance of this goal, it will take many years to develop such a combination.

Given the desperate need to improve MDR-TB treatment as early as possible, all new drugs in the pipeline should also be tested for use in MDR-TB. Once tested in MDR-TB, they might bring some improvement, if only to shorten MDR-TB treatment by a few months. This does not preclude that the new drugs can be used in the future for an improved first-line therapy. Staff at the US drug regulatory agency (the Federal Drug Administration, or FDA) have even indicated that such trials could lead to faster drug approval.[26]

There are also huge gaps in our understanding of how best to treat drug-resistant TB even with existing drugs. Due to lack of controlled trials comparing different treatment regimes, a controversial debate continues among experts on the number and types of drugs required.

Progress in diagnostic development is likewise insufficient: Although two methods were newly recommended by WHO in 2008 (liquid culture and line probe assay), these are still highly complex to perform.

Conclusions

Significant commitment is needed at the national level to scale up MDR-TB treatment as part of routine TB care to the greatest extent possible. Until now, MDR-TB treatment has been provided mainly in a centralized fashion, an approach that will not be feasible in high burden countries. In South Africa, some have called for isolation of potential transmitters as a means of control,[27] but the South African Medical Research Council warned that coercive measures would risk driving the MDR/XDR problem underground.[28] Also, the long delays until diagnosis is suspected, then confirmed and treatment started, means that most transmissions will have already occurred long before isolation is possible.[29] One way to reduce unacceptable delays is to decentralize patient management, as is now widely accepted for HIV care, while improving clinic and community infection control measures. Such an approach would also benefit from community-based support measures that exist within decentralized HIV programmes.[30]

Only newer drugs and better tests can overcome the challenges of MDR-TB treatment. There are two ways that this must be moved forward.

One concerns the need to accelerate the development of those tools currently in the pipeline. All drug developers involved in TB should be compelled to test their compounds also in MDR-TB patients, in order to improve the dismal treatment options available. In June 2008, stakeholders from communities, non-governmental organizations (NGOs), governments, donors, industry, and academia met in Cambridge, Massachusetts, and declared the formation of a movement to conduct the most important priority clinical trials to test strategies to shorten and improve treatment for drug-resistant TB, and to prevent drug-resistant TB.[31]

The other is to attract more actors and funding to R & D. The adoption of a Global Strategy and Plan of Action for Public Health, Innovation and Intellectual Property at the 2008 World Health Assembly marked a breakthrough for WHO and its member states to start playing a much stronger role in priority setting and providing funding and incentives for needs-driven R & D. This breakthrough must now be harnessed to realize the right to health for MDR-TB patients.

*   I wish to thank Ellen 't Hoen for helpful input into this paper.

1   World Health Organization (WHO) *Global Tuberculosis Control 2008* (Geneva: WHO, 2008), WHO/HTM/TB/2008.393.

2   MDR-TB is defined as resistance to at least isoniazid and rifampicin. XDR-TB is defined as MDR-TB that is also resistant to at least one fluoroquinolone and one or more injectable TB drugs.

3   F. Cobelens, E. Heldal, M. Kimerling et al. 'Scaling up Programmatic Management of Drug-Resistant Tuberculosis' 5(7) *PloS Medicine* (2008), at 1037–1042.

4   S. S. Munsiff, S. D. Ahuja, D. J. Li and C. R. Driver, 'Public-Private Collaboration for Multidrug-Resistant Tuberculosis in New York City' 10 *International Journal for Tuberculosis and Lung Disease* (2006), at 639–648.

5   H. S. Cox, S. Kalon, S. Allamuratova et al. 'Multidrug-Resistant Tuberculosis Treatment Outcomes in Karakalpakstan, Uzbekistan: Treatment Complexity and XDR-TB Among Treatment Failures' 2(11) *PloS One* (2007) e1126.

6   C. Hewison, V. Sizaire, S. Kalon et al. 'Development of extreme drug resistance in multidrug-resistant tuberculosis patients' 11(11) *International Journal for Tuberculosis and Lung Disease,* supplement 1 (2007) at S63, 38th World Conference on Lung Health of the International Union against Tuberculosis and Lung Diseases, abstract PC-71846–10.

7   Diana Weil, WHO, in presentation at MSF workshop, Oslo, September 2007, on file with author.

8   M. Raviglione 'Preface' in WHO, *Guidelines for the Programmatic Management of Drug-Resistant Tuberculosis* (Geneva: WHO, 2006), WHO/HTM/TB/2006.361, available at http://whqlibdoc.who.int/publications/2006/9241546956_eng.pdf.

9   Paul Farmer, *Infections and Inequalities* (Berkley: University of California Press, 1999).

10 Ibid.

11 C. Mitnick, L. Bayona and E. Palaciosis et al. 'Community-Based Therapy for Multidrug-Resistant Tuberculosis in Lima, Peru' 348(2) *New England Journal of Medicine* (2003), at 119–127.

12 Paul Farmer and Jim Yong Kim, 'Community Based Approaches to the Control of Multidrug Resistant Tuberculosis: Introducing "DOTS-plus"' 317 *British Medical Journal* (1998), at 671–674.

13 Raviglione, *supra* note 8.

14 World Health Organization (WHO) 'The Global Plan to Stop TB 2006–2015 / Stop TB Partnership' (Geneva: WHO, 2006), available at http://www.who.int/tb/publications/global_plan_to_stop_tb/en/index.html; WHO, 'Stop TB Partnership: The Global MDRTB & XDR-TB Response Plan 2007–2008' (Geneva: WHO, 2007), available at http://www.who.int/entity/tb/publications/2007/mdr_xdr_global_response_plan.pdf

15 Paul Hunt, UN Special Rapporteur on the right to the highest attainable standard of health, 'Human Rights Guidelines for Pharmaceutical Companies in Relation to Access to Medicines (Draft for Consultation)', 19 September 2007, available at http://www2.essex.ac.uk/human_rights_centre/rth/projects.shtm.

16 MSF, *Help Wanted: Confronting the Health Worker Crisis to Expand Access to HIV/AIDS treatment* (Johannesburg, MSF, 2007), available at http://www.msf.org.za/docs/Help_Wanted_FINAL.pdf.

17 J. A. Singh, M. Govender and E. Mills, 'Health and Human Rights 2: Do Human Rights Matter to Health?' 370 *The Lancet* (2007), at 521–527.

18 Hogerzeil H, Samson M, Casanovas J et al. 'Is access to essential medicines as part of the fulfilment of the right to health enforceable through the courts?' 368 *The Lancet* (2006), at 305–311.

19 S. Levy and B. Marshall, 'Antibacterial Resistance Worldwide: Causes, Challenges and Responses' 10(12) *Nature Medicine* (2004), at 122–129.

20 P. Trouiller et al. 'Drug Development for Neglected Diseases: A Deficient Market and a Public-Health Policy Failure' 359 *The Lancet* (2002), at 2188–2194.

21 MSF, *Development of New Drugs for TB Chemotherapy: Analysis of the Current Drug Pipeline* (Geneva: MSF, 2006), available at http://www.accessmed-msf.org/fileadmin/user_upload/diseases/tuberculosis/TBPipeline.pdf.

22 *Global Strategy and Plan of Action on Public Health, Innovation and Intellectual Property,* Sixty-first World Health Assembly, WHA61.21, 2008, available at http://www.who.int/gb/ebwha/pdf_files/A61/A61_R21-en.pdf.

23 C. Feuer *Tuberculosis Research and Development: A Critical Analysis of Funding Trends,* 2005–2006 (New York: Treatment Action Group, 2007).

24 M. Casenghi, S. Cole and C. Nathan, 'New Approaches to Filling the Gap in Tuberculosis Drug Discovery' 4(11) *PloS Medicine* (2007) e293.

25 S. Glickman, E. Rasieland, C. Hamilton et al. 'Medicine: A Portfolio Model of Drug Development for Tuberculosis' 311 *Science* (2006) 1246–7.

26 C. Mitnick, K. Castro, M. Harrington, L. Sacks and W. Burman, 'Randomized Trials to Optimize Treatment of Multidrug-Resistant Tuberculosis' 4(11) *PloS Medicine* (2007) e292.

27 J.A. Singh, R. Upshur, N. Padayatchi, 'XDR-TB in South Africa: No Time for Denial of Complacency' 4(1) *PloS Medicine* (2007), at 19–25.

28 'World Report: XDR Tuberculosis Spreads Across South Africa' 369 *The Lancet* (2007), at 729.

29 E. Goemaere, N. Ford, D. Berman et al. 'XDR-TB in South Africa: Detention is Not the Priority' 4(4) *PloS Medicine* (2007), at 771–2.

30 E. Goemaere, *MDR and XDR in High-Prevalence HIV Settings: An Epidemic Requiring a Paradigm Shift* (Cape Town: MSF, 2007), available at http://www.msf.org.za/docs/MDR_XDR_TBinhigh_prevalenceHIVsettings.pdf.

31 *The Cambridge Declaration: Towards Clinical Trials for Drug-Resistant Tuberculosis,* Cambridge, Massachusetts, USA, 12 June 2008, available at www.msfaccess.org.

For having kindly permitted us the use of his photographs, we thank James Nachtwey / VII.

These photographs by James Nachtwey form part of a broader project to use photographs to create awareness about extremely drug-resistant tuberculosis (XDR-TB) and stop the worldwide XDR-TB epidemic. See further http://www.xdrtb.org.

The New Global War on Malaria

Jeffrey D. Sachs and Raymond G. Chambers

The global control of malaria has followed a tortuous path during the past half century. There have been great and lasting successes but also tremendous failures of will and policy reversals. The world is girding up again for a new assault on the disease, the first concerted attempt in decades to bring the disease under control, and the first time in history that Africa is at the very epicentre of the global commitment. There are good chances for success in the next five years and beyond, but any progress in short-term control will have to be complemented by dramatically increased research and development for new solutions.

Ecological roots of the control challenge

As the late, great entomologist Andrew Spielman of Harvard University always emphasized, "malaria is a disease of place". That is, transmission is heavily dependent on the local geography. The first thing to understand about the control challenge, therefore, is the role of geography. Most importantly, for understandable reasons, the range of malaria transmission has shrunk during the past century. One hundred years ago, malaria was transmitted in temperate, sub-tropical, and tropical conditions. Today, the disease is almost entirely concentrated in the tropics, with tropical sub-Saharan Africa accounting for roughly 90% of the disease and deaths. The shrinking range of coverage is shown in Figure 1, where the map displays how the range of transmission has narrowed from its widest extent to a narrower band around the equator in the course of the past century.

Figure 01: The Declining Range of Transmission during 1900–2002[1]

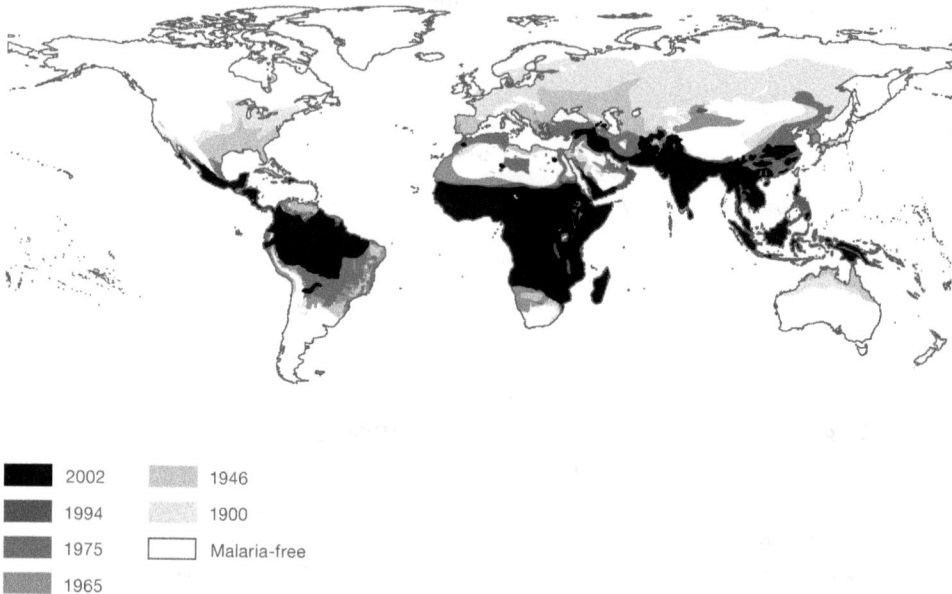

■ 2002	▨ 1946		
■ 1994	▨ 1900		
■ 1975	☐ Malaria-free		
■ 1965			

Human malaria is a constellation of four closely related diseases (with a fifth strain recently identified). All are caused by the protozoan Plasmodium, and all are transmitted by the female mosquito of the genus Anopheles. One of the protozoan strains, *Plasmodium falciparum*, is life threatening, while the others are usually not fatal though they may be seriously debilitating. This paper focuses on the control of *P. falciparum*. Unless otherwise noted, "malaria" refers therefore to *P. falciparum*.

Malaria transmission depends intimately on ecological conditions as well as on the nature of human settlements and human control efforts. There are three major ecological conditions:

1. Ambient temperature;
2. Precipitation (as a determinant of breeding sites for the mosquitoes); and
3. The species of Anopheles mosquito.

It is important to understand each of these ecological factors to understand the challenge of malaria control.

Malaria is transmitted between humans when a female Anopheles takes a blood meal from one infected person, thereby taking up the parasite into the mosquito, and then takes another blood meal some 14 days later from another person, thereby transmitting the parasite to that individual. The period between the two bites is known as "sporogony". The higher the ambient temperature, the shorter the biological period of sporogony, and the faster the mosquito becomes infective. If sporogony takes too long because the ambient temperature is too low, then the mosquito dies before transmitting the infection to another human being. In general, the ambient temperature must be at least 18 degrees Celsius to support transmission.

Precipitation matters for transmission because rainfall provides the collections of water that serve as the breeding sites for the mosquito larvae. A long dry season, for example, can break malaria transmission. The species of Anopheles matters mainly due to the propensity of the mosquito species to bite humans, as opposed to cattle or other animals. The proportion of blood meals taken on human blood as a share of all blood meals is called the Human Biting Index (HBI). When the HBI is near 1 (meaning that all feeding is on humans, and none on cattle or other animals), then the mosquito species is a powerful transmitter of the disease. When the HBI is near zero (meaning that most bites are on animals rather than humans), then the species is a weak transmitter of the disease. In fact, since the disease is transmitted only when two blood meals in a row are taken on humans, the probability of transmission is proportional to the HIB raised to the squared power.

It turns out, much to its bad luck, that African mosquito species are nearly complete human biters (HBI close to 1), while in Asia, for example, the HBI is around 0.3. In Africa, the probability of transmission is therefore proportional to $1 \times 1 = 1$, while in Asia the probability of transmission is proportional to $0.3 \times 0.3 = 0.09$, or roughly one-tenth of the transmission probability in Africa.

More generally, we can say that tropical Africa has all the factors for intense malaria transmission: High ambient temperatures year round; enough rainfall to support year round, or near year round breeding; and nearly complete human biters. The result is that Africa's ecology puts Africa in a unique situation, with the world's worst malaria transmission – by virtue of its ecology.

The ecological conditions conducive to malaria transmission can be summarized in a single statistic called Vector Competence (VC). In a study a few years ago, one of us (Sachs) worked with a number of colleagues in entomology and geographic information systems to map the VC in all parts of the world.[2] Figure 2 shows the result. We see that Africa has by far the world's most favourable ecology for malaria transmission (and hence least favourable from the point of view of the human beings living there!). Africa's ecological conditions are matched only by parts of Papua New Guinea. Other tropical regions (with high year-round temperatures) are, by and large, also favourable ecologies, but with mosquito species that have lower human biting rates.

Figure 02: Malaria Ecology Index[3]

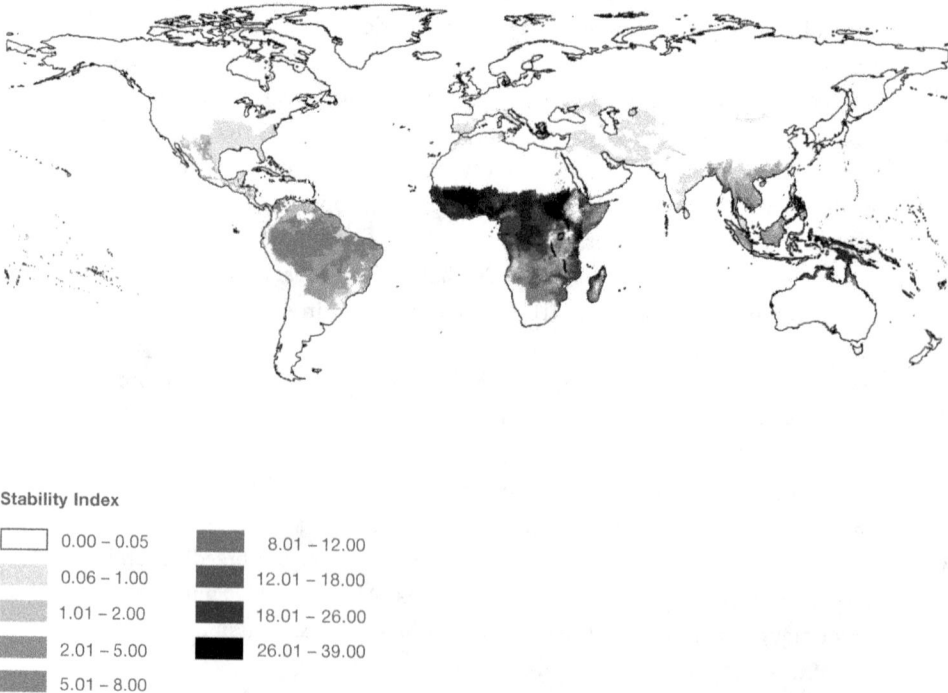

Stability Index

0.00 – 0.05	8.01 – 12.00
0.06 – 1.00	12.01 – 18.00
1.01 – 2.00	18.01 – 26.00
2.01 – 5.00	26.01 – 39.00
5.01 – 8.00	

Ecology and disease control

Epidemiologists summarize the challenge of controlling an infectious disease by the Basic Reproduction Number (BRN) of the disease, sometimes denoted as Ro. The BRN measures a key concept: How many people will a single infected individual infect if placed in a susceptible (but uninfected) population. If that number is greater than 1, then the disease propagates in a growing chain reaction. If, on the other hand, a single infected individual on average infects less than 1 other person, then the infection dies out on its own. The key to control is to take steps to ensure that the BRN is less than 1.

Consider the following example. Suppose that in a natural condition, a region has a BRN equal to 2. That is, a newly arrived individual infected with malaria is likely to infect two other people. Each of those will infect two others, and so forth. The infection, once introduced, would tend to spread rampantly in the population. Now suppose that control measures are taken to limit transmission. For example, the health services improve so that each infected individual is treated – and cured of infection – much more rapidly once symptoms become evident. This not only saves the infected individual, but cuts down on transmission as well, since the infected individual spends far less time being a "reservoir" for infection of others. When the mosquito bites the cured individual, the mosquito no longer picks up the parasites for transmission to others. Similarly, the use of insecticides or the introduction of screen doors rather than open doors might sharply cut down on the number of mosquito bites per person per day.

This too could cut BRN, perhaps below 1. Indeed, if BRN is reduced from 2 to less than 1, then nature itself will take its course and snuff out an infection. Each person is then likely to transmit the disease to fewer than even 1 other person. It is not necessary to track down and stop every single infection. It is merely necessary to prevent enough infections such that the Basic Reproduction Rate is less than 1.

Now, here's the catch, which helps to explain Africa's special predicament. Suppose that there are two locations, one with a BRN equal to 2 and the other with a BRN equal to 20 (by virtue of temperature, breeding site, and mosquito species). In each place, a special control effort is introduced which cuts down mosquito bites by half, and which speeds up the treatment and cure of infected individuals. In each case, the BRN falls by two thirds. In the first location, the BRN falls to 0.67, and the disease no longer creates a self-reinforcing epidemic. Indeed, it dies away on its own once BRN <1. In the second location, the BRN falls to 6.67, still much greater than 1. The disease transmission remains intense, though less than earlier. The actual proportions infected with malaria may change little, since the BRN remains far above 1.

A brief history of control from an ecological perspective

The biological pathways of malaria transmission were unknown until the late 19th Century and early 20th Century, when the great work of scientists including Charles Louis Alphonse Laveran, Patrick Manson, Ronald Ross, and Giovanni Battista Grassi deciphered the complex life cycle and transmission mechanisms of malaria. Until then, the disease was generally attributed to the bad air of swamps and low-lying areas, and hence, mal (bad) – aria (air). The new science uncovered the process by which the pathogen is ingested by a blood-feeding female mosquito and then transmitted to a human being in a later blood meal by the mosquito.

This discovery gave rise to the modern era of malaria control, and the main tools of control were quickly recognized. These included:

1. Human behaviour, notably avoiding places and times of the day where anopheles mosquitoes take blood meals;
2. environmental controls to reduce breeding sites, including drainage of swamps and other breeding sites, the use of chemical larvicides, and the use of fish that feed on mosquito larvae;
3. treatment of malaria patients with quinine, not only curing the patients but also shortening the period of infectivity of the patient and thereby the transmission to others;
4. bed netting, screen doors, and other mechanical barriers between the mosquitoes and humans to reduce biting rates; and
5. the use of insecticides and repellants, such as pyrethrum-based insecticides.

There were several notable accomplishments in the first half of the 20th Century. The island of Cuba was the site of the first comprehensive mosquito control campaign in 1901, after the occupation by the United States (US) following the Spanish-American War. General William Gorgas led this effort, a prelude to his efforts in the Panama Canal Zone during 1905–1910 to clear mosquitoes to enable construction of the Canal. In the US South, the Tennessee Valley Authority undertook malaria control actions in the 1930s. The Rockefeller Foundation supported Fred Soper on a remarkable campaign to rid Brazil of *A. gambiae*, which had been introduced from Africa into the mining regions of the Amazon. Soper used pyrethrum spraying and larvicides in a successful campaign. The greatest breakthroughs in control efforts came during and after World War II, however, with the discovery and mass production of the insecticide Dichloro-Diphenyl-Trichloroethane (DDT), and the discovery and synthesis of chloroquine as an effective treatment of illness. These two tools allowed an enormous advance in control efforts.

The progress of malaria control was largely dictated by four considerations:

1.   The Basic Reproduction Number of the site in pre-control conditions, dictating the extent of control needed to interrupt transmission;
2.   the physical geography of the location, which determines the ease of mosquito control;
3.   the economic development level of the site, affecting the frequency of mosquito-human contacts and bites; and
4.   the economic importance of the target site, determining the human and financial resources devoted to the control effort.

Thus, malaria control was favoured in the following conditions:

____ Temperate zones, where temperatures were sufficiently cool to limit sporogony and thereby keep the basic reproduction number near 1.
____ Islands (such as Cuba), making the control of the mosquito populations easier and with much less risk of reintroduction from areas outside of the control area.
____ High-priority regions, such as the Panama Canal Zone, where enormous human and material resources could be devoted to transmission control.
____ Ecologically favourable areas, such as the Brazilian Amazon, where control is undertaken against a newly introduced species of mosquito rather than an endemic (naturally occurring) species in the area.
____ Richer areas, where economic development (e.g. urbanization and/or improved homes with screen doors and windows) leads to reduced contact between Anopheles mosquitoes and human populations.

A powerful example of favourable ecological conditions was the US South. As a sub-tropical region with cool nights and winters, temperatures were often below the threshold rate of 18 degrees Celsius for transmission. Thus the Basic Reproduction Number was little above 1 in the pre-control environment, and transmission was seasonal rather than year round. Small declines in mosquito abundance or biting rates would suffice to break transmission. Such declines ensued in the period of the 1930s and 1940s, often before formal malaria control measures were undertaken. The declines resulted from improved housing, including the introduction of screen doors and windows; the drainage of swamp-lands and other breeding sites as part of local development efforts; and the increasing urbanization, which reduced breeding sites of the mosquito and biting rates (notably since Anopheles do not generally thrive in the polluted water sites of cities).

The discovery of DDT as an effective pesticide in 1939 gave rise to the vision of malaria eradication. It was felt by public health experts that the new insecticide made possible the eradication of the disease, if DDT were used simultaneously and intensively throughout the world. From the start, it was hypothesized that there would be a short window of opportunity until the mosquito developed DDT resistance. WHO launched the Malaria Eradication Programme in 1955. Ironically, despite being called a "global" programme, the effort completely bypassed sub-Saharan Africa, where it was felt that high transmission rates (that is, high BRNs) made control through DDT unfeasible.

The WHO eradication effort lasted between 1955 and 1966. It has been recorded in history as a failure, though in fact it had remarkable successes in ridding many regions of malaria transmission, or at least in dramatically reducing the fatality rates associated with the disease in those regions. The successes, once again, followed the basic logic of disease ecology. Where the basic reproduction number was low enough, i.e. close to 1, control efforts could break transmission. Where the BRN was far above 1, control efforts would rarely suffice to break transmission. Therefore, successes tended to be achieved in areas where the combination of relatively cooler temperatures, dry months (i.e. without breeding sites), and specific Anopheles species with sufficiently low human biting rates, made possible the interruption of malaria. This included most of the sub-tropical regions of the world, around the Mediterranean, the Black Sea, and large parts of the Americas and Asia. Islands were also especially favoured, as described above. Africa, as mentioned earlier, was bypassed.

During 1969–1976, the WHO led an intensive study of malaria control in a holo-endemic African site in Garki, Nigeria. An intensive effort was made there to break transmission through a combination of environmental controls, including DDT spraying, and case management of patients. This famous study was also recorded as a failure because it failed to break transmission despite an intensive effort. Ironically, though, the Garki trial was enormously successful at reducing illness and mortality. If the goal of the study had been defined as "malaria control", rather than malaria elimination, it would have been treated in history as a success, rather than remembered as a failure. This misinterpretation was very costly in public health thinking, because it erroneously led to the unfounded conclusion that malaria control efforts in sub-Saharan Africa "would not work".

By the 1970s, malaria control efforts were being radically scaled back. The eradication program was deemed a "failure" since global transmission was not broken. Not only did DDT resistance develop, as long feared, but the findings of environmentalist Rachel Carsons and others that DDT entered the animal food chain as a persistent chemical, with cumulative and adverse ecological effects higher in the food chain, led to an enormous environmental backlash against the use of DDT in malaria control. This was another misunderstanding. The public backlash against DDT did not distinguish between the heavy applications of DDT used in the open fields as a crop pesticide, versus the very low doses of DDT used in thin-film residual spraying inside households for malaria control with negligible environmental harms.

The 1980s saw a serious backsliding in malaria control efforts in many places, and a surge of malaria deaths in Africa. The first-line, low-cost treatment with chloroquine increasingly lost efficacy as wide-spread chloroquine resistance developed in regions of high drug use, especially in Africa and Southeast Asia. The end of DDT use in many places led to a recovery of Anopheles populations and a resurgence of transmission. Still, to summarize the conditions at the end of the 1980s, the picture was mixed rather than bleak:

—— Many regions in the temperate and sub-tropical regions enjoyed continued success in preventing a return of malaria transmission, following the successful interruption of transmission during the preceding decades.

—— Many regions, for instance in Latin America, continued to use DDT and other insecticides with effective results, even in areas where some DDT resistance was noted.

—— Fatality rates generally remained lower than pre-control era rates, even in places where transmission returned following a period of interruption. There was, however, always the risk of epidemic rebounds in such locations, especially as populations had lost acquired immunity during the interruption period.

—— Sub-Saharan Africa faced the worst situation of all, since comprehensive control efforts had never been tried (despite the evidence of successful reduction of morbidity and mortality in the Garki experiment) and the low-cost treatment with chloroquine was rendered increasingly ineffective due to drug resistance.

Beginning in 1992, the WHO once again introduced a global malaria control programme. This time, however, the focus was put on effective case management (i.e. treatment) to reduce mortality, and on a more limited effort of prevention than during the eradication period. The four pillars of the control strategy included: Early diagnosis and prompt treatment; selective and sustainable prevention efforts; early detection and control of epidemics; and strengthened local capacities in basic and applied malaria research. Despite these intentions, however, few additional financial and human resources were devoted to malaria control, especially in sub-Saharan Africa. By the end of the 1990s all signs were pointing to an alarming increase in disease burden and mortality rates in Africa, as public health investments withered under the weight of reform and chlorquines declined continued.

The roll-back malaria era since 1998

Dr. Gro Harlem Brundtland became Director General of the World Health Organization in 1998 with a commitment to reverse the dramatic deterioration of malaria control in Africa. She launched a new "Roll Back Malaria Initiative" alongside UNICEF, the World Bank, and UNDP to combine more intensive case detection and treatment, integrated vector control, and epidemic surveillance and control measures. Gradually, with considerable delays in mobilizing the needed funds and political will, the Roll Back Malaria effort has gained traction, and has made possible the adoption of new bold, yet realistic, targets of malaria control in Africa.

Two new technological developments considerably brightened the prospects for malaria control since the late 1990s. The first was the rise of insecticide-treated bed nets as a major measure of disease prevention. Bed nets have been in use for a century, but the treatment of bed nets with insecticides is only recent. Studies have shown that half or more of the protective effect of the bed nets lies not in the mechanical barrier afforded by the net (which often fails anyway because of holes, tears, or simply the mosquito's ability to get around the barrier), but in the dual role of the insecticide in repelling the mosquito or killing it through contact when the mosquito alights on the net. Insecticide-treated nets themselves have experienced a true revolutionary breakthrough when nets were engineered in which the insecticide would last through many years of use and repeated washing, rather than requiring the re-treatment of the nets with insecticides. Long-lasting insecticide-treated nets, effective for 4–6 years without retreatment, provide the most powerful single prevention tool at the household level.

The second breakthrough was the introduction of new low-cost alternatives to chloroquine. Several alternative anti-malaria medicines have been introduced, but many have also rapidly lost their efficacy through the rapid development of resistance by the pathogen. The key breakthrough in the past decade is the development and widespread adoption of Artemisinin-based Combination Therapies (ACTs), in which the drug artemisinin is combined with another anti-malarial medicine, with the objective of protecting both drugs against the development of resistance through their use in combination. Artemisinin is the discovery by Chinese scientists of the active molecular agent of a traditional herbal medicine for malaria control using the wormwood plant (Artemisia annua).

The WHO Commission on Macroeconomics and Health,[4] which one of us (Sachs) directed, called strongly for the scaled up effort on malaria control. The Commission reported the evidence that malaria not only takes an enormous human toll in Africa, but also contributes to an enormous economic loss and is a barrier to economic growth. Investments in malaria control thus offer an enormous return in lives saved and improved, and in economic benefits for Africa. This logic and evidence contributed to the decision by the African countries to adopt new and bold continent-wide targets at a malaria summit in Abuja, Nigeria, convened by President Olesegun Obasanjo in April 2000. The summit established the Abuja Targets for malaria control, to halve mortality by the year 2010, and to achieve 60% coverage of bed net prevention and prompt case treatment by the year 2005. This summit marked the invigoration and empowerment of Africa's political leadership in the control challenge.

The Abuja Declaration, the recommendations of the WHO Commission on Macroeconomics and Health, and the drama of the AIDS pandemic, all added a sense of urgency to the control of malaria, AIDS, and tuberculosis (TB). In the course of the work of the WHO Commission, Sachs called for the establishment of a global fund for AIDS at the International AIDS Conference in Durbin, South Africa, in July 2000. UN Secretary General Kofi Annan expanded that call in a path-breaking and world-changing address at the Abuja AIDS Summit in April 2001, where he first called for a Global Fund for AIDS, TB, and Malaria. In May 2001, the Secretary General's proposal for a Global Fund was endorsed by the US Government. Several other donor countries quickly joined the new Fund. It began operations in 2002. From the start it has played a crucial role in the scaling up of malaria control efforts, especially by providing funding for long-lasting insecticide bed nets (LLINs) and for artemisinin-combination therapies (ACTs).

The case for comprehensive malaria control, especially in sub-Saharan Africa (accounting for 90% of worldwide cases of *P. falciparum* and deaths), gained momentum in the next six years. The US Government joined the effort through a new President's Malaria Initiative (PMI) launched in 2005. The UN Millennium Project[5] strongly recommended a mass distribution of LLINs, along the lines of the pioneering distribution efforts led by the United Nations Children's Fund (UNICEF) and the International Federation of Red Cross and Red Crescent Societies (IFRC). This recommendation was endorsed by the UN General Assembly in September 2005. The World Bank adopted a Booster Programme for Malaria to speed disbursements. Various NGOs, most notably Malaria No More (MNM) and the United Nations Foundation's Nothing But Nets (NBN) project, have alerted the broad US and European publics to the potential and the importance of malaria control. The Millennium Villages Project (MVP), a partnership of the UN, the NGO Millennium Promise, and the Earth Institute, demonstrated the efficacy of combining the free mass distribution of bed nets with the mass availability of ACTs. Across sites in the MVP, malaria has been sharply reduced. Several other success stories, led by other projects, have also been recorded, leading to rising hopes for the success of comprehensive control. Public awareness has also risen sharply as mass media (such as the popular "American Idol" show) have taken on the cause of malaria control, notably through the mass distribution of bed nets.

Global control on the path to eradication

Comprehensive malaria control has come within reach, leading the Secretary General Ban Ki-moon to launch a bold initiative on World Malaria Day, 25 April 2008, to achieve 100% coverage of malaria control interventions (bed nets, indoor spraying in some locations, and rapid diagnostics, combined with effective case management with early diagnosis, community health workers, and free availability of ACTs).[6] His call to action is supported by the Roll Back Malaria Partnership, and is described in the Global Malaria Action Plan of RBM.[7] It is envisioned as a key step on the way to the eventual eradication of malaria, a step which will require the development of an effective malaria vaccine. Policy, therefore, will proceed in two parallel tracks: The first uses the current technologies (including LLINs, ACTs, indoor residual spraying, and rapid diagnostic tests) to bring malaria transmission, morbidity, and mortality to low levels; the second promotes the development of new tools, notably a vaccine.

The Global Malaria Action Plan sets out the basic modalities and estimated costs for comprehensive control, putting the costs at around USD 2–3 billion per year in sub-Saharan Africa, to be covered mostly by external donors. The aim is to cut deaths from malaria by at least half compared with 1990, and to bring deaths to "near zero preventable" levels by 2015. The budget guidelines of RBM are in conformity with the estimates recently published by McCord, Teklehaimanot, and Sachs (2007)[8] which also estimate the costs at USD 3 billion per year. These costs include LLINs (100% coverage), medicines, community health workers, indoor residual spraying (partial coverage), and diagnostic tests.

The basic modality for delivery will be through the leadership of the public sector of each country, supported by international financing and national budgets. In each country, the government and civil society will make a comprehensive national plan, and submit it for funding support to the Global Fund and other donors including the World Bank, the US PMI, and philanthropic donors who will be partners with the official donors. Countries have embraced the Secretary General's call for universal coverage of essential interventions by 31 December 2010 and are considering the date a deadline for results, not an aspirational goal. Round 8 of the Global Fund, for instance, saw an over 75% success rate in sub-Sahara Africa for malaria control proposals, each of which aimed for universal coverage. Coverage of nets will generally be free, and medicines for free or at very highly subsidized rates. The goal is to achieve a dramatic drop in malaria deaths to nearly zero by 2015 and beyond. Transmission of the disease will still occur, but at far lower levels than today, and the infections will be treated systematically to prevent serious illness and deaths.

Fighting malaria will also be a boon for other diseases. There is mounting evidence that dual infection with HIV and malaria fuel the spread of both diseases in sub-Saharan Africa (Abu-Raddad, Patnaik and Kublin, 2006). When people with AIDS contract malaria, it causes a surge of HIV virus in their blood, making them more likely to infect a partner. At the same time, people with weakened immune systems, compromised by HIV, are more likely to contract and die from malaria. Reducing malaria infections will therefore help protect against HIV-transmission and reduce mortality rates in people living with AIDS. An example from Uganda shows that the use of cotrimoxazole prophylaxis and insecticide-treated nets (ITNs) among HIV infected children is associated with a dramatic reduction in the risk of malaria.[9]

In addition to the humanitarian case for fighting malaria, a related economic case for rapid scale-up has been well established.[10] It is estimated that malaria costs the continent of Africa an estimated USD 12 billion a year in direct health costs and lost productivity, and much more through lost economic growth.[11] Making the investment in a thorough malaria control strategy would repay itself several-fold in higher gross domestic product (GDP) in Africa, through a reduction of health costs, increased productivity, and accelerated economic development. To quote from the 2008 Global Malaria Action Plan:

> "Malaria usually affects some of the poorest, most marginalized populations in the world. Minimizing the burden enables individuals to continue to go to work and school as well as lessening time away from work caring for the sick. This promotes economic growth and can diminish the cycle of poverty. These investments in malaria control can have a significant positive impact on a region's economy. Some analyses have estimated the annual economic burden of malaria to be at least USD 12 billion per year of direct losses, plus many times more than that in lost economic growth. This means that if USD 2.3 billion is needed annually to control malaria in Africa, then every USD 1 invested into malaria control could enable more than a USD 5 gain."

Conclusions

The year 2008 marked three anniversaries: The sixtieth year of the Universal Declaration of Human Rights (1948), the thirtieth year of the Alma-Ata Declaration of Health for All (1978), and the mid-point of the fifteen-year period of the Millennium Development Goals (2000–2015). It is fitting, therefore, that it also marks the emergence of a new global consensus on the dramatic scaling up of malaria control, aiming at the eventual eradication of the disease once an effective vaccine is added to the arsenal. Proven cost-effective prevention and treatment tools, combined with recent increases on malaria-control funding, are enabling countries across the continent to significantly decrease the deaths and financial burden of malaria. We know what we can do, what will work, and yet how much more we have to do. Investing in rapid scale-up of malaria interventions will save millions of lives, produce billions of dollars, and build the platform from which other diseases can be attacked. Having this knowledge and the resources to stop the deaths of 3000 children every day is an obligation. These children have a right to these life-saving resources. We are looking at an historic opportunity to end a public health crisis, one we cannot afford to miss.

1   S.I. Hay, C.A. Guerra, A.J. Tatem, A.M. Noor, R.W. Snow, 'The Global Distribution and Population at Risk of Malaria: Past, Present and Future' 4 *The Lancet: Infectious Diseases* (2004), at 327–336.

2   Anthony Kiszewski, Andrew Mellinger, Andrew Spielman, Pia Malaney, Sonia Ehrlich Sachs and Jeffrey Sachs, 'A Global Index Representing the Stability of Malaria Transmission' 77(5) *The American Journal of Tropical Medicine and Hygiene* (2004), at 486–498.

3   Kiszewski et al., *supra* note 1.

4   World Health Organization (WHO), *Macroeconomics and Health: Investing in Health for Economic Development: Report of the Commission on Macroeconomics and Health* (Geneva: WHO, 2001).

5   UN Millennium Project, *Investing in Development: A Practical Plan to Achieve the Millennium Development Goals* (New York: United Nations, 2005); UN Millennium Project, Coming to Grips with Malaria in the New Millennium, (New York: Task Force on HIV/AIDS, Malaria, RB and Access to Essential Medicines, Working Group on Malaria, 2005).

6 'United Nations Secretary-General Ban Ki-moon announces vision for universal coverage to end malaria deaths', Press Release, 25 April 2008, available at http://www.un.org/News/Press/docs/2008/sgsm11531.doc.htm.

7 *Roll Back Malaria – Global Malaria Action Plan*, available at http://www.rollbackmalaria.org/gmap/index.html.

8 Awash Teklehaimanot, Gordon C. McCord, and Jeffrey D. Sachs, 'Scaling Up Malaria Control in Africa: An Economic and Epidemiological Assessment' 77(Suppl 6) *The American Journal of Tropical Medicine and Hygiene* (2007), at 138–144.

9 M. R. Kamya, A. F. Gasasira, J. Achan, T. Mebrahtu, T. Ruel, A. Kekitiinwa, E. D. Charlebois, P. J. Rosenthal, D. Havlir and G. Dorsey, 'Effects of trimethoprim-sulfamethoxazole prophylaxis and insecticide-treated bednets on the risk of malaria among HIV-infected Ugandan children' 21(15) *AIDS 2007* (2007), at 2059–66.

10 J. L. Gallup and J. Sachs 'The Economic Burden of Malaria' 64 *American Journal of Tropical Medicine and Hygiene* (2001), at 85–96.

11 Extrapolated from a loss of USD 12 billion of direct costs compared to the cost of achieving control in SSA: ibid. J. Sachs and P. Malaney, 'The Economic and Social Burden of Malaria' 415 *Nature* (2002), at 680–685.

Bioethics and Genomics

George J. Annas*

Genomics, the study of an individual's entire genome, is often viewed as a potential medical saviour not just through "personalized" medicine in the developed world,[1] but also through application of genomic technology in the resource-poor world.[2] There is extensive literature on the bioethical issues involving genomics in both Europe and the United States (US), and bioethics has been used to frame the relationship between "Genomics and World Health" by the World Health Organization (WHO) as well.[3] Although the WHO has adopted a health and human rights perspective, in their 241 page report on genomics and world health, human rights are mentioned only once, and then in the context of genetic enhancements, that is, using genetic manipulations to try to make "better babies" or simply better humans:

> "Societies have a moral obligation grounded in equity or justice and human rights to ensure access to health care for their citizens. A fundamental part of the moral imperative of health care is its role in maintaining normal function, and in turn helping to secure equality of opportunity for persons that serious disease and disability undermine. Genetic enhancements of normal function, on the other hand, do not serve justice in this way and if and when they become possible, will almost certainly not be regarded as part of the social obligation to provide health care to all members of society."[4]

Put another way, the Advisory Committee on Health Research (ACHR) concludes that only some members of society, the elites, need have a right to the new genetics, and physicians who care for this elite can do so without worrying about medical ethics. Whether one finds appeals to the "norm" of humanity or species function persuasive as lines that circumscribe the "right to health" or not, genetic technologies will certainly change the way we think about ourselves and our species, and thus how we think about the right to health, including access to health care, and bioethics. This chapter aims to explain why genetics and bioethics seem to be naturally paired in global health, and why, nonetheless, a human rights framework – which focused more directly on equality including its mirror, non-discrimination, and the right to health itself – could prove more useful to meeting the basic goals of social justice.

Bioethics, most often referred to simply as medical ethics, deals primarily with decisions made in the doctor-patient relationship, and secondarily with the researcher-subject relationship. It is in this latter context that bioethics and genomics have been most widely discussed. The risks of genomic research, for example, are the subject of chapter six ('Potential risks and hazards of the applications of genomics and their control') of the Report of the WHO's ACHR. The chapter highlights three areas that present special risks: Germline genetic alterations; the establishment of genetic databases; and the application of genomics to biowarfare. The authors conclude that it is premature and dangerous to attempt germline genetic alterations; that nothing can stop the establishment of population-based gene banks (but that rules to protect privacy and guard against discrimination are required); and that the scientific community should take the risk of biowarfare applications of the new genomics seriously. The WHO report concludes on mixed notes of hope and caution: The "new and rapidly evolving" field of genomics "offers considerable possibilities for the improvement of human health" but "the full extent of its possible hazards are not yet fully appreciated."[5]

A Canadian group followed up the WHO report with an exercise designed to identify the new biotechnologies most likely to be helpful to improving the health of people living in developing countries. Their report, based on expert assessment using a Delphi methodology, put two genomic-based technologies at the top of their final list, and a related technology third. First, modified molecular technologies for affordable, simple diagnosis for infectious diseases; second, recombinant technologies to develop vaccines against infectious diseases; and third, technologies for more efficient drug and vaccine delivery systems.[6] The thesis of the Canadian report is that "biotechnology can help to bridge rather than deepen existing divides between the developed and developing world."[7] On the other hand, the authors recognize that there is no technological fix for health, and that we will require a balanced approach: "Biotechnology will never be a panacea to current health inequities, but the evidence demonstrates that it is rightly considered part of the solution."[8] On this subject, WHO's ACHR arrived at a similar conclusion: "None of these advances will be of any value unless the developing countries can evolve the health care systems on which these new advances can be based."[9]

All this is still pretty vague. Of course we all hope that the new genomics will help bridge the gap between the rich and the poor, and the developed world and the underdeveloped world, as it improves the lives and health of those it touches directly. But none of this will be automatic, and WHO's ACHR was right to highlight the dark side of genomics to health and development. The ACHR could have gone much further in this regard, and would have, had they employed a human rights framework instead of the more limited bioethics framework in their analysis. Here is how (I think) it should be done in the contexts of equality and the right to health.

Equality, genomics, and the risk of genism

Equality based on human dignity is at the core of a human rights approach to health. For example, a country's obligation to "respect" and "protect" the right to health requires governments to "refrain from denying or limiting equal access to all persons" and to "ensuring equal access to health care ..." The new genetics can be seen as scientific validation of human equality in that it demonstrates that we all share substantially identical genomes; but it can also be used to foster prejudice and discrimination, and thus to undercut the right to health. This human tendency to create divisions, which at least some people would describe as genetic, is well illustrated by an incident in late 2007 when the co-discoverer of the structure of DNA, James Watson, scandalized the world when he ignorantly told a British newspaper, "I'm inherently gloomy about the prospect of Africa because all our social policies are based on the fact that their intelligence is the same as ours, whereas all the testing says not really."[10]

Watson later apologized and acknowledged that there is no scientific evidence to support his statement about differences in intelligence among races. *Nature* magazine editorialized that Watson's remarks were "rightly ... deemed beyond the pale", but also warned: "There will be important debates in the future as we gain a fuller understanding of the influence of genetics on human attributes and behaviour. Crass comments by Nobel laureates undermine our very ability to debate such issues, and thus damage science itself."[11]

Our superficial perceptions of each other have often fostered racism in the past. Simply defined, racism is "the theory that distinctive human characteristics and abilities are determined by race." The hunt for genes, especially in groups identified by racial classifications, could lead to "genism" (a term not yet officially recognized, but one which could be defined as "the theory that distinctive human characteristics and abilities are determined by genes") based on DNA sequence characteristics with resulting discrimination as pernicious as racism. Watson's ignorant remark was not one of an old-time racist, but of a new-style "genist".

The great hope of human genomics has been that it will scientifically demonstrate that humans are all essentially the same, and that this demonstration will inhibit our penchant for making arbitrary distinctions among humans. And genomics has already accomplished the science part. After the draft of the human genome was announced in 2000, for example, Chris Stringer of London's Natural History Museum observed: "We are all Africans under the skin."[12] The same point was made by other geneticists in different words, one noting that "race is only skin deep"[13] and another, that "there is nothing scientific about race: No genes of any sort pattern along racial lines."[14] Craig Venter, the leader of the private genome mapping effort, concluded: "Race is a social concept, not a scientific one. We all evolved in the last 100 000 years from the same small number of tribes that migrated out of Africa and colonized the world."[15]

This is all to the good, and geneticists deserve high praise for getting this antiracism message out to the public early. Unfortunately, the message of genetics, while undercutting racism, can simultaneously invigorate its evil brother, genism. This is how it works. Eric Lander, the genomics leader from the Massachusetts Institute of Technology noted in 2000 that, although we are all 99.9% genetically identical, that 0.1% of difference is made up of three million spelling variations in our genomes.[16] Each of these genetic variations could be used as a pseudoscientific basis for discrimination based on genetic endowment.

Genome leaders have recognized this, and have called for legislation to prohibit genetic discrimination in employment, health insurance, life insurance, and disability insurance. This is reasonable, but genetic discrimination can only happen if private genetic information is shared – and to protect genetic privacy, we must not only ban genetic discrimination, but also regulate the collection of DNA samples, their analysis, and their storage. There is some irony in the fact that James Watson's genome is one of the few that has been sequenced. After his offensive remarks, an analysis of Watson's own genome was published that disclosed that he has, according to Dr. Kari Stefansson of DeCode Genetics, 16 times the number of genes considered to be of African origin than the average white European, or about the same amount of African DNA that would show up if one great-grandparent were African.[17] This does not, except to a genist, mean that Watson is African – but it should help demonstrate that genes alone tell us very little about the social construct we call race, and little about full-bodied humans.

The WHO's ACHR was right to worry about the proliferation of "DNA banks" and the lack of agreement on how to protect the genetic privacy of those whose DNA is stored and analysed in this context. An especially disturbing example of a human rights violation spurred by genomics is provided by the, now defunct, Human Genome Diversity Project, which sought to collect DNA samples form some 700 of the world's isolated ethnic groups, sometimes referred to as the world's "vanishing tribes". In the project's view, it was more important that science seize the opportunity to collect DNA from these peoples than that any action be taken to actually help the peoples themselves. The indigenous peoples around the world properly and forcefully rejected this project, and insisted that their human rights be placed above this dubious and reductionistic project.[18] Nonetheless, this project has re-emerged in another guise under the rubric of the National Geographic Project and the sponsorship of the *National Geographic*.[19]

It is true that "we are all Africans under the skin." It is also true, nonetheless, that if we decide to search for genetic differences in the 0.5% of our DNA that is different, we will find them and use them against each other. Philosopher Eric Juengst put it well: "No matter how great the potential of population genomics to show our interconnections, if it begins by describing our differences it will inevitably produce scientific wedges to hammer into the social cracks that already divide us."[20]

Preventing genism from taking over where racism left off, by substituting molecular differences for skin colour differences, will not be easy. Two actions, however, seem necessary. First, genetic privacy must be protected.

To help protect an individual's bodily integrity and security, no-one's genes should be analysed without express authorization, and, of course, no "genetic identity cards" should be permitted. Second, to help protect equality and the principle of non-discrimination, pseudoscientific projects that purport to identify genetic differences between "races" should be rejected.

The prospect of genetic genocide

The WHO's ACHR may seem to have spent too much time and emphasis on addressing the use of genetics to "enhance" human beings, specifically by making changes at the embryo level that could produce "better babies". But they were right to highlight this area, and that, although the technique is not currently possible, it is a subject that deserves far wider attention, especially in the human rights community. James Watson, this time from statements he made at a 1998 conference on Engineering the Human Germline, again provides an introduction to our discussion:

> "It seems to me the question we are going to have to face is, what is going to be the least unpleasant? Using abortion to get rid of nasty genes from families? Or developing germline procedures with which … You can go in and get rid of a bad gene … And the other thing, because no one has the guts to say it, if we could make better human beings by knowing how to add genes, why shouldn't we do it? What would be wrong with it? … if you could cure what I feel is a very serious disease – stupidity – it would be a great thing for people who are otherwise going to be born seriously disadvantaged."[21]

Screening genomes to detect differences creates more opportunities for discrimination. Using the new genetics to try to make a "better human" by genetic engineering goes beyond discrimination to elimination by raising the prospect of genetic genocide. This inflammatory language is justified. The project to make a better baby by genetic engineering begins with attempts to "cure" or "prevent" genetic diseases, but will almost inevitably lead to attempts to "improve" or "enhance" genetic characteristics to create the superhuman or posthuman. It is this project that, if successful (a large scientific "if") creates the prospect of genetic genocide as its likely conclusion. This is because, given the history of humankind, it is extremely unlikely that we will see the posthumans as equal in rights and dignity to us, or that they will see us as equals. Instead, it is most likely either that we will see them as a threat to us, and thus seek to imprison or simply kill them before they kill us. Alternatively, the posthuman will come to see us (the garden variety human) as an inferior subspecies without human rights to be enslaved or slaughtered pre-emptively.

It is this potential for genocide based on genetic difference that makes species-altering genetic engineering a potential weapon of mass destruction, and makes the unaccountable genetic engineer a potential bioterrorist. This suggestion has been seen as overblown by some who favour the development of germline genetic alterations, but, given the history of humanity, the burden of proof should be on those who want to try to alter humans, rather than on those who oppose such a move.[22] It has been suggested by others that germline genetics is unnecessary to produce a de facto two species result. James Evans, for example, has noted that simply depriving the poor of personalized genomic medicine "runs the risk of creating a genetically defined underclass which, because of inheriting more than a fair share of disease-susceptibility genes, is unable to afford adequate [medical] care."[23]

What should be done?

Bioethics has been called on to save us from the potential harms of the new genetics, but with its focus on individual decisions made in the context of the doctor-patient relationship, it cannot help us confront either global or species-wide issues. Although bioethics can help, and UNESCO's new Universal Declaration on Bioethics and Human Rights is a step in the right direction of integrating human rights and bioethics, the language and practice of international human rights itself provides the most powerful approach to global governance of the new genetics.

In 2001 I suggested, with my co-authors Lori Andrews and Rosie Isasi, that the threat by cults and others, operating on the margins of human society, to clone a human being created an opportunity for the world to act preventively in ways that have been either extremely difficult or impossible. Specifically, I believed it was reasonable and responsible to suggest that UNESCO's Universal Declaration on the Human Genome and Human Rights, and the overwhelming repulsion of peoples and governments around the world to the plan to clone humans, could be followed by a formal treaty on The Preservation of the Human Species.[24] Such a treaty would ban species-endangering experiments, including cloning and germline genetic alterations. This does not mean that these techniques could never be used, but that no individual or corporation would be given the moral warrant to put the entire human species at risk without a worldwide discussion and a modification in the treaty. To the extent that it is concluded that the fear of genetic genocide is too extreme or overblown, the treaty could be time limited and expire automatically after the human species has gone, for example, 100 years without a genocide.

Species-endangering experiments (including the creation of new genetically-based bioweapons) directly concern all humans and should only be authorized by a body that is representative of everyone on the planet. These are the most important decisions our species will ever make. And they are of special concern to the human rights community. It is not that the human species is perfect the way it is (far from it), or that changes in humanity driven by evolution are not inevitable (they are). Rather it is that to the extent that human rights law is grounded in our understanding of what it means to be human, changing the nature of humanity at least puts at risk our understanding of human rights themselves.

We have a tendency to simply let science take us wherever it will. But science has become so powerful, both in terms of making our lives better and raising the risk of species suicide, that we can no longer abdicate our mutual responsibility to each other as fellow members of the human species.

Conclusion

It is currently completely illusory to believe, either that the new genetics are likely to do more good than harm to people in resource-poor countries, or that bioethics provides useful guidance to deal with genomic research in developing countries. We need a much wider, global framework, and a more inclusive language – human rights is suggested – to both promote social justice and inhibit discrimination. We must work together to promote genetic privacy, prevent the genetic engineering of humans, and promote and protect universal human rights-based on dignity and equality. Without action on the species level, genism based on pseudoscience will eclipse racism as the most destructive disease on the planet.

* Portions of this chapter are adapted from a presentation at the UN World Conference Against Racism, Durban, South Africa, 31 August – 7 September 2001, UNESCO Forum on the Future, and 'Genism, Racism, and the Prospect of Genetic Genocide' 6 *Pacific Ecologist* (2003) 43–45.

1 For example, Maxwell Mehlman, *Wondergenes* (Indiana: Bloomington, 2003).

2 University of Toronto Joint Center for Bioethics, 'Top 10 Biotechnologies for Improving Health in Developing Countries' (Toronto: University of Toronto, 2005).

3 WHO, 'Genomics and World Health: Report of the Advisory Committee on Health Research' (Geneva: WHO, 2002).

4 Ibid., at 169.

5 Ibid., at 122.

6 *Supra* note 2, at 6.

7 Ibid., at 8.

8 Ibid., at 86.

9 *Supra* note 3, at 105.

10 As quoted in Editorial, 'Watson's Folly' 449 *Nature* (2007), at 948.

11 Ibid.; C. Milmo, 'Fury at DNA Pioneer's Theory: Africans are Less Intelligent than Westerners', *The Independent*, 17 October 2007, at 24.

12 As quoted in 'Genetics and Geneology: We are All Africans', *The Times* (London), 17 November 2000, at 1.

13 Natalie Angier, 'Race is only Skin Deep', *New York Times*, 22 August 2000.

14 Sharon Begley, 'Race is only Skin Deep So It Isn't a Basis for Health Recommendations', *Wall Street Journal Europe*, 1 August 2003, at 1.

15 Natalie Angier, 'Race is an Unscientific Concept, Experts Say', *New York Times*, 30 August 2000.

16 Ibid.

17 J. Schwartz, 'DNA Pioneer's Genome Blurs Race Lines', *New York Times*, 12 December 2007, A24. It should be noted that scientists now believe there is closer to a 0.5 percent variation than a 0.1 percent variation in human genomes.

18 National Research Council, *Evaluating Human Genetic Diversity* (Washington, D.C.: National Research Council, 1997).

19 For more on this project see https://www3.natio nalgeographic.com/genographic/.

20 E. Juengst, 'Groups as Gatekeepers to Genomic Research: Conceptually Confusing, Morally Hazardous, and Practically Useless' 8 *Kennedy Institute of Ethics Journal* (1998) 183–200.

21 Quoted in Gregory Stock and John Campbell (eds.) *Engineering the Human Germline: An Exploration of the Science and Ethics of Altering the Genes We Pass to Our Children* (New York: Oxford University Press, 2000), at 79. Watson has also consistently argued against any sort of international agreement on genetic engineering: For example, "I think it would be complete disaster to try and get an international agreement. I just can't imagine anything more stifling. You end up with the lowest possible denominator. Agreement among all the different religious groups would be impossible. About all they'd agree upon is that they should allow us to breathe air … I think our hope is to stay away from regulations and laws whenever possible." (Ibid., at 87).

22 G. J. Annas, L. Andrews and R. Isasi, 'Protecting the Endangered Human: Toward an International Treaty Prohibiting Cloning and Inheritable Alterations' 28 *American Journal of Law & Medicine*, (2002) 151–178. Updated in George J. Annas, *American Bioethics: Crossing Human Rights and Health Law Boundaries* (New York, Oxford University Press, 2005), at 43–58.

23 J. P. Evans, 'Health Care in the Age of Genetic Medicine' 298 *Journal of the American Medical Association* (2007), at 2670–72.

24 *Supra* note 22, and see George J. Annas, 'The ABCs of Global Governance of Embryonic Stem Cell Research: Arbitrage, Bioethics and Cloning' 39 *New England Law Review* (2005), at 489–500; and R. Isasi and G. J. Annas, 'Arbitrage, Bioethics, and Cloning: The ABCs of Gestating a United Nations Cloning Convention' 35 *Case Western Reserve Journal of International Law* (2003), at 397–414.

06

MULTILATERAL INSTITUTIONS AND RESPONSES

Governance and the Response to AIDS: Lessons for Development and Human Rights

Peter Piot, Susan Timberlake and Jason Sigurdson

Because of how Human Immunodeficiency Virus (HIV) is transmitted, whom it affects, and the devastation it wreaks, Acquired Immunodeficiency Syndrome (AIDS) has challenged societies to confront some of their greatest prejudices, fears and injustices. These relate not only to the obvious issues of sex, sexual orientation and drug use, but also to issues frequently kept under the table – discrimination, gender inequality and economic inequality. AIDS has challenged the international community to reconsider how it assists, and governments how they want to be assisted. It has challenged us all to think more deeply about the "right to health", both in terms of its critical dependence on the realization of other human rights, and our recent refusal to continue to accept the health-related disparities between high and low-income countries. It has challenged how development work is done, with communities no longer willing to wait for discretionary handouts but demanding to be in the centre and at the table, advocating, designing and delivering the HIV prevention, treatment and care that enable them to live, as well as reduce the burden of illness. The challenges of HIV and AIDS have meant that communities, nations, and the international community must learn how to do governance differently, both governing and being governed, in ways that produce results and protect, respect and fulfil human rights.

What is governance? Broadly defined, it is the capacity to regulate oneself and/or a community – a large one, as in international; a medium one, as in national; and a small one, as in local. In human rights terms, it is the capacity to regulate oneself while fulfilling the human rights principles of responsibility, accountability, transparency, non-discrimination, participation and inclusion. Perhaps one of the very few "silver linings" of the AIDS cloud has been that the scale and nature of the disease has required the international community, governments and local communities (and individuals) to govern themselves differently.

What are the elements of this "new" governance? They are:

1. An empowered civil society with the necessary skills and resources for advocacy, influence and programming, demanding accountability but also accountable to the broader communities they represent and serve;
2. Strong national leadership, processes and institutions for managing a participatory, multi-sectoral, human rights-based and evidence-informed AIDS response; and
3. An international system that is responsive to and aligns behind national priorities, advancing shared international commitments to AIDS, health, development and human rights and producing results for those most affected.

Governance has advanced in the context of AIDS due to the complexity of both the causes and consequences of the epidemic. We have learned in the response that there is no "quick fix" or "one solution", though there continue to be many who believe these exist. Responding effectively requires the coordinated and long-term commitment and action of many people and institutions, within countries and internationally. It requires leadership and the courage to speak out on difficult subjects. It requires a commitment to evidence and effectiveness over ideology. It demands the active participation of people living with HIV in all decisions that affect their lives and their communities. It requires that we address the deep structural determinants of vulnerability, as well as the broad range of impacts on individuals, communities and nations.

How we have arrived at where we are today in governing the response to AIDS has taken enormous struggle, and our greatest achievements are under threat. As countries move towards their 2010 targets on universal access to HIV prevention, treatment, care and support, and intensify efforts to reach the Millennium Development Goals, we should take stock of what has been achieved in building community, national and global capacity for governance in the AIDS response. These achievements have profound implications for human rights and development broadly, and if carried forward with new partners and expanded coalitions, have the potential to transform the face of international assistance and development to empower the poor and vulnerable to overcome the many injustices that threaten health, life and human potential,[1] including and beyond AIDS.

Governance and the community response

Civil society was the first to respond to the early signs of AIDS at the outset of the 1980s. It was ad hoc and far from a "governed" or coordinated response – rather it comprised communities trying to understand and cope with what they were seeing and experiencing. In the United States and Europe, important organizations like Gay Men's Health Crisis, the San Francisco AIDS Foundation, Terrence Higgins Trust, and AIDES, were formed to provide care, support and prevention information for those affected and infected. In Uganda, the community came together and formed the AIDS Support Organization (TASO) in 1987 which became a model for community response.

Community organizations were faced with more than just the health consequences of AIDS. They were up against the public fear and moralizing that was spreading as fast as HIV itself. People living with, or suspected of having, HIV faced discrimination in the workplace, in hospitals, with landlords, and within their families. (They still do today.) Community organizations built their work – and their own governance capacity – necessarily running not only care and support activities but also a growing advocacy agenda, based on the needs and rights of their members that many either wanted to jail or forget. People living with, and affected by, HIV, worked with determination and courage to ensure that they would not be pushed aside or left unheard. In 1983, a group gathered in the United States as the "advisory committee of people with AIDS" produced the Denver Principles. This group condemned attempts to label people living with HIV as "victims" or to scapegoat them. The Principles articulated the right to quality treatment and care, as well as the responsibility that people have to their sexual partners, and asserted the right to participate in AIDS forums and be involved as decision-makers.[2] The Denver Principles were an important

precursor to the formal adoption of the principle of the Greater Involvement of People Living with HIV, recognized at the Paris AIDS Summit in
1994.[3] Many challenges remain to make the "GIPA principle" meaningful
and real, but it nonetheless represents a radical departure from treating
ill people as passive victims and recipients of charity. GIPA is a major human rights and health accomplishment, embracing the principles of non-
discrimination, participation, and inclusion. At the same time, it has demonstrated that empowered actors are the ones who can best improve their
health and that of their communities.

From the start, the greatest contribution to the response to AIDS, and
the most effective force in calling for accountability, has been from civil society. Not only was "taking the lead" a necessity in terms of dealing with indifference on the part of government, it was also needed to challenge calls
for punitive, "law and order" responses that appear to "get tough on AIDS",
but in reality only exacerbate stigma and do nothing to address risk, vulnerability or impact. Countries imprisoned people living with HIV, segregated them, and adopted restrictions on entry and residence in a vain attempt to keep HIV outside their borders, even if it was already clear that
the virus was widespread, hard to detect, and beyond public health "con-
tainment" strategies. Community mobilization and coalition-building was
supported by positive and principled leadership, coming from leaders such
as Justice Michael Kirby, who warned against simplistic solutions in the
fight against AIDS, as well as the threat of a new virus – "HUL: Highly useless laws."[4] Indeed, the solutions would be complex. Civil society took up
care and support, prevention education, issues of stigma and discrimination, and pushed their governments for more leadership and more action.
Groups like the Treatment Action Campaign in South Africa have shown
how community mobilization, treatment literacy and strategic litigation
can come together to spur action, even in an environment of denial.[5]

Governance and the international response

In the early days, it became clear that AIDS was more than an isolated
phenomenon and would require shared understanding and an international response. But on what principles should this international response
be based? The first meeting to assess the global AIDS situation was convened in November 1983, and marked the beginning of the World Health
Organization's (WHO) surveillance on AIDS. Four years later, in 1987, WHO

Director-General Halfden Mahler appointed Jonathan Mann to establish the Global Programme on AIDS. Mann quickly realized that discriminatory and punitive measures would not result in protection of public health; rather they would alienate and lose the very people on whose behaviour change public health depended. Thus, the Programme was founded on the need for a human rights-based approach to AIDS.

Mann actively engaged political leaders through the World Health Assembly and other fora to spur national commitment and action. Mann accompanied Mahler to New York to address the United Nations General Assembly on the issue of AIDS in October 1987. At that session, UN Secretary-General Javier Pérez de Cuéllar stated that AIDS "cannot be prevented from crossing borders, and any effort by a country to ... isolate itself from all others offers only a delusion of protection. ... We must unequivocally establish that our battle is against AIDS, and not against people ... Those who suffer should not be made to suffer more. Those endangered by illness should not be penalized by society."[6] The General Assembly adopted a resolution calling on WHO to continue to "direct and co-ordinate the urgent global battle against AIDS."[7] A few months later the World Health Assembly adopted a resolution on discrimination and AIDS,[8] calling on WHO Member States "to protect the human rights and dignity of HIV-infected people and people with AIDS, and of members of population groups, and to avoid discriminatory action against and stigmatization of them in the provision of services, employment and travel." The Global Programme supported inter-country conferences to raise awareness, and national AIDS committees were set up in more than 100 countries. WHO supported training of laboratory workers and assisted a limited number of countries to mobilize support for three to five-year AIDS plans. Despite these gains, generating positive political leadership was difficult, given the need to confront major taboos. The Global Programme on AIDS still had far to go to cultivate the critical mass of political will and donor support to make a significant breakthrough.[9]

It was increasingly clear that an expanding AIDS epidemic quickly reveals political and administrative weak points at national and community levels.[10] The range of entry points to engage in order to prevent the transmission of HIV, as well as the range of impacts in highly affected countries, illustrated that AIDS was more than a health issue – being effective meant tackling the epidemic through health, education, employment, social security, law and law enforcement, public administration and finance. This

complexity was in part the motivation for the creation of the Joint United Nations Programme on HIV/AIDS – UNAIDS – in 1996. Originally com-
prising six UN programmes and agencies (now ten),[11] UNAIDS was to mar-
shal the diverse perspectives and strengths of different UN programmes
and agencies. It was also unique in the history of the UN that the UNAIDS
governing body – the UNAIDS Programme Coordinating Board – includes
seats at the table for civil society, meaning that people directly affected by
HIV are part of the governance of the Joint Programme itself. In 2001, at
the creation of the Global Fund to Fight AIDS, Tuberculosis and Malaria,
the need for broad engagement and partnership was also recognized with
inclusion on the Global Fund Board of representatives of donor and recipient governments, non-governmental organizations, the private sector and
affected communities.

The early years of UNAIDS were largely focused on advocacy, working
with and supporting governments and civil society, bringing an ever-great-
er array of partners on board in the response, and bringing HIV out of the
shadows. From its inception, UNAIDS engaged with the United Nations
Commission on Human Rights (succeeded by the Human Rights Council),
urging its members to recognize how critical it was, and is, to address the
intersections between lack of human rights protection and vulnerability to
HIV. UNAIDS also urged governments to take steps to realize the right of
women to be free from sexual violence; the rights of children and adolescents to have access to age-appropriate sexual education, including about
HIV; the right to care and support for children orphaned by AIDS; and the
rights of prisoners to HIV prevention information and services.

In response to a call from the Commission,[12] UNAIDS, together with the
Office of the UN High Commissioner for Human Rights, hosted the Second
International Consultation on HIV/AIDS and Human Rights in September
1996, bringing together governments, national AIDS programmes, people
living with HIV, human rights activists, and UN agencies and programmes.
International experts in the consultation produced the International Guidelines on HIV/AIDS and Human Rights.[13] Though controversial because they
address the most difficult issues head-on, the Guidelines have become a foundational resource for national responses, outlining concrete steps states can
take to protect human rights in the context of AIDS, and realize the human
rights of those vulnerable to and living with HIV. While the Guidelines address critical human rights issues, they also fundamentally advocate for good
governance – an effective, transparent and participatory national framework

(Guideline 1), community involvement in all phases of programme design, implementation and evaluation (Guideline 2), law reform and protection of vulnerable groups (Guidelines 3, 4 and 5), access to legal support services (Guideline 7), creation of a supportive and enabling environment for women, children and vulnerable groups (Guideline 8) and support to human rights monitoring and enforcement mechanisms (Guideline 11).

As advocacy and partnerships expanded on many fronts, the political environment began to change significantly around 2000. That year, the United Nations Security Council held a session focused on AIDS – the first time it addressed a health issue – confirming that AIDS was a challenge of global proportions, belonging to foreign policy as well as domestic agendas. In 2001, Heads of State of the Organization of African Unity (OAU, now the African Union) issued a consensus declaration on HIV/AIDS, tuberculosis and other diseases. At that OAU summit, then United Nations Secretary-General Kofi Annan called for a "war chest" of USD 7 to 10 billion to fight AIDS and other diseases linked to poverty, noting that new lifesaving medicines for people living with HIV were out of reach for more than 90% of the people who needed them.[14] These developments were the beginning of a new type of governance to address a health issue at the international level. Governments, with the UN and regional organizations in support, were coming to realize their responsibility and accountability for the AIDS epidemics in their midst.

From international commitment to accelerated country action

The United Nations General Assembly Special Session on HIV/AIDS (UN-GASS) followed shortly after, in June 2001, and was a defining moment in global and national political commitment to the AIDS response. What made it such a defining moment was not the event itself, but rather the intensification of national commitment to programmatic action; the significant increase in funding both internationally and nationally that followed; and the issuance of a set of time-bound targets – a framework of accountability – in the form of the Declaration of Commitment on HIV/AIDS[15] (2001). Agreeing to report on their delivery under the Declaration of Commitment and using the Guidelines on Construction of Core Indicators[16] developed by UNAIDS, 103 countries (55%) submitted country progress reports in 2003, increasing to 137 countries (72%) in 2005, and 147 countries in 2007. Supported by the process, civil society has participated actively in the development of official government reports or undertaken independent "shadow reports" on country progress.

The Declaration of Commitment has provided an important accountability framework in the context of a comprehensive AIDS response. It includes commitments regarding HIV prevention, treatment, care and support, but also commitments regarding leadership, financial resources, and specific commitments to strengthen and enforce legislation, regulations and other measures to eliminate all forms of discrimination against people living with HIV, as well as to protect the rights of women and members of vulnerable groups in the context of the epidemic.[17]

The reports under the Declaration of Commitment are both a powerful incentive and an important resource for good governance. It has been a goal of UNAIDS to support countries to be able to report, that is, to develop monitoring and evaluation capacity; to disaggregate data by sex, age and marital status; to track funding receipts and expenditures; and to evaluate programme effectiveness. The content of the reports highlights progress as well as gaps, nationally and globally. On financing, funding for AIDS-related activities in low and middle-income countries reached USD 10 billion in 2007 – a 12% increase over 2006 and a ten-fold increase within a decade. Governments have been remarkably forthcoming on some of the gaps. On issues of legal protections for people living with HIV and vulnerable groups, one-third of countries report that they still lack such protections. 57% of countries also report that they have laws and policies that impede access to AIDS services.[18] Usually these concern laws that criminalize homosexuality, drug use and sex work, requiring governments to consider the larger impact of such laws. While we may recognize successes, there is still much to be done.

It is significant that in 2008 "*universal access* to HIV prevention, treatment, care and support" is the focus of our collective efforts.[19] It was not always the case. AIDS has taught us that community and international activism is essential if we are to make progress on human rights and good governance. It was activism that pushed the G8 group of countries to make universal access to HIV treatment a goal of the international community,[20] and continued activism that led to the commitment being endorsed at the 2005 World Summit[21] and at the High Level Meeting on HIV (2006) in the Political Declaration on HIV/AIDS.[22]

While the 2001 UNGASS was significant, there was still scepticism among many officials about the ability to make HIV treatment available in low and middle-income countries. In 2001, scarcely 200 000 people were on antiretroviral therapy, and nearly exclusively in high-income countries, with the exception of Brazil – a country which demonstrated exceptional leadership by making treatment available as of 1996. At the UNGASS, all donors (except for France and Luxemburg), all African countries and all Asian countries were opposed to mentioning the words "antiretroviral therapy"and to including a target or a goal on treatment for people living with HIV. After a night of debate in the UN General Assembly, all that went into the Declaration of Commitment on the subject was vague and compromised language. Governments and donors pushed back against the notion that people living with HIV in low and middle-income countries were citizens "worth the cost", and that the rights to life, health and development include breaking out of the "structural violence"[23] that makes us all accept limited funding to save lives (though not to take lives – given the annual USD 1.2 trillion expenditure on war).[24] Civil society and communities of activists, on the other hand, pushed us past this "governance block" into greater responsibility, accountability and non-discrimination. Without their efforts, many of the estimated 3 million people currently on treatment in low and middle-income countries would not be alive today.

Increased resources and greater commitment fundamentally changed the nature of the response at country level. While positive, it also made assistance – and governance – increasingly challenging with great problems involving lack of clarity about responsibilities and roles, donor priorities and processes displacing national ones, and proliferation of reporting lines and management systems. Whose response to AIDS was it anyway? The extremity of the situation forced governments and the international community to develop a new form of AIDS response. This has taken the form of increased harmonization and cooperation under the banner of the "Three Ones": One national AIDS framework, one national AIDS coordinating authority, and one national monitoring and evaluation system.[25] The Three Ones is about government taking responsibility for its response to AIDS and being held accountable for it. It is about donors and the UN system recognizing and supporting government responsibility and accountability. Finally, it is about ensuring that all those responding to AIDS are brought within a recognized framework, both to benefit from, and add to, that framework, and hence contribute coherently to the response. Again, it is where the response to AIDS has interwoven human rights principles into a new fabric of governance.

This fabric of governance also has direct and indirect pay-offs for human rights protection and realization in the context of AIDS. The direct pay-offs involve institutionalizing an inclusive and participatory approach through one national AIDS framework. When there is a national AIDS framework that is truly multi-sectoral (including a programme of work addressing law, law enforcement, discrimination, access to justice, gender equality), a coordinating authority that works closely with ministries of justice and interior, national human rights institutions, and networks of people living with HIV, and a monitoring and evaluation framework that disaggregates data by relevant categories, and includes monitoring of stigma and discrimination, then governance is greatly strengthened towards human rights ends.

The indirect pay-off of harmonization and alignment for human rights is about producing results for those most affected ("making the money work for human rights", so to speak).[26] It requires considerable investment to strengthen epidemiologic and behavioural surveillance, monitoring and evaluation systems – all parts of good governance in the AIDS response – to ensure that evidence-informed programming is responding to the dynamics of the local epidemic (the "know your epidemic and response" approach) and hence addressing the health and the human rights of those most vulnerable to and affected by HIV. All of this goes to responsiveness to national priorities – with the international community having to let governments take the lead, but in the context of commitments that all governments have undertaken. The devil is in the details, of course, but this is where we need to be going. As noted in an article by Kent Buse and colleagues, "Improved systems of mutual accountability are required to ensure that governments and donors undertake the required actions to meet previously stated commitments if Universal Access is to become more than the latest rhetoric emanating from the international AIDS community."[27]

Future governance challenges

While we have good reason to celebrate how the response to AIDS has helped transform and improve the way we respond to critical health, development and governance issues, there are those who want to reorient this approach. First, the rights-based approach to AIDS is (again) under threat by those who advocate a top-down, punitive approach: Mandatory testing, mandatory disclosure, criminalization of HIV transmission, criminalization of key populations at risk, deportation of HIV-positive migrants, stigma, shame, and so on. If these troubling approaches take hold, we not only risk losing effective responses to the epidemic, but also participation, inclusion and accountability for all, i.e. non-discriminatory responses.[28]

Hard-won gains in the response are also under threat by those who want to "put HIV in its place".[29] Rather than calling for all health and development challenges to receive the same level of concern, funding and programmatic attention as AIDS has received, there are those who want to shift to health-system strengthening and reduce AIDS funding they view as "disproportionate" (read: Too much) vis-à-vis other diseases. This is not a time for infighting on how to divide up the pie – it is time to push for a much bigger pie, in a world that in 2007 spent only USD 103.7 billion on official development assistance.[30] The fact remains that we are still far short of halting and turning back the epidemic, nor are we at a place where we can say that the estimated 33 million people living with HIV around the world today can be assured of sustainable access to the prevention, treatment, care and support they will need over the course of their lives.

We need to be clear that, as we head towards the 2015 target for achieving the Millennium Development Goals, we do not undo the achievements of the AIDS response, including in governance, but rather we put all health, human rights, and development challenges in their rightful place on the global governance agenda. That means mobilization of all those who can contribute to solutions (especially those whose rights are not being realized), and the promotion of leadership, responsibility and accountability of all partners.

This will require governments and donors to learn another lesson from the response to AIDS: Responses to health and other social issues must seek to address as much as possible the structural factors driving these. These structural factors usually involve a failure to realize or protect human rights which is manifested by a failure of a social system. Strengthening health systems is critical for improving health, including in relation to AIDS. It is in fact a part of realizing the highest attainable standard of health, but it will not happen without similar attention, as has been the case with AIDS, to government and donor responsibility and accountability in terms of national budget allocations, development assistance, and the imperative to attend to the most vulnerable and disadvantaged. Nor will it solve all the health problems of the users of the health systems if they are not empowered to engage in, and sustain, health-seeking behaviour and healthy lifestyles.

Expanding capacity for good governance in AIDS and beyond

Ensuring effective and human rights-based governance of the response to AIDS will require significant investment in a new generation of leadership – from health professionals, to civil society, to civil servants, to educators, to scientists, to lawyers and judges, to parliamentarians – with the knowledge, commitment and skills needed to take on the diverse and complex development and human rights challenges that sustain vulnerability to HIV infection and impact. It will also require new coalitions facing common challenges and shared opportunities – for example, in the research and development field, finding new mechanisms to reward innovation in the public and private sectors.[31] Perhaps most importantly, it means that civil society will need much greater capacity and means to translate human rights into concrete demands.[32]

This means more programmatic attention to supporting human rights and access to justice in the response to AIDS, including for example "know your rights" campaigns, provision of legal aid, campaigns against harmful gender norms and violence against women, campaigns against stigma and discrimination, and programmes working with police and health care workers in terms of non-discrimination, and the need to ensure access to HIV information and services with protection of informed consent and confidentiality.[33] Making sure that human rights are addressed in more programmatic terms will require the human rights community to engage more effectively in costing, budgeting, monitoring and evaluation, ensuring that human rights obligations are more than an advocacy agenda. This is an essential skill set and an important contribution to the governance of a truly comprehensive response to AIDS.

Effective governance to halt and turn back the AIDS epidemic will require vision and resolve on some of the most difficult and protracted development challenges. Expanded partnerships with development and human rights practitioners beyond the health field will be critical. We need to force a change in mindset, translating the vision of a life in dignity outlined in the Universal Declaration of Human Rights 60 years ago into the realities of communities and individuals. Just as we see a functioning justice system as essential for the rule of law, and fair electoral systems as a fundamental for upholding democracy, so too must we see health, education, and social insurance systems as core institutions for the protection of the economic, social and cultural rights of all.[34] And as we have learned in the response to AIDS, all of this will require resources: more high-income countries reaching the target of 0.7% of their Gross Domestic Product for development assistance, more low and middle-income countries investing greater domestic resources in health, education, employment, gender equality and social programmes.

Conclusions

The response to AIDS to date has shown that effective governance and real results for those most affected requires leadership at all levels of government, in multiple sectors. Equally important, it requires sufficient resources and an active and empowered civil society, all in a broad framework of accountability for the health and human rights of everyone. Where the response has moved the furthest, it is because civil society has been empowered to claim their rights and push for accountability for human rights commitments – some of the most important ingredients for good governance.

As a health, development and human rights challenge, the greatest contribution of the response to AIDS has been putting people in the centre. It is not only the space for people to speak to the urgency of the situation, but one where they can affirm their needs and rights, and organize the resources of their community and beyond to respond effectively – honouring the commitments made in the Declaration of Commitment on HIV/AIDS. It is a response that ultimately must have its foundations in the Universal Declaration of Human Rights and two Covenants on human rights[35] that together form the International Bill of Rights. This is what the art of governance must be, in the domestic context but also internationally, and beyond the world of AIDS.

Arriving at where we are today has taken enormous struggle. We must take steps to ensure that our greatest achievements in addressing AIDS are not only protected, but built upon. As countries move towards their 2010 targets on universal access to HIV prevention, treatment, care and support, and as they intensify efforts to reach the Millennium Development Goals, we need to build a new generation of leadership at community, national and global levels dedicated to maintaining and strengthening the response to AIDS, and all health and development challenges. This is not the time to reduce, but the time to expand, taking international development and human rights to the next level in ways that empower the poor and vulnerable to overcome all threats to health, life and human potential, including and beyond AIDS.

1   Mark Heywood, 'Human Rights – do we believe in them and what if we do?', Speech to the Civil Society Hearing of the High Level Meeting on AIDS, *Action for Universal Access 2010: Myths and Realities, 10 June 2008*, available online at http://webcast.un.org/ramgen/ondemand/ga/62/2008/ga080610am1.rm?start=00:07:10&end=00:13:56.

2   The Denver Principles (1983), available online at http://data.unaids.org/pub/ExternalDocument/2007/gipa1983denverprinciples_en.pdf.

3   The Paris Declaration (1994), Paris AIDS Summit, 1 December 2004, available online at http://data.unaids.org/pub/ExternalDocument/2007/theparisdeclaration_en.pdf.

4   Justice Michael Kirby, 'The New AIDS Virus-Ineffective and Unjust Laws', 1 *Journal of Acquired Immune Deficiency Syndromes* (1998).

5   Zackie Achmat and Julian Simcock, 'Combining Prevention, Treatment and Care: Lessons from South Africa', 21(4) *AIDS* (2007) 511–520.

6   'General Assembly pledges support for war against AIDS', 25(1) *UN Chronicle* (1988) 30–33.

7   'Prevention and control of acquired immunodeficiency syndrome (AIDS)', United Nations General Assembly Resolution 42/8, 26 October 1987.

8   'Avoidance of discrimination in relation to HIV-infected people and people with AIDS', World Health Assembly Resolution 41/24, Geneva, 13 May 1988.

9   Michael Merson, 'The HIV-AIDS Pandemic at 25 – The Global Response', 354(23), *New England Journal of Medicine* (2006) 2414–2417.

10 Peter Piot, Sarah Russell and Heidi Larson, 'Good Politics, Bad Politics: The Experience of AIDS', 97(11) *American Journal of Public Health* (2007) 1934–1936.

11 At its founding, UNAIDS was comprised of United Nations Development Programme (UNDP), the United Nations Children's Fund (UNICEF), the United Nations Population Fund (UNFPA), the World Health Organization (WHO), the United Nations Educational, Scientific and Cultural Organization (UNESCO) and the World Bank. The Office of the United Nations High Commissioner for Refugees (UNHCR), the World Food Programme (WFP), the United Nations Office on Drugs and Crime (UNODC) and International Labour Organization (ILO) have joined as co-sponsors, bringing the total to ten.

12 Commission on Human Rights, Fifty-Second Session, Resolution 1996/43, 19 April 1996.

13 UNAIDS and OHCHR, *International Guidelines on HIV/AIDS and Human Rights: 2006 Consolidated Version* (Geneva: UNAIDS, 2006), available online at http://data.unaids.org/Publications/IRC-pub07/jc1252-internguidelines_en.pdf.

14 Kofi Annan, Speech to the African Union, 26 April 2001, Abuja, Nigeria.

15 *Declaration of Commitment on HIV/AIDS* (2001), UN Document A/RES/S-26/2, available online at http://www.un.org/ga/aids/docs/aress262.pdf.

16 UNAIDS, *Monitoring the Declaration of Commitment on HIV/AIDS: Guidelines on Construction of Core Indicators – 2008 Reporting* (Geneva: UNAIDS, 2007) available online at http://data.unaids.org/pub/Report/2007/jc1318_core_indicators_manual_en.pdf.

17 *Declaration of Commitment on HIV/AIDS*, paras. 58–61.

18 *Declaration of Commitment on HIV/AIDS and Political Declaration on HIV/AIDS: Midway to the Millennium Development Goals*, Report of the United Nations Secretary-General, 2008, UN Document A/62/780.

19 See notes 20 to 22 below.

20 G8 Gleneagles Communique on Africa, 6–8 July 2005, available online at http://collections.europarchive.org/tna/20080205132101/www.fco.gov.uk/Files/kfile/PostG8_Gleneagles_Communique,0.pdf.

21 2005 World Summit Outcome, United Nations General Assembly Resolution 60/1, available online at http://www.un.org/summit2005/documents.html.

22 United Nations General Assembly Resolution 60/262, available online at http://data.unaids.org/pub/Report/2006/20060615_HLM_Political Declaration_ARES60262_en.pdf.

23 Paul Farmer, *Pathologies of Power: Health, Human Rights, and the New War on the Poor* (Berkeley: University of California Press, 2005).

24 Reuters, 'Global military spending hits USD 1.2 trillion – study', 11 June 2007, available online at http://www.alertnet.org/thenews/newsdesk/L11802421.htm.

25 In the 2005 World Summit Outcome, Governments committed themselves to "working actively to implement the 'Three Ones' principles in all countries, including by ensuring that multiple institutions and international partners all work under one agreed HIV/AIDS framework that provides the basis for coordinating the work of all partners, with one national AIDS coordinating authority having a broad-based multisectoral mandate, and under one agreed country-level monitoring and evaluation system …".

26 Considerable work has been done on issues of human rights and aid effectiveness, including by the Development Assistance Committee of the Organization for Economic Co-operation and Development (OECD/DAC). See for example the 'Action-oriented Policy Paper on Human Rights and Development', OECD Document DCD/DAC(2007)15/FINAL, available online at http://www.danidadevforum.um.dk/NR/rdonlyres/CB3847BF-E2F6-4076-B3C3-BF7A7D467761/0/DACAOPPen.pdf. See also Office of the UN High Commissioner for Human Rights, *Frequently Asked Questions on a Human Rights-Based Approach to Development Cooperation* (New York and Geneva: OHCHR, 2006), available online at http://www.ohchr.org/Documents/Publications/FAQen.pdf.

27 Kent Buse, Michel Sidibe, Desmond Whyms, Ini Huijts and Steven Jensen, *Scaling-up the HIV/AIDS Response: From Alignment and Harmonization to Mutual Accountability*, (London: Overseas Development Institute, 2006), available online at http://www.odi.org.uk/publications/briefing/bp_aug06_hivscalingup.pdf.

28 Justice Edwin Cameron, 'Opening remarks and recap of previous day', UNAIDS Secretariat and UNDP International Consultation on the Criminalization of HIV Transmission, Geneva, 2 November 2007, available online at http://data.un aids.org/pub/Presentation/2007/20071112_edwin _cameron_remarks_en.pdf.

29 For example, see Roger England, 'Are we spending too much on HIV?', 334(7589) *British Medical Journal* (2007) 344, available online at http://www.bmj.com/cgi/content/extract/334/7589/344.

30 See OECD, 'Debt Relief is down: Other ODA rises slightly', available online at http://www.oecd.org/document/8/0,3343,en_2649_34447_40381960_1_1_1_1,00.html.

31 Commission on Intellectual Property Rights, Innovation and Public Health, *Public Health, Innovation and Intellectual Property Rights: report of the Commission on Intellectual Property Rights, Innovation and Public Health* (Geneva: World Health Organization, 2006), available online at http://www.who.int/intellectualproperty/documents/thereport/ENPublicHealthReport.pdf.

32 Joint United Nations Programme on HIV/AIDS and the Canadian HIV/AIDS Legal Network, *Courting Rights: Case Studies in Litigating the Human Rights of People Living with HIV* (Geneva: UNAIDS, 2006), available online at http://data.unaids.org/pub/Report/2006/jc1189-courtingrights_en.pdf.

33 UNAIDS Reference Group on HIV and Human Rights, 'Statement on Human Rights & Universal Access to HIV Prevention, Treatment, Care & Support', 6 June 2008, available online at http://data.unaids.org/pub/BaseDocument/2008/20080606_rghr_statement_universalaccess_en.pdf.

34 Paul Hunt, 'Report of the Special Rapporteur on the right of everyone to the enjoyment of the highest attainable standard of physical and mental health', 31 January 2008, UN Document A/HRC/7/11.

35 International Covenant on Economic, Social and Cultural Rights (1966) and the International Covenant on Civil and Political Rights (1966).

Human Rights Implications of Governance Responses to Public Health Emergencies: The Case of Major Infectious Disease Outbreaks

Gian Luca Burci and Riikka Koskenmäki*

Introduction

At the Fiftieth Anniversary of the Universal Declaration of Human Rights in December 1998, the Director-General of the World Health Organization (WHO) stated that "health security is a notion which encompasses many of the rights enlisted in the [Universal] Declaration", including the right "to live and work in an environment where known health risks are controlled."[1] Only a few years later, the multi-country outbreak of severe acute respiratory syndrome (SARS) in 2003, and the looming possibility of a catastrophic outbreak of pandemic influenza, prompted unprecedented attention to the threat of worldwide spread of emerging and re-emerging infectious diseases. These developments underlined the fact that an individual's health security must be founded upon global health security.[2]

The rapid international spread of SARS highlighted the insufficiency of domestic measures to tackle diseases that recognize no borders.[3] It also revealed the lack of preparedness of many countries, both developed and developing, to address large-scale public health emergencies.[4] Increased recognition of the need for an effective international prevention and control mechanism led to the revision of the WHO International Health

Regulations (IHR) in 2005.[5] The IHR are the key international legal instrument designed to help protect all states from international public health risks and emergencies.

This chapter discusses human rights implications of selected governance responses, at both national and international levels, to public health emergencies. It focuses on major infectious disease outbreaks with potential to spread internationally, and on the IHR as the main international instrument for their control. While multiple state and non-state actors may be involved in responses to public health emergencies, this discussion focuses on responses by states at the national and international levels.

International human rights bodies and scholars have studied the limitations that can be imposed on the rights and freedoms of individuals for the purpose of controlling infectious diseases.[6] There has not been a comparable level of scrutiny regarding the impact of national and international disease prevention and control measures on the right to the highest attainable standard of health (hereafter "the right to health").[7] This chapter seeks to further understanding of such impact and links. For the purpose of this contribution, we will use as a normative reference for the right to health Article 12 of the International Covenant on Economic, Social and Cultural Rights (ICESCR),[8] as clarified by the Committee on Economic, Social and Cultural Rights in its General Comment No. 14 of 4 July 2000 (hereafter "General Comment").[9]

Human rights implications of governments' responses at the national level

States have the duty to take measures to prevent and control epidemic and endemic diseases. This obligation exists under Article 12 of the ICESCR, as a step to achieve the full realization of the right to health, as well as under the IHR.[10] Disease control requires epidemiological surveillance, implementation of immunization programmes and other disease control strategies, including pharmaceutical and non-pharmaceutical interventions during outbreaks. In addition to activities at the national level, disease control requires cooperation with other states and international agencies.[11]

Preparing for public health threats of unknown origin, such as SARS or Ebola hemorrhagic fever, is however particularly challenging since pharmaceutical interventions may not be available, at least during the first stages of the outbreak. Even when medication is available, states may face difficult questions such as ensuring access to treatment and prioritizing scarce resources in the face of widespread and acute needs of their populations. Non-pharmaceutical interventions, mostly applied in health emergencies where medication is not available (e.g. during the SARS outbreak) include testing and screening; notification and reporting of cases; mandatory medical examinations; social distancing;[12] isolation of persons with infectious conditions; and contact tracing and quarantine of persons who have been exposed to a public health risk.[13]

The widespread use of these measures during the SARS outbreak[14] and related advice by WHO,[15] drew renewed attention to the challenge of striking the proper balance between the protection of public health on the one hand and respect for individual rights and freedoms on the other.[16] It is well established that states are entitled to limit the exercise of certain human rights, or to derogate from some of their human rights obligations in particular circumstances. In serious communicable disease outbreaks, for example, states are permitted to apply health measures that may "limit" or "restrict" the right to freedom of movement (in case of isolation or quarantine), the right to physical integrity (in case of compulsory testing, screening, examination and treatment), or the right to privacy (in case of compulsory contact tracing or patient retrieval), under certain conditions.[17] The Siracusa Principles provide guidance concerning the question of when interference with human rights may be justified in order to achieve a public health goal. The Principles make clear that any limitation must be provided for by law and carried out in accordance with law; serve a legitimate aim and be strictly necessary to achieve that aim; be the least restrictive and intrusive means available; and not be arbitrary or discriminatory in the way it is imposed or applied.[18]

The burden of proof for assessing the legality and justifiability of measures limiting human rights for a common good normally falls on those who impose such restrictions.[19] State practice of resorting to such measures during the SARS outbreak makes an interesting study for assessing whether the above-mentioned human rights framework was actually followed. D. P. Fidler has noted that measures taken by states differed significantly, even in similar circumstances. While some states used compulsory and tightly monitored isolation and quarantine measures, others, by contrast, relied more on voluntary measures or no such measures at all.[20] These differences in policy, which may in part be explained by different factual circumstances, including the scientific knowledge available, as well as cultural and social contexts, raise questions concerning the application to the measures in question of the International Covenant on Civil and Political Rights (ICCPR), or comparable regional instruments, as well as the interpretive guidance contained in the Siracusa Principles. In particular, the question of whether such normative frameworks provide sufficient guidance on these complex issues is of central importance.

One of the important lessons of the SARS outbreak is the need for health emergency preparedness, including relevant legislation, policies, plans and programmes, in line with human rights law.[21] All such strategies should be established and implemented through transparent and accountable processes, as the active and informed participation of individuals and communities in decision-making that bears upon their health is part of the right to health.[22] The strategies should address the rights of those affected and pay particular attention to the needs of the most vulnerable groups. For example, legal authority for quarantine and isolation, including that of recalcitrant individuals, needs to be established with clear criteria, including scientific assessment of public health risk and effectiveness of envisaged measures, due process guarantees and use of the least restrictive alternatives.[23] Legislation is also needed for protecting privacy in different contexts, for due process requirements and compensation when infected property may need to be destroyed, and for ensuring non-discriminatory practices and equal treatment, among other things. The strategies should also ensure that individuals can access a full range of information on health issues affecting themselves and their communities.[24] The enactment of such policies, plans and legislation are essential tools for a balanced and accountable implementation of the right to health.[25]

Another important lesson from the SARS outbreak is the crucial role of well functioning national health systems for the control of epidemic diseases, capable of providing urgent medical care and relief.[26] Ensuring equitable access to health facilities, goods and services is essential for implementing the right to health but remains a challenge for many states, even in the absence of particular health emergencies.[27] Strengthening of health systems should thus be a high priority and based, according to the UN Special Rapporteur on the right to health, on a right-to-health approach.[28] The implementation of the core capacity requirements under the IHR provides an opportunity to reinforce work on surveillance and response capacities of health systems.[29]

Human rights implications of the WHO International Health Regulations

The IHR were initially adopted by the World Health Assembly in 1951,[30] and revised several times thereafter. They represent the culmination of a process of international cooperation begun in the mid-nineteenth century, which WHO was expected to continue and rationalize through centralized collective decision-making.[31] Under the WHO Constitution, regulations become legally binding for all member states unless they opt-out by a certain deadline.[32] This process and the constitutional basis of their legal effects make WHO regulations innovative international instruments, meant to address urgent regulatory needs in crucial public health areas.[33]

The IHR became progressively marginalized during the 1980s and 1990s, in particular since they were based on a number of assumptions that were overtaken by the development of public health and international law during that period.[34] The revision of the IHR languished, however, until 2003 when the collective scare caused by SARS and pandemic influenza made revision a top priority for the Organization. The World Health Assembly eventually adopted the revised IHR in May 2005 and they entered into force in June 2007. The IHR have 194 States Parties – the entire membership of WHO plus the Holy See – making them a truly global instrument.[35]

The IHR, as revised in 2005, are a complex and innovative instrument that opens a new era in international health law. The main features of the revised IHR include:

1. Expanded scope to address virtually all urgent and serious public health risks, regardless of origin or source, that might be transmissible across international borders – whether by travellers, trade, transportation or the environment. The IHR's scope of application goes well beyond the natural spread of infectious diseases, abandoning almost completely the approach based on a finite list of diseases. The IHR is consequently applicable to the public health aspects of diseases from biological, chemical or radionuclear sources, including in case of deliberate release of such agents;[36]

2. Detailed obligations requiring States Parties to develop national capacities for the surveillance of, and response to, diseases and events falling under the IHR and to report them to WHO;[37]

3. The central role of WHO in interacting with States Parties, providing information and supporting their prevention and control activities. In this

context, WHO may rely on information obtained from non-governmental sources, as provided in the Regulations;[38]

4. The Director-General of WHO may under certain circumstances determine that an event constitutes a "public health emergency of international concern" and issue temporary recommendations to respond to it, thus guiding the international response to grave public health risks as in the case of SARS.[39] The dramatic expansion of the scope and application of the IHR raises delicate issues as to their interaction with many other international rules, from trade and transportation to environmental protection and nuclear incidents.[40]

A major distinguishing feature of the revised IHR is that, unlike the predecessor Regulations, they contain provisions seeking to ensure that measures are applied consistent with human rights and freedoms, aiming to strike a balance between the protection of public health, interference with international traffic and trade,[41] and the protection of fundamental human rights.[42] While the protection of human rights is not an explicit component of the IHR's objectives, it figures prominently among their principles (Article 3) and thus provides fundamental interpretative guidance for their implementation.[43] Notwithstanding the reference to "persons" in that principle and the articles concerning WHO's recommendations, other IHR provisions mostly focus on "travellers",[44] thus significantly restricting their scope of protection ratione personae. The most important protective measures in the IHR include the requirement to apply the least intrusive and invasive medical examination that achieves the public health objective (Articles 17, 23, 31 and 43)[45] and the need for prior express informed consent except in special circumstances (Article 23). States Parties must treat travellers undergoing health measures with respect for their dignity and human rights, and provide certain facilities to minimize their discomfort (Article 32). The Regulations provide some protection as to confidentiality and lawful use of personal data collected under the IHR (Article 45) and introduce, most importantly, a general requirement of transparency and non-discrimination in the application of health measures (Article 42).

The aforementioned IHR provisions may seem narrow or skewed in favour of potentially coercive public health measures, and according to some commentators, they leave some important gaps.[46] At the same time, the IHR recognize in general terms that they and other international agreements should be interpreted so as to be compatible with each other, and the IHR clarify that the former shall not affect the rights and obligations of States Parties under the latter (Article 57). Consequently, over and above the specific protections summarized above, human rights obligations of States Parties may arguably prevail over incompatible IHR-based obligations. It has been suggested that, at the very least, the limitation or restriction of rights granted under the ICCPR in the implementation of the IHR should be subject to the balancing and interpretative test contained in the Siracusa Principles (explained above).[47] It is worth noting that the Principles state that "due regard shall be had to the International Health Regulations of the World Health Organization",[48] strengthening the importance of the IHR as a reference for achieving a balance between respect for human rights and protection of public health. The IHR have also been given the credit of contributing "to existing law on restricting human rights for health purposes" by providing greater detail for some of these principles.[49]

WHO provides guidance to states on measures in response to disease outbreaks, including those potentially affecting human rights and freedoms. For example, WHO advises countries neighbouring an area affected by cholera against the establishment of quarantine measures or a *cordon sanitaire* at borders; the introduction of travel restrictions, including requirement that travellers have proof of cholera vaccination; or the screening of travellers.[50]

In this connection, one may wonder whether the outbreak of an infectious disease with a potentially very serious public health impact – for example the virulence and lethality of current strains of avian influenza – may be invoked by States Parties to the ICCPR as a ground for the proclamation of a "public emergency which threatens the life of the nation" under Article 4. Even though the drafters of the Covenant probably had political situations in mind, the effects of an infectious disease may be equally devastating on the physical integrity of the population and the functioning of indispensable national institutions.[51] Furthermore, it may be questioned whether an event that has been determined to constitute a "public health emergency of international concern" by the Director-General of WHO under the IHR, could also qualify as a "public emergency" under the Covenant.

Even though explicit concerns about the protection or promotion of the right to health were absent from the negotiations on the revised IHR, an analysis of the IHR against the content and context of the right to health as articulated in General Comment No. 14 on the right to health reveals a number of synergies that could assist States Parties in pursuing the progressive realization of that right. The following aspects should be stressed in this regard:

1.   Article 12 paragraph 2(c) of the ICESCR spells out "the prevention, treatment and control of epidemic ... diseases" as an example of a core obligation of the Parties to the Covenant. Through the very fact of implementing the IHR, therefore, States Parties take steps in fulfilling an important component of the right to health.

2.   The General Comment on the right to health gives much importance to the enactment of policies and strategies as essential tools for a balanced and accountable implementation of the right to health.[52] This planning approach is also prominent in the case of the IHR, particularly through the obligation of States Parties in Articles 5 and 13 and Annex 1 to develop and implement plans of action to ensure the required core capacities to detect, report and respond to relevant public health risks.[53]

3.   Ever since the 1978 Alma-Ata Declaration on Primary Health Care,[54] national health systems and their main components have been seen as the primary elements for the delivery of equitable public health outcomes and for fulfilling the right to health.[55] It is significant that the IHR follow and strengthen this approach by abandoning the traditional focus on ports and airports in favour of a more holistic vision to strengthen the components of national health systems crucial for the prevention of the international spread of disease. If based on a realistic and accountable process, including in terms of available resources, such an approach may usefully complement, and be integrated into, national health systems policies.[56]

4.   Both the implementation of the IHR, and the realization of the right to health, rely substantially on international cooperation. The General Comment identifies a joint and individual responsibility of ICESCR Parties to cooperate, inter alia, in the international control of epidemic diseases, with particular regard to the needs of developing countries.[57] In view of the nature of infectious disease control as a global public good,[58] and the deep interdependence between states in this regard, there is arguably a collective responsibility of all States Parties to the ICESCR to cooperate in good faith with each other and with WHO in preventing and responding to the international spread of disease. The IHR provide a specific legal framework to enable such cooperation, which, at the same time, is instrumental in fulfilling a core dimension of the right to health. WHO in particular should play an important role in this respect, both directly and through the network of

experts and institutions that it coordinates. WHO is not a financial institution and its main functions in this context would consist of technical advice and support, and the provision of reliable information and guidance. Among the networks at the disposal of WHO, particular mention should be made of the Global Outbreak Alert and Response Network (GOARN). GOARN is a technical collaboration of existing institutions and networks that pool human and technical resources for the rapid identification, confirmation and response to outbreaks of international importance. It enables WHO to rapidly mobilize highly specialized teams of experts from institutions around the world to support countries affected by an outbreak of infectious disease. GOARN has played a crucial role in several critical situations such as the 2007 outbreak of Ebola hemorrhagic fever in the Democratic Republic of the Congo.[59]

Concluding remarks

As evidenced by the successful response to the SARS outbreak, responses at both national and international levels – and through the interplay of different governmental and non-governmental actors – are essential requirements for public health emergency governance. While the IHR establish an international framework for this cooperation, formidable challenges remain, in particular as concerns resources for enabling States Parties to implement their capacity-building obligations at the national level. With the inclusion of human rights protection in their crucial provisions, the IHR underline the synergy between preparedness and response to health emergencies, on the one hand, and protection of fundamental rights on the other, both at the national and international levels.[60]

* The opinions expressed are solely those of the authors and do not necessarily represent the views of the World Health Organization.

1 Address by Dr. Gro Harlem Brundtland, Director-General of the WHO on the Fiftieth Anniversary of the Universal Declaration of Human Rights, Paris, France, 8 December 1998, available at http://www.who.int/director-general/speeches/1998/english/19981208_paris.html.

2 'Global Health Security: Epidemic Alert and Response', World Health Assembly resolution WHA 54.14, 21 May 2001; WHO, *World Health Report 2007: A Safer Future*, (Geneva: WHO, 2007), available at http://www.who.int/whr/2007/whr 07_en.pdf. Global health security looks, through the public health lens, at "the collective health of populations living across geographical regions and international boundaries". Health security, at an individual level, includes universal access to adequate health care, access to education and information, the right to food in sufficient quantity and of good quality, the right to decent housing and to live and work in an environment where known health risks are controlled. Individuals' health security is affected by global health risks.

3 On the SARS outbreak, see for example, WHO, *SARS: How A Global Epidemic Was Stopped* (Geneva: WHO, 2006), available at http://whqlibdoc.who.int/wpro/2006/9290612134_eng.pdf; and D. P. Fidler, *SARS, Governance and the Globalization of Diseases* (New York: Palgrave Macmillan, 2004).

4 See e.g. T. Kian and F. Lateef, 'Infectious Diseases Law and Severe Acute Respiratory Syndrome – Medical and Legal Responses and Implications: The Singapore Experience' 7 *Asia Pacific League of Associations for Rheumatology Journal of Rheumatology* (2004), at 123–129.

5 The initial WHO International Sanitary Regulations of 1951 were revised and renamed the International Health Regulations (IHR) in 1969. The 58th World Health Assembly adopted the most recent revision of the Regulations on 23 May 2005. The text of the IHR (2005) is attached to World Health Assembly resolution WHA58.3 and is available at http://www.who.int/gb/ebwha/pdf_files/WHA58/WHA58_3-en.pdf. The revised IHR entered into force on 15 June 2007.

6 See, for example, WHO, *25 Questions & Answers on Health & Human Rights* (Geneva: WHO, 2002) and Lawrence Gostin, 'When Terrorism Threatens Health: How Far Are Limitations on Human Rights Justified', 31 *Journal of Law, Medicine & Ethics* (2003), at 521–528.

7 See, however, most notably, D. P. Fidler, *International Law and Infectious Diseases* (Oxford: Oxford University Press, 1999), at 179–197.

8 International Covenant on Economic, Social and Cultural Rights (ICESCR), adopted by UN General Assembly Resolution 2200A (XXI) of 16 December 1966.

9 Committee on Economic, Social and Cultural Rights, *General Comment No. 14 (2000) on the right to the highest attainable standard of health*, UN Doc. E/C.12/2000/4, 4 July 2000 (hereafter "General Comment No. 14").

10 ICESCR, Article 12(2)(c). According to the Committee on Economic, Social and Cultural Rights, the obligation is of comparable priority as the ICESCR's core obligations, i.e. a "minimum essential level[s]" of obligations for all states. General Comment No. 14, *supra* note 9, at paras. 43 and 44(c). See also IHR, in particular Articles 2, 5(1), 13(1) and Annex 1.

11 General Comment No. 14, *supra* note 9, paras. 16 and 40. For further analysis with regard to the IHR, see discussion below.

12 Social-distancing measures have been defined as "[a] range of community-based measures to reduce contact between people (e.g. closing schools or prohibiting large gatherings). Community-based measures may also be complemented by adoption of individual behaviours to increase the distance between people in daily life at the worksite or in other locations (e.g. substituting phone calls for face-to-face meetings, avoiding hand-shaking)." WHO, *Ethical considerations in developing a public health response to pandemic influenza*, WHO/CDS/EPR/GIP/2007.2 (Geneva:

WHO, 2007), p. IX, available at http://www.who.int/csr/resources/publications/WHO_CDS_EPR_GIP_2007_2/en/index.html.

13 See on different measures in the context of pandemic influenza preparedness, ibid.

14 For an overview of the measures see J. W. Saspin, L. O. Gostin, J. S. Vernick et al., 'SARS and International Legal Preparedness' 77 *Temple Law Review* (2004) 155–173, at 158–163.

15 For advice issued by WHO in March–June 2003 relating to the SARS outbreak, see http://www.who.int/csr/sars/travel/en/index.html.

16 See e.g. Sofia Gruskin, 'SARS, Public Health and Global Governance: Is there a Government in the Cockpit: A Passenger's Perspective on Global Public Health: The Role of Human Rights' 77 *Temple Law Review* (2004) 313–333 at 322; and Fidler, *supra* note 3, at 152.

17 See ICCPR, Articles 12 and 17, and General Comment No. 14, *supra* note 9, at paras. 28–29 and 34.

18 United Nations Economic and Social Council, UN Sub-Commission on Prevention of Discrimination and Protection of Minorities, 'Siracusa Principles on the Limitation and Derogation of Provisions in the International Covenant on Civil and Political Rights', Annex, UN Doc E/CN.4/1985/4 (1985) (hereafter "Siracusa Principles"). See also, for example, Susan Marks and Andrew Clapham, *International Human Rights Lexicon* (Oxford: Oxford University Press, 2005), at 206.

19 General Comment No. 14, *supra* note 9, at para. 28.

20 Fidler, *supra* note 3, at 153.

21 For legal preparedness in particular see WHO, *Ethical considerations in developing a public health response to pandemic influenza, supra* note 12, p. 9, and J. W. Saspin, L. O. Gostin, J. S. Vernick et al., *supra* note 14, at 155–173.

22 General Comment No. 14, *supra* note 9, at para. 14. See also S. Gruskin and B. Loff, 'Do Human Rights have a Role in Public Health Work?' 360 *The Lancet* (2002), at 1880.

23 Lawrence O. Gostin, 'Public Health Strategies for Pandemic Influenza: Ethics and the Law' 295(14) *Journal of the American Medical Association* (2006) 1700–1704, at 1703.

24 General Comment No. 14, *supra* note 9, at para. 12.

25 See, inter alia, ICESCR, Article 2 and General Comment No. 14, *supra* note 9, paras. 36, 43 and 53.

26 See also accompanying text to notes 54–56 below.

27 General Comment No. 14, *supra* note 9, at para. 12.

28 Paul Hunt, 'Report of the Special Rapporteur on the right of everyone to the enjoyment of the highest attainable standard of physical and mental health', UN Doc. A/HRC/7/11, 31 January 2008.

29 IHR, Articles 5 and 13, and Annex 1. See also accompanying text to notes 54–56 below.

30 International Sanitary Regulations, adopted on 25 May 1951, reproduced in WHO *Technical Reports Series* No. 41, Geneva 1951, available at http://whqlibdoc.who.int/trs/WHO_TRS_41.pdf.

31 See, for example, D. P. Fidler, 'The Globalization of Public Health: the first 100 years of international health diplomacy' 79(9) *Bulletin of the World Health Organization* (2001) 842–849.

32 Articles 21 and 22 of the WHO Constitution, reproduced in WHO, *Basic Documents* (Fifty-sixth edition, Geneva: WHO, 2007), at 1, available at http://www.who.int/gb/bd.

33 For discussion see e.g. Laurence Boisson de Chazournes, 'Le pouvoir réglementaire de l'Organisation Mondiale de la Santé à l'aune de la santé mondiale: réflexions sur la portée et la nature du Règlement Sanitaire International de 2005' in *Droit du pouvoir, pouvoir du droit : mélanges offerts à Jean Salmon* (Bruxelles: Bruylant, 2007) 1157–1181.

34 Most notably, the IHR (1) only covered a limited list of diseases that had become scourges of the past; (2) they set maximum measures that states may apply to persons and conveyances, rather than relying on a contextual risk assessment – which placed them in conflict with international trade rules; and (3) they did not support WHO's active role in surveillance, coordination and cooperation.

35 A list of the States Parties to the IHR and related information is available at http://www.who.int/ihr/states_parties/en/index.html.

36 See IHR, Article 1(1) (in particular the expansive definitions of "disease", "event", "public health risk") and Article 2, according to which the pur-

pose and scope of the Regulations are "to prevent, protect against, control and provide a public health response to the international spread of disease in ways that are commensurate with and restricted to public health risks, and which avoid unnecessary interference with international traffic and trade."

37 See IHR, Articles 5, 6, 13 and Annex 1.

38 See IHR in particular Articles 5(4), 9, 11 and 13(3).

39 IHR, Article 1(1) provides that "'public health emergency of international concern' means 'an extraordinary event which is determined, as provided in these Regulations: (I) to constitute a public health risk to other States through the international spread of disease and (II) to potentially require a coordinated international response'". See also IHR, Articles 12, 15–18, 48.

40 See, for example, information document prepared by the WHO Secretariat, 'Review and Approval of Proposed Amendments to the International Health Regulations: Relations with other International Instruments', Intergovernmental Working Group on Revision of the International Health Regulations, A/IHR/IGWG/INF.DOC./1, 30 September 2004, available at http://www.who.int/gb/ghs/e/e-igwg.html.

41 IHR, Article 11 defines the term "international traffic" as "the movement of persons, baggage, cargo, containers, conveyances, goods or postal parcels across an international border, including international trade."

42 For human rights related provisions in the IHR, see e.g. D. P. Fidler, 'From International Sanitary Conventions to Global Health Security: The New International Health Regulations' 4(2) *Chinese Journal of International Law* (2005) 325–392, Table 2; and B. Plotkin, 'Human Rights and Other Provisions in the Revised International Health Regulations (2005)' 121 *Public Health* (2007) 840–845.

43 IHR, Article 3(1) reads as follows: "The implementation of these Regulations shall be with full respect for the dignity, human rights and fundamental freedoms of persons".

44 Defined in Article 1(1) of the IHR as "a natural person undertaking an international voyage."

45 Under Article 17, the WHO Director-General al-

so has an obligation to consider health measures "that, on the basis of a risk assessment appropriate to the circumstances, are not more ... intrusive to persons than reasonably available alternatives that would achieve the appropriate level of health protection."

46 D. P. Fidler, *supra* note 42; and Lawrence O. Gostin, 'The New International Health Regulation: An Historic Development for International Law and Public Health' 34(1) *The Journal of Law, Medicine and Ethics* (2006) at 85–94. The lack of the least intrusive measures approach in case of involuntary vaccination or other prophylaxis, isolation and quarantine, and the absence of specific due process requirements with regard to the application of public health measure are seen as important gaps by these authors.

47 H. L. Lambertson, 'Swatting a Bug without a Flyswatter: Minimizing the Impact of Disease Control on Individual Liberty under the Revised International Health Regulations' 25(2) *Penn State International Law Review* (2006) 531–555 at 554, and the Siracusa Principles, *supra* note 18.

48 Ibid., at para. 26.

49 States' determination of potential additional measures that may affect rights of persons in accordance with Article 43 of the IHR must be based, inter alia, on scientific principles and available evidence of a risk to health. As noted by B. von Tigerstrom, this criterion is more specific than the relevant provisions concerning limitation of human rights for public heath purposes under international human rights treaty law. For analysis, see B. von Tigerstrom, 'The Revised International Health Regulations and Restraint of National Health Measures' 13 *Health Law Journal* (2005) 35–76 at 63–64.

50 WHO statement relating to international travel and trade to and from countries experiencing outbreaks of cholera. 16 November 2007, available at http://www.who.int/cholera/choleratravelandtradeadvice161107.pdf.

51 Siracusa Principles, Part II, *supra* note 18.

52 General Comment No. 14, *supra* note 9, at paras. 36, 43 and 53.

53 Interestingly, D. P. Fidler considers that the surveillance and response capacity obligations in the IHR are more demanding than those under article 12 of the ICESCR because the IHR States Parties are required to have the capacities in place generally after the five-year grace period following the entry into force of the IHR as foreseen in the Regulations. The ICESCR's right to health is, by contrast, to be progressively realized. See further, Fidler, *supra* note 42, at 373.

54 'Primary Health Care: Report of the International Conference on Primary Health Care' (Geneva: WHO, 1978) in particular the definition of primary health care at 3.

55 WHO has recently stated that "a health system consists of all organizations, people and actions whose primary intent is to promote, restore or maintain health". WHO, *Everybody's Business; Strengthening Health Systems to Improve Health Outcomes* (Geneva: WHO, 2007) at 1. The report identifies the building blocks of a health system as health services, health workforce, health information systems, medical products, health financing, as well as leadership, governance and stewardship. Ibid., at 3.

56 The UN Special Rapporteur on the right to health has reviewed this complex issue in 2008, recommended a right-to-health approach to strengthening health systems, and singled out planning, governance and accountability as aspects in particular need of strengthening. Paul Hunt, 'Report of the Special Rapporteur on the right of everyone to the enjoyment of the highest attainable standard of physical and mental health', UN Doc. A/HRC/7/11, 31 January 2008.

57 General Comment No. 14, *supra* note 9, at paras. 16 and 40.

58 See, for example, J. Giesecke, 'International Health Regulations and Epidemic Control' in R. Smith, R. Beaglehole, D. Woodward, and N. Drager (eds.) *Global Public Goods for Health: Health Economics and Public Health Perspectives* (Oxford: Oxford University Press, 2003) 196–211.

59 For more information on GOARN, see http://www.who.int/csr/outbreaknetwork/en/.

60 Lance Gable, 'The Proliferation of Human Rights in Global Health Governance' 35 *Journal of Law, Medicine & Ethics* (2007) 534–544 at 539.

Trade and the Right to Health

Sarah Joseph*

There are numerous intersections between the activity of trade, that is the passage of goods or services between countries, and the enjoyment of the right to the highest attainable standard of health. Trade can facilitate access to goods that promote the right, such as new medicines, as well as goods that harm human health, such as cigarettes. In this chapter, the effect of certain international trade rules on the enjoyment of the right to health is summarized.

Regulation of international trade

Global trade is regulated by a network of trade agreements. The World Trade Organization (WTO), which has 153 members at the time of writing, supervises obligations under its various treaties. Its agreements are generally designed to diminish and regulate trade barriers, which promote more efficient and beneficial trade relations between states (which can help generate friendlier relations), as well as greater commercial certainty. The WTO also serves as a forum for the negotiation of further reductions in trade barriers. There are also regional trade agreements, such as the Treaty of Maastricht for the European Communities (EC), the North American Free Trade Agreement (NAFTA) for the United States of America (US), Canada and Mexico, and MERCOSUR[1] for Brazil, Argentina, Uruguay and Paraguay. Finally, there are bilateral trade treaties, which lower trade barriers between two states.

Various elements of such agreements can impact on the enjoyment of the right to the highest attainable standard of health. These impacts are discussed below, with a particular focus on WTO rules, given that they represent the global benchmark.

Intellectual property agreements

Numerous trade agreements impose minimum standards of intellectual property protection upon parties. Within the WTO, intellectual property protection is regulated under the Agreement on Trade Related Aspects of Intellectual Property, the "TRIPS" agreement. TRIPS was preceded in 1993 by the inclusion of similar intellectual property protections in NAFTA. Since the advent of TRIPS in 1994, intellectual property protection has formed a component of numerous bilateral trade agreements.

Intellectual property rights reward monopoly rights to the creators (e.g. authors or inventors) of new products. Such regimes are said to encourage research, development and innovation, as they ensure that inventors can enjoy commercial benefits from their endeavours before being exposed to competition.

Intellectual property protection actually restricts competition, so intellectual property clauses are somewhat anomalous in trade agreements, which are normally designed to decrease trade barriers. Intellectual property rights nevertheless arguably facilitate trade. As traders are less concerned about pirating, global intellectual property rights promote foreign investment and technology transfer.

However, as intellectual property laws confer monopoly rights, they generally inflate prices. This circumstance is problematic as goods that are essential for the enjoyment of human rights, such as new medicines, can be priced out of the reach of poor people.

Under TRIPS, WTO Member States are obliged to confer patent rights which last 20 years. While developed states had to comply with TRIPS immediately, developing states were permitted some time lag before full compliance was required. Most time extensions have now run out.

Thus, prices are likely to be artificially inflated for that 20 year period, as patent holders seek to maximize returns on their investment. For example, the costs of drugs which combat the HIV virus are enormous. A month's worth of Atripla, a relatively new anti-HIV drug, costs USD 1300 a month.[2] Such prices are only affordable in industrialized countries due to government subsidies, which are not available in the developing world. Clearly, it is impossible for most people in the developing world, where most HIV cases arise, to pay such prices. The result is a health divide: HIV remains a death sentence for most sufferers in the developing world, whereas it can be managed for many years by sufferers in the developed world who have access to alleviating medication.

TRIPS does allow for compulsory licenses. A compulsory license arises when a government licenses a manufacturer to produce generic versions of a patented product, regardless of the wishes of the patent holder. Governments may issue compulsory licenses so long as certain conditions are complied with, including the payment of fair remuneration to the patent holder. A condition that commercial negotiations with the patent holder precede the issuing of compulsory licenses may be waived in times of national emergency. Therefore, TRIPS provides some leeway for governments to ensure the availability of cheap patented medicines.

In 2001, a hearing began in Pretoria, whereby 39 pharmaceutical companies brought an action against the South African government to prevent the passage of legislation which was designed to facilitate access to cheaper medicines. The companies claimed that the legislation would breach South Africa's TRIPS obligations. In April 2001, the companies dropped the case, which had provoked outrage around the world, given that South Africa had (and has) one of the highest HIV rates in the world. In the same year, the US threatened to bring a WTO case against Brazil to challenge its compulsory licensing laws, which had been designed to ensure the availability of low cost HIV drugs. As with the companies in South Africa, the US's threat attracted considerable criticism, and it ultimately retreated from this action. Finally, in the same year, the anthrax scare took place in the US. In response, the US and Canada threatened to issue compulsory licenses to ensure the availability of Cipla, an anti-anthrax drug. This stance provoked controversy as it seemed that industrialized countries were adopting double standards. They pressured developing nations to refrain from compulsory licenses despite massive health crises, while proposing compulsory licenses in response to a local scare that killed three people.[3]

This confluence of events in 2001 ensured that the impact of TRIPS on access to drugs was a major issue at the WTO Ministerial conference in Doha in December 2001. The Member States accordingly adopted the Doha Declaration on the TRIPS agreement and public health. In this Declaration, it was confirmed that TRIPS "can and should be interpreted and implemented in a manner supportive of WTO members' right to public health and, in particular, promote access to medicines for all". In particular, the right of states to issue compulsory licenses was reaffirmed, and "public health crises, including those relating to HIV/AIDS, tuberculosis, malaria and other epidemics" were recognized as national emergencies for the purposes of issuing a TRIPS compliant compulsory license. Furthermore, the least developed states were given until 2016 before they are required to respect pharmaceutical patents.

Another breakthrough arose in 2003. One general restriction in TRIPS on compulsory licenses is that the license should be issued "predominantly for the supply of the domestic market." This provision was problematic, as numerous developing states have no capacity to manufacture generic pharmaceutical products. Such states could not import compulsorily licensed products because other states were prohibited from producing such goods primarily for export. In 2003, the WTO waived the territorial restriction on compulsory licenses for pharmaceutical products in certain circumstances. The waiver remains in place, pending ratification of a formal TRIPS amendment designed to enshrine the rules of the waiver.

Under the waiver, the territorial restrictions on compulsory licenses may only be lifted to facilitate the export of generic drugs to the least developed countries in respect of pharmaceuticals to combat epidemics. There are extensive procedural prerequisites concerning notice by both exporter and importer to the WTO's TRIPS Council regarding use of the waiver. Safeguards must be in place to ensure that the relevant pharmaceuticals are not diverted to another market.

The Doha Declaration and the waiver have somewhat alleviated the deleterious impact of TRIPS on access to medicines. However, they have not completely solved the problem.[4] For example, it is uncertain about the extent of the application of the Declaration and the waiver to health crises beyond epidemics; the TRIPS initiatives may do little to enhance access to drugs for sufferers of cancer or heart disease, or other lethal non-communicable diseases. Indeed, the US threatened trade sanctions against Thailand in 2007 for its proposal to issue compulsory licenses with regard to medication for heart disease and cancer.[5] Furthermore, by December 2008, only Rwanda had notified the WTO of an intention to make use of the waiver as an importing state.[6] It may be that even generic drugs are too expensive for some states; that there is insufficient commercial incentive for generic manufacturers to produce drugs for such impoverished consumers; that pressure is being applied behind the scenes to discourage use of the scheme; or that there are delays in amending local legislation. Alternatively, the availability of the new scheme may be prompting pharmaceutical corporations, who feel threatened by compulsory licensing schemes, to make their products available to the least developed states on a cheaper, or even cost-free, basis.[7] Indeed, numerous corporations have adopted such a strategy.[8]

There are also concerns over the health impact of other free trade agreements. In particular, "TRIPS-plus" provisions, which impose even stricter intellectual property obligations than TRIPS on states, such as stricter controls on compulsory licenses, may be found in numerous US bilateral free trade agreements, such as those it has concluded with Colombia, Peru, and Jordan. Furthermore, TRIPS-plus provisions have been imposed as conditions on states acceding to the WTO, such as China and Cambodia. For example, Cambodia's WTO accession agreement requires it to protect data from clinical trials for five years, an obligation not imposed in TRIPS itself, which means that producers of generic copies will have to conduct trials from scratch, raising costs and generating delays, as well as ethical concerns.[9]

A final concern with the patent system is that it creates the wrong incentives for pharmaceutical companies. The system in some ways discourages research which could have an enormously beneficial health impact. For example, the global market for products designed to combat hair loss and acne is highly profitable. In comparison, the global market for a malaria or tuberculosis cure is not as lucrative, as sufferers are generally poor people in developing states. Therefore, the patent regime can encourage companies to focus on profitable yet less useful products, rather than on making breakthroughs regarding more beneficial products to combat lethal yet neglected diseases. In the same way, the patent regime encourages companies to focus on products which alleviate symptoms, rather than on cures and vaccines: There is a more profitable market in sick people who continue to buy a product to ease their suffering, than in people who are cured and no longer need any medicine. In this respect, Professor Thomas Pogge has proposed that a new system for rewarding companies according to the "health impact" of their innovations be devised, in order to promote proper incentives for research in the pharmaceutical field.[10] It would be appropriate for such a scheme, if it was to come into being, to be supervised by a global international body, such as the WTO or perhaps the World Health Organization.

Restrictions on trade on health grounds

As noted above, international trade rules are generally designed to break down or at least regulate trade barriers. Therefore, trade rules restrict the extent to which states can limit imports in order to protect public health.

The trade rules in the General Agreement on Tariffs and Trade (GATT), an agreement that predates but is now encompassed within the WTO, target protectionism, that is favourable treatment of local industries compared to overseas industries. Therefore, provisions that are discriminatory, even if they are allegedly imposed to promote public health, are only allowed in exceptional circumstances.

The *Thai Cigarettes* dispute was a case decided under the auspices of the GATT, prior to the advent of the WTO. Thailand had restricted the importation of foreign cigarettes, which led to a complaint by the US. Thailand contended that its restrictions on foreign imports were justified because chemical and other additives contained in US cigarettes might make them more harmful than Thai cigarettes, and because competition in the tobacco industry would lead to the use of better marketing techniques, wider availability of cigarettes, reductions in prices, and improvements in quality, all of which would probably lead to an increase in total consumption. Thailand did not wish to impose a complete ban on cigarettes as that measure might have led to an increase in the consumption of narcotic drugs. The GATT Panel however found the restrictions to be discriminatory, as they did not apply to domestically produced cigarettes, and were therefore in breach of GATT rules.[11]

Similar reasoning applied in *US-Gasoline*, the first cases decided by WTO dispute resolution bodies, where "clean air" regulations applied differentially to US gasoline, and imported gasoline. Despite the apparent environmental and health motivations behind the law, the WTO Appellate Body found that the law was prohibited under WTO law due to its discriminatory impact.[12]

In contrast, France's ban on asbestos products, clearly imposed for health reasons, was found to comply with WTO law in *EC-Asbestos*.[13] The ban was not found to be discriminatory as the asbestos products were deemed to be distinguishable from domestic substitutes which did not contain asbestos, therefore no impermissible "discrimination" arose in France's differential treatment of the two types of products.

Brazil-Tyres concerned a Brazilian restriction on the import of retreaded tyres, that is reconditioned used tyres.[14] The EC challenged the ban as a breach of WTO law. Brazil argued that the import of retreaded tyres, which have a shorter life than new tyres, led to a greater accumulation of waste tyres, which were breeding grounds for mosquitoes and mosquito-borne diseases, and also led to dangerous tyre fires. It was not apparently possible to dispose of the tyres in an environmentally friendly way. The WTO Appellate Body found that the ban was justified for health and environmental reasons. However, the ban was still found to breach WTO rules as they were discriminatory. First, non-reconditioned tyres could be imported. Second, reconditioned tyres from MERCOSUR countries, which were exempt from the ban under regional trade arrangements, were discriminatory. Thus, Brazil could maintain its ban so long as it extended it appropriately.[15] However, it might not be so easy for Brazil to extend the ban to MERCOSUR countries, due to its apparent obligations (according to a MERCOSUR tribunal) to allow the import of tyres under MERCOSUR.

One WTO agreement, the Agreement on the Application of Sanitary and Phytosanitary Measures (SPS), regulates the extent to which states can implement measures to protect human, animal and plant life and health from pests, diseases and food additives and contaminants. SPS provisions apply regardless of whether a measure discriminates against overseas products, and thus has a broader application than the GATT. It therefore imposes greater restrictions on the ability of states to adopt health measures in respect of the trade in agricultural products compared to other products.

In the *Beef Hormone* case, the EC banned the sale of meat produced with certain hormones.[16] It justified the ban on the basis of the precautionary principle; the health effects of the hormones were not fully known so the EC argued that it was justified in taking a precautionary approach and banning them outright until scientific studies could confirm the extent of any health effects. The US challenged the ban under the SPS. The EC ban was found to breach the SPS, as the WTO Appellate Body found that the ban was not based on an adequate risk assessment. The Appellate Body found that the precautionary principle could not override the EC's SPS obligations in this respect.

In all of the above cases, dispute settlement bodies under the WTO (or its predecessor GATT) had to consider the respective health and trade impacts of a measure. There is nothing inherently wrong, even from a human rights point of view, in the fact that trade law restricts the ability of states to adopt health measures. It would otherwise be quite possible for states to adopt spurious "health" measures which simply disguise protectionist measures, which would threaten the viability of the world trade regime and its economic and diplomatic benefits. Furthermore, health advocates would be pleased with the *Asbestos* decision.

However, a significant concern is whether the WTO dispute resolution bodies, which are staffed by trade experts and where argument is dominated by trade experts, sufficiently take non-trade issues, such as health, into account in making their decisions. Perhaps the test of discrimination was too strict in *Thai Cigarettes* and *Brazil Tyres,* as it was arguably unfeasible or legally difficult to adopt non-discriminatory provisions with similar health benefits. In *Beef Hormone,* the hormone ban was found to breach WTO law even though the hormones might possibly harm human health.[17] Furthermore, the right to health per se was not raised by any of the parties or dispute resolution bodies in any of the above cases, which indicates it was not in fact taken into account. It would be preferable, from a human rights point of view, for human rights concerns such as health to be more fully integrated into WTO decision making and standard setting, to ensure that they are not routinely, even if unintentionally, overridden by commercial imperatives.[18]

Conclusion

A state's duties under international trade law can potentially conflict with its duties regarding the right to health under international human rights law. States should be mindful of the latter duties when negotiating and ratifying trade deals. Furthermore, as noted by the United Nations Special Rapporteur on the right of everyone to the enjoyment of the highest attainable standard of physical and mental health: "States should respect the enjoyment of the right to health in other jurisdictions, and ensure that no international trade agreement or policy adversely impacts upon the right to health in other countries."[19] Therefore, states must be also mindful of the obligations of other states regarding the right to health; they should not seek to promote a trade deal, or enforce existing trade rules, in a way that undermines the enjoyment of that right in those other states.

* This chapter is part of the outcomes for an Australian Research Council grant on Human Rights and the WTO.

1 MERCOSUR stands for the Southern Common Market (*Mercado Común del Sur* in Spanish).

2 Daniel Costello, 'HIV treatment becoming profitable', *Los Angeles Times*, 21 February 2008.

3 See generally, Sarah Joseph, 'Pharmaceutical Corporations and Access to Drugs: The "Fourth Wave" of Corporate Human Rights Scrutiny' 25 *Human Rights Quarterly* (2003) 425, at 442–445.

4 See generally, Oxfam, 'Patients versus Patents: Five years after the Doha Declaration' (Oxfam Briefing Paper 95, 2006), available at http://www.oxfam.org/en/policy/briefingpapers/bp95_patent_svspatients_061114.

5 Kevin Outterson, 'Should access to medicines and TRIPS flexibilities be limited to specific diseases?' 34 *American Journal of Law and Medicine* (2008) 279, at 282.

6 Canada notified the WTO that it would manufacture and export generic anti-HIV drugs to Rwanda.

7 Adam McBeth, 'When Nobody Comes to the Party: Why Have No States Used the WTO Scheme for Compulsory Licensing of Essential Medicines?' 3 *New Zealand Journal of International Law* (2006) 1, at 23–30.

8 See for example, http://www.diflucanpartnership.org/en/welcome/Default.aspx regarding Pfizer's initiatives.

9 See United Nations Development Program, *Asia Pacific Human Development Report 2006: Trade on Human Terms* (Colombo: UNDP, 2006), at 133.

10 Thomas Pogge, 'Medicines for the World: Boosting Innovation without Obstructing Free Access', available at http://www.law.monash.edu.au/castancentre/events/2008/pogge-lecture.html.

11 See *Thailand – Restrictions on Importation of and Internal Taxes on Cigarettes – Report of the Panel Adopted on 7 November 1990*, WTO Doc DS10/R – 37S/200, paras. 21, at 27–28.

12 See Appellate Body Report, *United States-Standards for Reformulated and Conventional Gasoline*, WT/DS2/AB/R, adopted 20 May 1996, DSR 1996: I, 3.

13 Appellate Body Report, *European Communities – Measures Affecting Asbestos and Asbestos-Containing Products*, WT/DS135/AB/R, adopted 5 April 2001, DSR 2001: VII, at 3243.

14 Appellate Body Report, *Brazil – Measures Affecting Imports of Retreaded Tyres*, WT/DS332/AB/R, adopted 17 December 2007.

15 See Hannes Schloemann, 'Brazil Tyres: Policy Space confirmed under GATT Article XX', *Bridges Monthly*, Year 12 No. 1, February 2008, available via www.ictsd.org.

16 See Appellate Body Report, *EC Measures concerning Meat and Meat Products (Hormones)*, WT/DS 26/AB/R, WT/DS48/AB/R, adopted 13 February 1998, DSR 1998: I, at 135.

17 See Caroline Dommen, 'Raising Human Rights Concerns in the World Trade Organization: Actors, Processes and Possible Strategies' 24 *Human Rights Quarterly* (2002) 1, at 17–21.

18 It is a matter of speculation as to why states are not using explicit human rights claims to bolster their arguments before the WTO. One reason may be that the bureaucrats that submit arguments before the WTO are not human rights experts; see Stephen Powell, 'The place of human rights law in World Trade Organization rules' 16 *Florida Journal of International Law* (2004) 219, at 220. Indeed, explicit reference to human rights language by states in the WTO is extremely rare. One example was a submission by Mauritius to the WTO Committee on Agriculture on negotiations regarding liberalization of agricultural trade, mentioning the right to food: see G/AG/NG/W/75 (30 November 2000).

19 See Paul Hunt, *Report of the Special Rapporteur: Mission to the World Trade Organization*, 1 March 2004, UN Doc. C/CN.4/2004/49/Add.1. See also Committee on Economic Social and Cultural Rights, *General Comment No. 14 on the right to the highest attainable standard of health*, 11 August 2000, UN Doc. E/C.12/2000/4, para. 39.

Developing Countries and the Promotion of the Right to Health in Multilateral Institutions: A Review of Developments in Trade and Health Institutions

Sisule F. Musungu

Introduction

The protection of human rights in developing countries is heavily influenced by external processes and the activities of international organizations and entities. These institutions, especially United Nations (UN) agencies and related organizations such as the Breton Woods Institutions, often have a direct and lasting role in the human rights situations of these countries. The impact on the respect, protection and fulfilment of economic, social and cultural rights, such as the right to the enjoyment of the highest attainable standard of physical and mental health (hereinafter "the right to health"), is particularly significant. At least two reasons explain why.

First, while civil and political rights attract significant public attention in developed countries, and hence, significant financial and other support towards their protection in developing countries, the same is not the case for economic, social and cultural rights. Many in developed countries, including influential academics, still entertain the notion that economic, social and cultural rights are "second generation rights". In some cases there is outright resistance to accepting that economic, social and cultural rights are human rights at all. It therefore falls to international organizations and non-governmental organizations (NGOs) to provide most of the external support for the promotion and protection of these rights. In other words, international assistance and cooperation to support the progressive realization of economic, social and cultural rights is more likely to come from international organizations such as the World Health Organization (WHO), in the case of the right to health, than bilateral development agencies.

The second reason relates to the impact of standards developed in multilateral institutions, such as the World Trade Organization (WTO), on economic, social and cultural rights. To start with, while key civil and political rights, such as due process rights, are explicitly recognized in the foundational instruments of such organizations as the WTO, economic, social and cultural rights are at best seen as distant aspirations. At the same time, however, efforts, for example, aimed at trade liberalization can have negative consequences for economic, social and cultural rights.

This chapter reviews the role, and the nature of responses, that developing countries have advocated in the areas of trade and public health with respect to the promotion of the right to health. This is both in terms of shaping international assistance and cooperation from the relevant multilateral institutions, as well as in terms of addressing the negative impact that international standards may have on the right to health. The developments reviewed are mainly those that have occurred in the WTO and WHO: It is in these institutions that there has been the most significant efforts by developing countries. These two institutions have also been chosen because they are the lead international organizations for trade and health, respectively.

The chapter is divided into four main parts. Following this introduction, the chapter first discusses the international dimensions of the right to health. This is followed, in part three, with a detailed discussion of the role and international responses promoted by developing countries with respect to access to essential medicines, essential health research and development (R&D), and the relationship between the right to health and trade more generally. The chapter concludes with some final remarks.

The international dimension of the right to health

The right to health enjoys unquestionable recognition at the international level. This recognition starts with Article 25 of the Universal Declaration of Human Rights (UDHR) and continues with Article 12 of the International Covenant on Economic, Social and Cultural Rights (ICESCR), which recognizes the right of everyone to the enjoyment of the highest attainable standard of physical and mental health. It is also highlighted in the

Constitution of the WHO and a number of other international human rights instruments including: The Convention on the Elimination of All Forms of Racial Discrimination (CERD);[1] the Convention on Elimination of All Forms of Discrimination Against Women (CEDAW);[2] and the Convention on the Rights of the Child (CRC).[3] These international instruments are complemented by regional instruments that also unequivocally recognize the right.[4] In practice, the right has been implemented in many countries through national constitutions. The justiciability of the right to health has also been well established at the national level.[5]

From a legal standpoint, the foundational legal instrument with respect to the right to health is the ICESCR. In addition to the recognition of the right under Article 12(1), the Covenant provides a non-exhaustive list of steps that are necessary to achieve the full realization of the right under Article 12(2). These include steps necessary for:

1.   Reducing stillbirth rates and infant mortality as well as for the healthy development of the child;
2.   improving all aspects of environmental and industrial hygiene;
3.   the prevention, treatment and control of epidemic, endemic, occupational and other diseases; and
4.   creating conditions which would assure to all medical service and attention in the event of sickness.

Deriving from its international recognition and the nature of the steps necessary to ensure its full realization, the right to health has at least four key aspects with significant international dimensions.

First, as is the case with all economic, social and cultural rights recognized under the ICESCR, it is foreseen that, in order to undertake the necessary steps for the progressive realization of the right to health, State Parties need to take individual action as well as action through international assistance and cooperation.[6]

Secondly, the ICESCR places significant emphasis on the economic and technical nature of the steps necessary for the progressive realization of the rights. In the context of developing countries, this presupposes important international financial and technical cooperation activities. As already noted, because of the dichotomy which is perceived between civil and political rights on the one hand, and economic, social and cultural rights on the other, such financial and technical cooperation activities to support the realization of the latter rights has tended to predominantly fall on international organizations.

Third, the necessity of taking steps to prevent, treat and control epidemics, in particular, requires international coordination and rule-making. Cases such as Avian Influenza and SARS are clear examples.[7]

Finally, the steps necessary to achieve progressive realization of the right to health are directly impacted by international standards and rules in a range of areas including trade.

It is in the context of these four international aspects of the right to health that we examine the role of developing countries in promoting the right in health and trade organizations with a specific focus on the WTO and the WHO.

Developing countries and the right to health in multilateral institutions: Recent developments in health and trade organizations

Developing countries, in global public opinion, are often associated with civil and political rights violations. This is, in large part, because of democratic and institutional weaknesses as well as conditions of poverty in these countries. In the context of international human rights mechanisms such as at the UN Human Rights Council, developing countries are also perceived to be less than enthusiastic to condemn the violation of civil and political rights in other UN Member States.

Though less perceptible in global public opinion, developing countries' populations also suffer significant violations of their economic, social and cultural rights. Similar reasons explain the situation, though poverty and economic conditions play a larger role than with respect to civil and political rights. The situation is, however, markedly different with respect to the role of developing countries in upholding economic, social and cultural rights in international processes. In recent years, the right to health especially has been brought into sharp focus in both the WHO and the WTO. In these two institutions, I would argue, developing countries have played a significant, positive role in promoting the right to health and in shaping responses that are critical in achieving its full realization.

The most important developments which illustrate the role of developing countries in shaping international responses relate to the debates and discussions on access to essential medicines, essential health R&D, or needs-driven R & D, and with respect to the relationship between the right to health and trade liberalization generally.

Right to health and access to essential medicines

The impact of intellectual property (IP) rights on access to essential medicines in developing countries has been at the centre of international debate and policy-making for almost a decade now. This debate first played out for several years at the WTO, but has recently been most notable at the WHO. We briefly examine how the right to health featured in both cases.

The right to health and access to medicines at the WTO

The controversy and discussions relating to the impact of IP rights, patents in particular, on access to medicines is not new, though it has been played out in world public opinion much more significantly in the last decade or so. In the context of the WTO, the impact of patenting and the need to protect public health was a central sticking point in the negotiations of the WTO Agreement on Trade-Related Aspects of Intellectual Property Rights (TRIPS).[8]

On the one hand, developing countries argued against minimum patent rights in the pharmaceutical sector on the basis that such monopoly rights would raise prices and put essential medicines out of the reach of their populations. This would impact the realization of the right to health. On the other hand, developed countries, in general, argued for stringent minimum rules in order to protect their pharmaceutical industries and on the basis that such protection was essential for innovation. These rules, in their view, would also promote the right to health.

In the final text of the TRIPS Agreement, developing countries succeeded in establishing the principle, in Article 8, that in implementing the TRIPS Agreement all WTO Members were entitled to adopt measures "to protect public health and nutrition".[9] Though not phrased in specific human rights language, this essentially meant that a space had been opened in the international IP rules to take domestic measures to realize the right to health and to address one of the key determinants of health – nutrition. This principle was complemented by a series of rules permitting specific exceptions, commonly referred to as TRIPS flexibilities.[10]

However, in attempting to implement the above principle and flexibilities, developing countries faced a number of challenges. These included hostility from developed countries to the use of the flexibilities to improve access to medicines, leading to a renewed contest at the WTO. It is the debate on the scope and use of flexibilities in the TRIPS Agreement for public health purposes that led to adoption of the Doha Declaration on the TRIPS Agreement and Public Health at the Fourth WTO Ministerial Conference in November 2001.[11] The Declaration, in essence, was aimed at clarifying the relationship between the TRIPS Agreement and public health.

In the debate leading to the adoption of the Declaration, developing countries and civil society organizations heavily relied on the right to health as a basis for their proposed interpretation of the relationship between the Agreement and access to medicines. As a result, the final language provided a significant boost to the accessibility component of the right to health. Specifically, in the Declaration, trade ministers, inspired, in part, by the strong argumentation on the right to health, affirmed that the TRIPS Agreement can and should be interpreted and implemented in a manner supportive of WTO Members' right to protect public health and, in particular, to promote access to medicines for all.[12]

In sum, it can be argued that both in the negotiations of the TRIPS Agreement and in the follow-on discussions on access to medicines, developing countries have succeeded in making a clear link between the right to health and the need for flexibilities in patent law. It is notable, however, that though references to the right to health were made in discussions, there is no direct mention of the right to health in the relevant WTO documents. This leaves the linkage to the right to health subject to continued disputation and diverging interpretations.[13]

The right to health and access to medicines at the WHO

In the wake of the Doha Declaration on the TRIPS Agreement and Public Health, the role of the WHO in ensuring that IP rights do not undermine the public health objectives came to the fore. Though WHO resolutions mentioning IP and its potentially negative consequences date further back, the Doha Declaration had a catalytic effect in the WHO. Consequently, in its Resolution on ensuring the accessibility of essential medicines in May 2002, the World Health Assembly welcomed the Doha Declaration and urged WHO Member States "to continue monitoring the implications on access to medicines of recent patent-protection laws and compliance with WTO's Agreement on Trade-Related Aspects of Intellectual Property Rights (TRIPS)."[14] This was followed in the succeeding years with intensified discussions culminating in the adoption, in May 2008, of the Global Strategy and Plan of Action on Public Health, Innovation and Intellectual Property Rights.[15] The Strategy is discussed in the next sub-section.

The main contention relating to access to medicines centred around WHO's competence to address IP related issues, especially its competence to provide technical assistance on these issues. In the main, developing countries argued that as the pre-eminent global health organization, WHO had the competence, and responsibility, to assist developing countries to ensure that the implementation or negotiations of IP rules did not negatively affect access to medicines. On the other hand, developed countries, the United States in particular, argued that WHO did not have a mandate on these issues including provision of technical assistance for the use of TRIPS flexibilities.

As a result, in the resolution on ensuring the accessibility of essential medicines, no mandate was given to the WHO Secretariat to support developing countries in their TRIPS implementation. Reference to the right to health was also absent. The situation has gradually changed as developing countries have continued to seek more specific responses and action from the WHO on these matters, basing many of their arguments on the right to health.

The right to health and essential health research and development

It has been argued that efforts to improve access to medicines and efforts to create incentives for R&D in the pharmaceutical sector – two interlinked objectives – can at times run contrary to one another.[16] While this is not necessarily correct, it is true to say that it is partly because of this perception that developing countries have been pitted against developed countries, both at the WHO and at the WTO. While developing countries have traditionally emphasized the impact of IP rights on affordability and access to medicines, developed countries have argued for the need for strong IP rights as a basis for innovation in the pharmaceutical sector. Both sides, explicitly and implicitly, have touted their position as the most conducive for promoting the right to health.

Although divergences remain, the work of developing countries in seeking the creation of the Commission on Intellectual Property Rights, Innovation and Public Health (CIPIH),[17] and ultimately, the adoption of the Global Strategy and Plan of Action on Public Health, Innovation and

Intellectual Property Rights (hereinafter "the Global Strategy on Essential Health R&D") have significantly helped address the controversy. The idea, promoted by developing countries, to examine the needs of access at the same time, and in the same strategy, with the needs for innovation and funding for R&D, will have important positive outcomes for the realization of the right to health.

The Global Strategy on Essential Health R&D "aims to promote new thinking on innovation and access to medicines as well as ... provide a medium-term framework for securing an enhanced and sustainable basis for needs-driven essential health research and development relevant to diseases which disproportionately affect developing countries ..."[18] This approach recognizes the right to health as the basis of WHO's action in this area, including recognition of WHO competence to provide technical assistance to developing countries. Such technical assistance is an important part of the international assistance and cooperation necessary to promote the full realization of the right to health in these countries.

In this context, the Strategy establishes two key principles which should transform the thinking in the WHO and its Member States regarding the organization's role in promoting the right to health where IP rights are concerned.

First, the Strategy provides that, because the WHO Constitution establishes its objective as being "the attainment by all peoples of the highest possible level of health", the organization must play a strategic and central role in the relationship between public health, innovation and IP rights.[19] Accordingly, WHO, including its regional and country offices, is required to strengthen its institutional competencies and relevant programmes in order to play its role in implementing the Strategy. This means that WHO will now be in a much stronger position to provide international assistance to developing countries in their efforts to realize the right to health by improving the development and provision of essential medicines.[20]

Secondly, and more importantly, the Global Strategy and Plan of Action for Essential Health R&D establishes the right to health as a core principle. In specific terms, the resolution provides that "The enjoyment of the highest attainable standard of health is one of the fundamental rights of every human being without distinction of race, religion, political belief, economic or social condition."[21] What this means is that the actions of WHO Member States and its Secretariat with respect to: Prioritizing R&D needs; promoting R&D; building and improving innovative capacity; transfer of technology; application and management of IP to contribute to innovation and promote public health; improving delivery and access; promoting sustainable financing mechanisms; and establishing monitoring and reporting systems, should be underpinned by the right to health.

The right to health and trade

Beyond the TRIPS Agreement, other WTO rules have also been identified as having important implications for the right to health. Of particular interest are the rules in the General Agreement on Trade in Services (GATS).[22] The main concern here is that trade liberalization in the health services sector in the manner foreseen in the GATS is shifting the thinking and health policy in developing countries towards privatization. The consequence is increased costs for health services.[23] This has negative impacts for the progressive realization of the right to health.

Unlike the case of TRIPS, however, the impact of GATS on access to health services has attracted much less attention in the WTO processes and debate. Much more has been done at the WHO where, in 2006, the World Health Assembly adopted a resolution on international trade and health.[24] Developing countries played a critical role in its passage and in linking it with important principles related to the right to health.

This resolution was mainly aimed and promoting policy coordination between national ministries and departments, and providing the WHO with the mandate to provide support to developing countries as well as to generate relevant evidence regarding the implication of trade for health. In particular, the resolution seeks to engage the WHO in supporting Member States (mainly developing countries) in framing coherent policies to address the relationship between trade and human rights, and to build their capacity to understand and respond to the impacts of trade, and trade agreements, on health, through relevant policies and legislation.

Though there is no specific reference to the right to health in the resolution, it is foreseen that its implementation would promote the right to health by ensuring that trade officials who negotiate trade agreements and are responsible for national implementation understand the implications of such agreements for the right to health. It would also ensure that there is a legislative framework to ensure that activities in the trade area are designed to support the full realization of the right to health. The emphasis on legislative action in the resolution fits well with the emphasis in Article 2(1) of the ICESCR, which recognizes adoption of legislative measures as a particularly appropriate means for progressive realization of economic, social and cultural rights.

Final remarks

The situation of the right to health in developing countries still leaves a lot to be desired. This is despite efforts by developing country governments, human rights and civil society organizations, as well as international institutions. The challenges and gaps, as well as the efforts (or lack thereof) of developing countries to achieve the full realization of the right to health are, however, increasingly being understood and are receiving significant attention. Various chapters in this book attest to this fact. Much less understood is the role that developing countries have played in promoting the right to health in multilateral institutions.

Focusing on health and trade institutions, the WTO and WHO in particular, this chapter has highlighted the role and nature of responses promoted by these countries in efforts to ensure that the right to health shapes and influences the manner in which IP and trade rules are designed and implemented, as well as the type of international assistance provided. In this, these countries have achieved significant progress both in the WTO and WHO. It is particularly notable that these countries have succeeded in:

1.   Placing the right to health at the centre of WHO's technical assistance in the area of access to medicines, essential health R&D and with respect to the relationship between trade and health; and
2.   establishing the right to health as an overriding principle in the implementation of the Global Strategy and Plan of Action for Essential Health R&D.

It is expected that, in light of these developments, there will be renewed importance given to the right to health in economic and development circles. These developments will also help shape the understanding of the right to health in a progressive way influencing how people, especially those concerned with trade and related issues, think about the right to health.

1 See Article 5(e).

2 At Article 11(1) (f) and 12.

3 See Article 24.

4 Examples include the European Social Charter (ESC), Article 11, and the African Charter for Human and Peoples' Rights (ACHPR), Article 16.

5 See, for example, the judgement in *Soobramoney v. Minister of Health* (Kwazulu-Natal), CCT 32 (1997), available at http://www.constitutionalcourt.org.za/uhtbin/cgisirsi/doAm2Altsx/MAIN/294410 011/9.

6 See Article 2(1) of the ICESCR.

7 See the chapter by Gian Luca Burci and Riikka Koskenmäki in this volume.

8 For a historical account of the TRIPS negotiations and debate on patenting and health see UNCTAD and ICTSD, *Resource Book on TRIPS and Development* (New York: Cambridge University Press, 2005). Also see J. Braithwaite and P. Drahos, *Global Business Regulation* (Cambridge: Cambridge University Press, 2000), for a flavour of the motivations behind the TRIPS Agreement and the role of the pharmaceutical industry in developed countries.

9 In general, the TRIPS Agreement required all developing countries to introduce minimum monopoly rights (patents) for the protection of pharmaceutical products and pharmaceutical manufacturing processes starting on 1 January 2000. Those developing countries, like India, which had previously excluded pharmaceutical products from patenting, for public health and industrial reasons, were required to offer such minimum protection by 1 January 2005.

10 For a discussion of these flexibilities and how they relate to access to medicines see e.g., Sisule F. Musungu, 'The TRIPS Agreement and Public Health' in C. Correa and A. Yusuf (eds.) *Intellectual Property and International Trade: The TRIPS Agreement* (Second Edition, The Netherlands: Kluwer Law International, 2008) 421–470.

11 The Declaration is contained in WTO document WT/MIN(01)/DEC/W/2, available at http://www.wto.org/english/thewto_e/minist_e/min01_e/

mindecl_e.htm. For detailed discussion of the Declaration including its antecedents, see, for example, C. Correa, 'Implications of the Doha Declaration on the TRIPS Agreement and Public Health', *Health Economics and Drugs, EDM Series No. 12* (Geneva: WHO, 2002) and F. M. Abbott, 'The TRIPS Agreement, Access to Medicines and the WTO Doha Ministerial Conference', *Occasional Paper 7* (Geneva: Quakers United Nations Office, 2001).

12 Paragraph 4 of the Declaration.

13 For a discussion on some of the interpretational challenges and issues see e.g., the Report on the mission of the Rapporteur on the Right to Health to the WTO, UN Document E/CN.4/2004/49/ Add.1 available at http://www.unhchr.ch/Huri docda/Huridoca.nsf/(Symbol)/E.CN.4.2004.49. Add.1.En?Opendocument.

14 See resolution WHA55.14 of 18 May 2002, available at http://ftp.who.int/gb/archive/pdf_files/ WHA55/ewha5514.pdf.

15 See Resolution WHA61.21 of 24 May 2008, available at http://www.who.int/gb/ebwha/pdf_files/ A61/A61_R21-en.pdf.

16 See, for example, J. O. Lanjouw, 'Intellectual Property and the Availability of Pharmaceuticals in Poor Countries' 3 *Innovation Policy and Economy* (2002).

17 Information about the Commission, including its final report, is available at http://www.who.int/ intellectualproperty/en/.

18 See paragraph 13 of the Global Strategy and Plan of Action on Public Health, Innovation and Intellectual Property Rights, available at www.who. int/gb/ebwha/pdf_files/A61/A61_R21-en.pdf.

19 Ibid., para. 15.

20 Element 5.2 of the Strategy sets out a number of specific actions in this area. See ibid.

21 Ibid., para. 16.

22 For useful literature on the subject see WHO publications on trade and health available at http:// www.who.int/trade/resource/tradewp/en/index. html.

23 For additional discussion on trade liberalization and the effects for the right to health and other

economic, social and cultural rights, see also J. Oloka-Onyango and D. Udagama, 'Globalization and its Impact on the Full Enjoyment of Human Rights', Progress Report of the Special Rapporteurs on Globalization, UN Doc. E.CN.4/sub.2/2001/10, available at http://www.unhchr.ch/Huridocda/Huridoca.nsf/(Symbol)/E.CN.4.Sub.2.2001.10.En?Opendocument; and Sisule F. Musungu, 'The Right to Health in the Global Economy: Reading Human Rights Obligations into the Pat-ent Regime of the WTO-TRIPS Agreement' in C. Heyns (ed.) *International Yearbook of Regional Human Rights Master's Programmes 2001*, (Pretoria: Centre for Human Rights, 2003), 197–198. See also the Report of the Special Rapporteur on the right to health, *supra* note 13.

24 This is resolution WHA59.26, available at http://www.who.int/gb/ebwha/pdf_files/WHA59/A59_R26-en.pdf.

07

THE ROLE OF THE HEALTH CARE PRACTITIONERS

Physicians and the Right to Health

Leonard S. Rubenstein[*]

Every day, physicians[1] confront the harms inflicted on their patients from infringements on their human rights. They see patients who are coping not only with illness and disease, but with deprivation, discrimination and violence that undermine their health. They witness the tragic impact of social policies that deny women the ability to control their reproductive lives and deny health services to people simply because they are immigrants or members of ethnic or racial minorities.

In poor countries, physicians agonize over their inability to provide the quality health care they are trained to offer because the facilities in which they work may lack the medical supplies, functioning laboratories, drugs, or clean water that are prerequisites to such care. In those wealthy countries that view health care as a commodity, physicians experience the frustration of not being able to offer care that is clinically necessary because a third-party payer denies reimbursement, or because the patient lacks insurance coverage at all. In all these settings, and many more, they can't help but be acutely aware of how the ideals of the profession to treat the sick cannot be realized, no matter how personally committed they are to their craft or to the patients and communities they serve.

Yet despite these experiences, and professional values that seem very much in harmony with the realization of the right to the highest attainable standard of health, physicians have not generally been in the forefront, and are often not involved at all, in striving to end the human rights violations that impede their own ability to care for the sick and to promote health. This chapter seeks both to identify the sources of that anomaly and to suggest ways in which the traditions of medicine can be used to transform the commitments and actions of physicians to advance the right to health.

Values and commitments

The values and ethical commitments of the medical profession, like those of human rights, begin with a belief in the dignity of every individual. Doctors are trained to promote and respect human life and health and the autonomy of the individual patient. Their central duty is to employ their professional skills to advance health. The World Medical Association's Declaration of Geneva, the modern version of the Hippocratic Oath, opens with a pledge "to consecrate my life to the service of humanity;" it continues with commitments to use one's skills "with conscience and dignity;" not to allow "considerations of age, disease or disability, creed, ethnic origin, gender, nationality, political affiliation, race, sexual orientation, social standing or any other factor to intervene between my duty and my patient;" and "not to use my medical knowledge to violate human rights and civil liberties, even under threat."[2] Another foundational document of the World Medical Association, the International Code of Medical Ethics, requires physicians to "strive to use health care resources in the best way to benefit patients and their communities."[3] Though not expressed in the same language, these values are consistent with those found in the Universal Declaration of Human Rights, which is grounded in a belief in the inherent dignity of every individual.[4]

True to the values of human rights, throughout history physicians have carried out this ethos not only in places of safety and security and where resources are abundant, but in very difficult and even dangerous environments. Many choose to work in impoverished regions of their communities or the world, or to serve prisoners and other marginalized people. Others provide medical services in the tumult of war, and in that role may act as witnesses as well as healers.[5] Some physicians follow the admonition of the 19th century physician Rudolph Virchow, the founder of modern pathology and a towering figure in medicine, to be engaged in the world and devote themselves to assuring that determinants of health like clean water and sanitation are available to all.

The apparent convergence of medical values and physician action to advance human rights, however, is often overstated; indeed, the examples just given often represent departures by individual physicians from mainstream medical communities' responses to human rights violations rather than an expression of them. The first and most obvious barrier to such a convergence is the inevitable conflicts of interest that arise as an outgrowth of any profession's concern with its financial, professional and career interests.

Collective action by physicians most often is directed at preservation of their power and autonomy, including enhancement of their incomes. Even in impoverished countries, where increased pay for physicians and other health care personnel is essential to assure quality care, and may help stem the brain-drain of medical personnel, self-interest is not always congruent with the realization of health rights if the increases are a product of user fees that decrease access of the poor to health care. Conflicts also arise in physicians' relationships with pharmaceutical companies,[6] and even from physicians' efforts to develop scientific and medical knowledge and new drugs, which can lead to discounting the rights of study participants.

A second barrier is that ethical commitments do not immunize physicians from the biases of the larger society that disrespect human rights. In some circumstances, indeed, ethical standards have been manipulated to accommodate these biases. For example, until recently, entities that set out regulatory and ethics standards for physicians allowed them to choose whom they wanted to treat. This rule, though apparently innocuous and respectful of physician autonomy, permitted physicians to refuse to treat patients who are members of a stigmatized minority. And, as late as 1997, years after apartheid ended in South Africa, staff of the licensing and disciplinary authority for physicians opined that racial discrimination by a physician in patient selection did not constitute misconduct.[7] Moreover, as studies in the United States have shown, even when physicians do not consciously engage in discrimination, their clinical decisions may be influenced by biases and stereotypes of the larger society about members of minority communities that lead to lower quality of care to members of those groups. [8]

Third, the ethic of promoting human dignity co-exists with another, often unstated, tradition of using professional skills to advance the interests of the state, even at the expense of human rights. Dating at least to the 18th century,[9] governments have found it useful to enlist physicians and other health professionals in policies and practices that advance state not patient interests and that violate human rights. Physicians have used their medical skills to aid torturers; support security goals in prisons and other places of detention; enforce social norms that devalue women or mistreat women through such practices as "virginity examinations"; and manipulate medical diagnoses to punish political dissidents.[10]

Finally, and perhaps most important of all, medical education and, indeed, medical ethics, take scant heed of human rights. As a result, as Paul Hunt, former Special Rapporteur for the Right to Health, reported to the

U.N. General Assembly, "To be blunt, most health professionals whom the Special Rapporteur meets have not even heard of the right to health. If they have heard of it, they usually have no idea what it means, either conceptually or operationally. If they have heard of it, they are likely to be worried that it is something that will get them into trouble."[11] The convergence between medical ethics and human rights can't take place if physicians aren't even aware of human rights or their potential role in their fulfilment.

The medical community has struggled, often with great success, to bring down these barriers to a true human rights stance. With active leadership from the World Medical Association, and certain national medical associations, like the British Medical Association and the South African Medical Association, the profession has, in recent years, sought to harmonize professional practices with human rights standards, and especially to end rationalizations for medical complicity in human rights violations. These efforts are reflected, for example, in now widely accepted ethical duties not to discriminate in clinical practice based on race, ethnicity, religion, sexual orientation or gender, and in ever-stronger protections against medical complicity in torture.[12] The British Medical Association has taken the further step of setting out human rights standards for clinical practice, producing a "toolkit" on human rights and clinical medicine.[13] It cites obligations that ensure that physicians provide the highest possible standard of care and treatment in a way that respects the fundamental dignity of each of their patients. This involves a number of interrelated factors including:

—— Being honest, polite and respectful to all patients without discrimination

—— Ensuring professional skills are maintained to the highest possible level

—— Respecting the autonomy and dignity of patients and their right to self-determination

—— Providing up-to-date and relevant information without discrimination to support patients' decision-making

—— Respecting patient confidentiality

—— Treating patients with the highest ethical standards

The toolkit, however, while a concise statement of obligations of clinicians to patients in a clinical setting, also illustrates what is perhaps the most profound constraint on physicians' role in advancing human rights: A divide between the realms of medical practice and human rights advancement. Medicine is fundamentally based on an ethic of service, while a human rights "ethic" stresses analysis and accountability through advocacy.

Physicians well know that poverty, deprivation, inequality and marginalization – key concerns in the human rights context – have a profound impact on health.[14] They can recognize how lack of resources, entrenched discrimination, and inequitable social policies limit their ability to help their patients and, more generally, undermine the health of the population; but they are trained to navigate within the system, indeed to conform to it, and offer the patient the best care they can within those constraints, rather than systematically challenging them.

Physicians are generally neither trained nor expected to seek to change social, economic and policy circumstances that lead to ill-health, and rarely see it as their duty to do so. Perhaps even more profoundly, they are not taught to be self-reflective about the ways in which clinical practices that take place within a patently unjust system may actually reinforce health inequalities.[15] Further, medical training and medical traditions may even result in some discomfort in engaging in the advocacy needed to ameliorate human rights violations that lead to ill health because doing so is often seen as inconsistent with the neutrality required for a profession whose interventions are grounded in science. Finally, an ethic of service imposes its own burdens, starting with the efforts required to care for patients adequately, especially where resources are scarce or workload demands are high, leaving little time for systemic concerns.

The human rights enterprise, by contrast, focuses on the inequalities, deprivations, and infringements that lead to ill health, demanding that these, along with other impediments to health, such as poor access to, or quality of, health services, be remedied. It is designed to hold governments to account for compliance with universal standards of performance and legal obligations imposed by treaty to assure all people the opportunity to live a healthy life. In the health context, a human rights approach starts with recognition of the responsibility of government to take necessary steps to prevent disease (e.g., surveillance, immunization, assuring clean water and sanitation, protection against forms of discrimination that lead to ill-health); and moves on to require the government to assure the existence of health services that are available (including having sufficient staffing and supplies); are physically, geographically and financially accessible; are culturally acceptable to all; are of high quality; and are effective in meeting the needs of poor and vulnerable people.[16] A human rights approach also demands that members of the affected populations are provided an opportunity to participate in the structure of health services and have access to mechanisms to hold the government accountable for compliance with its obligations. Finally, it requires governments to play a legislative, monitoring and oversight role, assuring, for example, that drugs are safe and effective, and toxic products are adequately regulated. The need for accountability for all these obligations, in turn, requires a different form of engagement than service; it is centred on analysis and advocacy.

Toward a medical role in realizing the right to health

Physician engagement in advancing the right to the highest attainable standard of health can begin with awareness of how violations of human rights affect their own ability to offer the quality treatment they aspire to give. This may require asking difficult and sometimes personally uncomfortable questions about the system in which the physician practices. For example, what are the human rights implications for physicians practicing in a system where discrimination against certain groups is embedded or institutionalized? Or when the societies in which they live, their own governments, or the institutions where they practice limit the care available to uninsured people, immigrants or refugees to emergency services? Or where the care system lacks the basic equipment, laboratory facilities and medications needed to diagnose and treat a condition, or even assure safe childbirth? Or where lack of transportation precludes impoverished people from even reaching a clinic? Or where they themselves practice in a privileged, resource-rich environment, but know that these resources are not available to millions of people in need? These questions in turn raise issues of complicity: When does lack of awareness or knowledge result in some involvement in a violation of the right to health?

Posing such questions represents a different way of thinking about health inequities and professional roles. Even in considering their own practice and their own patients, it casts aside the idea that human rights are "extra-curricular" to practice, but rather it suggests that human rights are central to medical practice. Paul Farmer put this in the simplest terms, suggesting that a physician operating in a clinic bereft of supplies needs to view the availability of sutures as a human right.[17] Training and support in this new approach, which links self-reflection with awareness of the

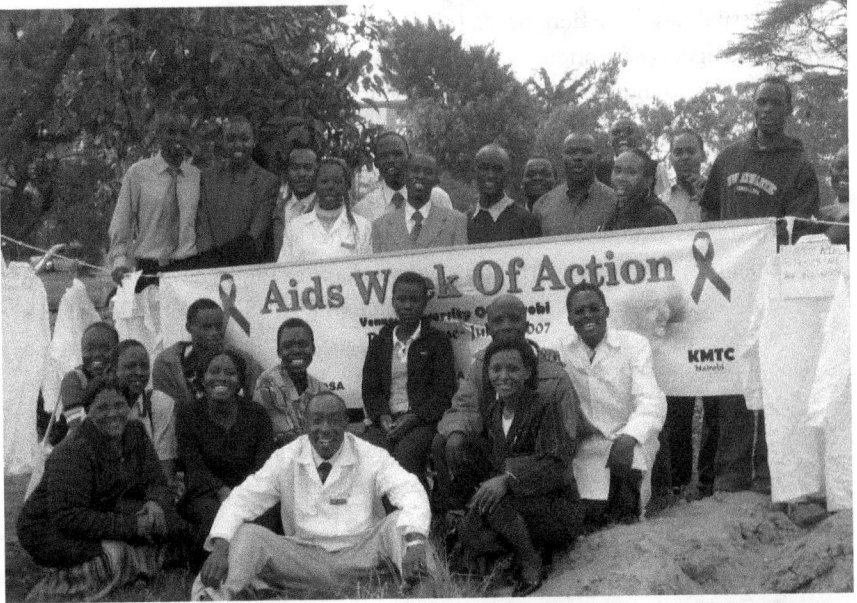

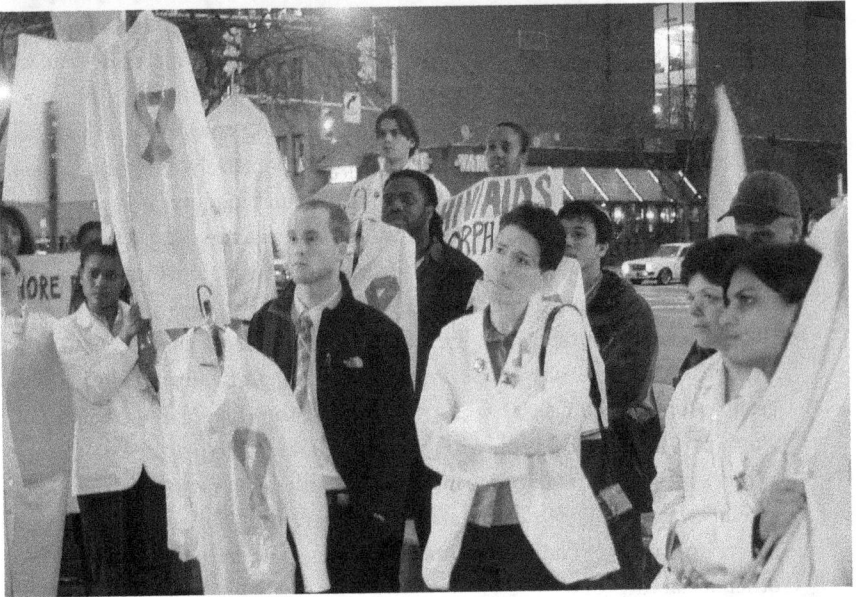

01

Students from University of Nairobi Medical School and the Kenya Medical Training College gather for the first campus-wide AIDS Week of Action, July 2007.

02

Medical Students at University of Rochester Medical Center in the US hold a rally in support of health workers in Africa on World AIDS Day, December 2006.

possibilities for action, needs to be a component of both medical training and ongoing education.

This foundation in inquiry and self-reflection can, in turn, lead to a transformation in the way physicians see themselves, not simply as service providers but rather as agents and advocates, along with patients and communities, in realizing the right to health. Physicians can appreciate that a rights-based approach requires physicians to view health as requiring more than technical interventions, recognizing, for example, as Jonathan Mann did two decades ago, that diseases like HIV/AIDS cannot be eradicated without attention to the marginalization and discrimination that increases vulnerability.[18] From there, it is not a leap to begin to take action to address the ways in which human rights violations affect the health of individuals and communities, whether these involve social determinants of health, inequities in access to health care and related social policies, or attitudes within the profession itself.

Achieving such a transformation, of course, poses enormous challenges, and physicians who are already burdened by their everyday responsibilities, and receive neither training nor support for new roles, cannot be expected to achieve it on their own. Medical leadership, including leaders in medical education, must show the way, through such means as introducing human rights in medical education and changing how physicians are socialized into the profession. This approach is not entirely new, as a variety of proposals for an ethical obligation to act against inequity in health have emerged, albeit not in human rights terms. One proposal urges that physicians become involved in advocacy for increased availability and access to care and to address social determinants of health that have a clear connection with health outcomes in the clinic.[19] Another urges that "all who provide health care must work to improve it."[20] A joint European-American group adopted a "Physicians' Charter", one of the three core principles of which is: "The medical profession must promote justice in the health care system, including the fair distribution of health care resources. Physicians should work actively to eliminate discrimination in health care, whether based on race, gender, socioeconomic status, ethnicity, religion, or any other social category."[21]

These obligations cannot be imposed solely on the individual, who is often powerless, acting alone, to alter the human rights circumstances of patients and communities. That is why collective action is needed. The International Working Group on Dual Loyalty and Human Rights recognized the limitations of what physicians and other health professionals can be expected to do on their own to advance human rights. But it urged them, instead of passively accepting the constraints on them in assuring equity in health, to act collectively to end policies and practices that prevent the health professional from providing core services to some, or all, patients in need.

The Working Group identified a number of relevant issues including: A state's failure to take steps needed to achieve the highest attainable standard of health for all; inequity in allocation of health resources or benefits; discrimination (or tolerance of discrimination) in health services; and denial of health information.[22] As the Working Group put it, "Rather than adjust one's behaviour to the constraints imposed by discrimination or the state's failure to develop a fair and equitable allocation of health resources, the health professional should act to change it."[23]

Recognizing that the changes needed to enable them to provide care consistent with their obligations was beyond their individual ability to affect, the Working Group urged collective action through their associations. Similarly, as Gruen and colleagues put it, "although individual action is laudable, collective action is a hallmark of professionalism."[24]

Though many physicians find the attention to awareness of human rights, much less action to realize rights, unusual or uncomfortable, they can look to the many precedents for physician action to advance human rights in recent decades. Indeed, the opportunities for physicians to advance human rights are limitless. Physicians, working collectively through associations or independent non-governmental organizations have fought threats to the human rights and health of individuals and communities from toxic chemicals, nuclear weapons, anti-personnel landmines, restrictions on reproductive services for women, the use of tobacco, and torture; and they have been outspoken in demanding access to quality health services for all, including people living in extreme poverty and disenfranchised groups like prisoners.[25] Their special skills give them important roles in documentation and analysis, and their voices, united with each other and with civil society, are powerful.

There are reasons for optimism that both the new self-concept and the new role can be embraced. In recent years the beginnings of a transformation toward a human rights orientation for the medical profession have begun to appear. The world's leading medical journals increasingly devote space to peer-reviewed articles on human rights subjects, ranging from the sources of global health inequities, to the treatment of asylum seekers and immigrants in highly developed societies, to torture, to developing an epidemiology of war that considers how to track mortality, rates of sexual violence, and atrocities in armed conflict. The World Medical Association has developed ever more detailed standards of conduct for physicians, premised on human rights.

The most exciting developments may be taking place in the poorest countries, where doctors, along with other health professionals, are forming human rights organizations and partnering with civil society organizations to join in the struggles of communities regarding health financing, stigma that affects health services, the shortage of health workers, and much more.[26] Organizations of physicians and other health professionals that are explicitly based on human rights have been formed in a dozen countries and an international consortium, the International Federation of Health and Human Rights Organizations, links them with one another.[27]

The medical profession remains a long way from overcoming the still-pronounced cautiousness and institutional conservatism stemming from an ethic of service that limits their willingness to confront and address the infringements of the right to health for individuals and communities. But at least the belief that you can only be a good doctor if you promote the right to health is within sight.

* The author appreciates the helpful comments of Dr. Holly Atkinson and Dr. Frank Davidoff on an earlier draft of this chapter.

1 This chapter focuses on physicians particularly, but much of the analysis applies to other health professionals as well.

2 World Medical Association, Declaration of Geneva, 1990, available at http://www.wma.net/e/policy/c8.htm.

3 World Medical Association, International Code of Medical Ethics, 2006, available at http://www.wma.net/e/policy/c8.htm.

4 Preamble, Universal Declaration of Human Rights (1948), available at http://www.un.org/Overview/rights.html.

5 J. Orbinski, C. Beyrer and S. Singh, 'Violations of Human Rights: Health Practitioners as Witnesses' 370 The Lancet (2007) at 698–706.

6 D. Rothman, 'Medical Professionalism: Focusing on the Real Issue' 342(17) North England Journal of Medicine (2000) at 1284–1286.

7 L. Rubenstein, and L. London, 'The Universal Declaration of Human Rights and the Limits of Medical Ethics: The Case of South Africa' 3 Health and Human Rights (1998) at 161–175.

8 Institute of Medicine of the National Academy of Sciences, Unequal Treatment, (Washington, D.C., National Academy of Sciences, 2003); Physicians for Human Rights, The Right to Equal Treatment (Cambridge, MA: Physicians for Human Rights, 2003), available at http://physiciansforhumanrights.org/library/documents/reports/report-rightequaltreat-2003.PDF

9 K. Geraghty, and M. Wynia, 'Advocacy and Community: The Social Roles of Physicians in the Last 1000 Years: Part II' 39022 MedGenMed E28 (2000).

10 Physicians for Human Rights and School of Public Health and Primary Health Care, University of Cape Town, Health Sciences Faculty, Dual Loyalty and Human Rights in Health Professional Practice: Proposed Guidelines and Institutional Mechanisms (Cambridge, MA: Physicians for Human Rights, 2003), available at http://physiciansforhuman

rights.org/library/documents/reports/report-2002-duelloyalty.pdf.

11 P. Hunt, Report of the Special Rapporteur of the right of everyone to the highest attainable standard of physical and mental health, 17 January 2007, UN Doc. A/HRC/4/28.

12 World Medical Association, Declaration of Tokyo, 2006, available at http://www.wma.net/e/policy/c18.htm.

13 British Medical Association and Commonwealth Medical Trust, The Right to Health: A Toolkit for Health Professionals (London: British Medical Association, 2007), available at http://www.bma.org.uk/ap.nsf/AttachmentsByTitle/PDFRighttoHealthtoolkit/$FILE/Righttohealth.pdf.

14 World Health Organization Commission on Social Determinants of Health, 'Interim Statement, Achieving Health Equity: From root causes to fair outcomes' (Geneva: WHO, 2007) available at http://whqlibdoc.who.int/publications/2007/interim_statement_eng.pdf; and P. Braverman and S. Gruskin, 'Poverty, Equity, Human Rights and Health' 81(7) Bulletin of the World Health Organization (2003) available at http://www.who.int/bulletin/volumes/81/7/en/Braveman0703.pdf.

15 American Association for Advancement of Science and Physicians for Human Rights, Human Rights and Health: The Legacy of Apartheid (Washington, D.C.: Physicians for Human Rights, 1998).

16 Committee on Economic, Social and Cultural Rights (CESCR), General Comment No. 14 on the right to the highest attainable standard of health, 11 August 2000, UN Doc. E/C.12/2000/4, available at http://www.unhchr.ch/tbs/doc.nsf/(symbol)/E.C.12.2000.4.En.

17 P. Farmer, 'Challenging Orthodoxies in Health and Human Rights', Address to American Public Health Association, 2006, available at http://www.pih.org/inforesources/essays/APHA_2006_keynote-Paul_Farmer.pdf.

18 J. Mann, 'Human Rights and AIDS: The Future of the Pandemic Health and Human Rights' in J. Mann, S. Gruskin, M. Grodin, and G. Annas

(eds.) *Health and Human Rights, A Reader* (New York and London: Routledge, 1999).

19 R. Gruen, S. Pearson, and T. Brennan, 'Physicians-Citizens: Public Roles and Professional Obligations' 291 *JAMA* (2004) at 94–98.

20 R. Smith, H. Hiatt, and D. Berwick, 'A Shared Statement of Ethical Principles for Those Who Shape and Give Health Care: A Working Draft' 130(2) *Ann Int Med* (1999) at 143–147, available at http://www.acponline.org/clinical_information/journals_publications/ecp/mayjun99/tavistock.htm.

21 'Medical Professionalism in the New Millennium: A Physician Charter' 136 *Ann Intern Med* (2002) at 243–46.

22 Physicians for Human Rights and School of Public Health and Primary Health Care, University of Cape Town, Health Sciences Faculty, *Dual Loyalty and Human Rights in Health Professional Practice: Proposed Guidelines and Institutional Mechanisms* (Cambridge, MA: Physicians for Human Rights, 2003), General Guideline 13, available at http://physiciansforhumanrights.org/library/documents/reports/report-2002-duelloyalty.pdf.

23 Ibid.

24 Gruen, *supra* note 19, at 97.

25 British Medical Association (BMA), *The Medical Profession and Human Rights* (London:, BMA, 2003).

26 See, for example, the Action Group for Health, Human Rights and HIV/AIDS, further information available at http://physiciansforhumanrights.org/hiv-aids/partnerships-in-africa/uganda/agha-inspiring-results.html; Kenya Health Rights Advocacy Forum, further information available at http://www.heraf.or.ke/; and Zimbabwe Association of Doctors for Human Rights, further information available at http://www.kubatana.net/html/sectors/zimo65.asp.

27 See further, http://www.ifhhro.org.

For having kindly permitted us the use of their photographs, we thank Physicians for Human Rights.

The Voice of Health Professionals in Achieving the Right to Health: The Action Group for Health, Human Rights and HIV/AIDS (AGHA) Uganda

Nelson Musoba and Sarah Kalloch*

Background

Every movement starts somewhere, and every journey has twists and turns. Ours is a movement of health workers, policy makers and health consumers in Uganda dedicated to addressing the many links between health and human rights. The Action Group for Health, Human Rights and HIV/AIDS (AGHA) started in July 2003 as an idea among four young energetic Ugandan health professionals who had just completed a course on health, human rights, social justice and equity at Makerere University. It has now become a nationwide movement bringing together doctors, nurses, lawyers, social workers, consumers of health services and other professionals throughout Uganda.

Since our beginning in 2003, AGHA has mobilized hundreds of members, conducted more than 15 health, human rights and advocacy trainings, brought human rights awareness to key health and policy making bodies, and started a movement of health workers for human rights. But the task has not been easy. This case study examines the evolution of AGHA: Our early years, how we grew our successful campaigns, and where we want to go next.

Why did we start AGHA?

We were four health professionals who had recently finished the course on health and human rights at Makerere University. Our earlier understanding of human rights advocacy was one of opposition and agitation – carrying placards and marching through the streets. Yet we were doctors and nurses, several employed by the government, and we wanted neither to protest, nor to riot. We simply wanted to share our medical expertise and human rights ideals with others, including policy makers. Together we decided that we needed to change the perception of human rights in Uganda – and bring health rights to the fore.

We met under the trees in the garden of Fairway Hotel in Kampala, trying to figure out how to help our health worker colleagues to see health from a human rights perspective. Our first inspiration was the work of Paul Farmer and Jonathan Mann. We decided to share their stories with our colleagues through a journal club at Mulago Hospital, the first and oldest teaching hospital in the country. In September 2003 we held our first meeting and, to our surprise, it was very well attended. Our colleagues were curious to find out what health and human rights really meant. What was originally planned as a 45 minute discussion turned into a two hour conversation and from that point on there was no turning back.

The beginning of AGHA – lots of energy, no office ...

Within three months of that first journal club, we were registered with the local non-governmental organization board, one step in a long and still ongoing process to build the organizational capacity we need to reach our dreams. In late 2003, we met with staff from Physicians for Human Rights (PHR), an NGO from the United States that was interested in starting a partnership in Uganda to nurture a network of health professionals dedicated to human rights. In September 2004, AGHA and PHR, with support from the Bill and Melinda Gates Foundation, officially joined forces to augment AGHA's current work and make the vision of a health worker movement for human rights a reality.

We were lucky: We had leadership, vision, excitement and a critical niche. Political space in Uganda was opening up, and money was flowing in from the international community to support global health initiatives. However, we had very limited organizational capacity. We had only enough funds to hire one staff person, open a small office, and hold a few trainings.

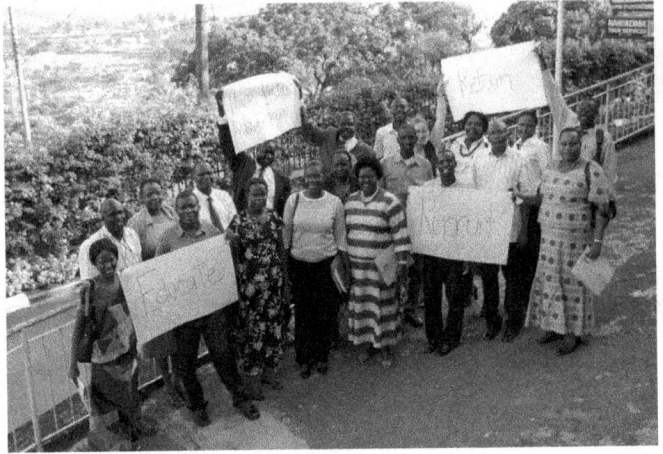

AGHA's first bank account was opened using personal contributions from the founder members. They also contributed furniture and other equipment for the first office, in addition to volunteering their time and skills to provide AGHA with the needed leadership and strategic direction – a major contribution from people who all had full time jobs. AGHA, with PHR support, began to build both a movement and an NGO at the same time – no small feat in Uganda, or anywhere in the world.

We needed to start slowly, as health workers interested in the movement had the same reaction as AGHA's founders, shying away from human rights and advocacy. We began to dispel the rumours and innuendo around human rights and advocacy through concerted outreach training and workshops in Kampala and three other rural districts, culminating in a national conference on AIDS and health advocacy. Slowly, we built support for action to key decision makers. The platform approved at our first conference formed the basis for a letter, signed by over 150 health workers from across the country, which was presented to a key Ministry of Health Commissioner and a Member of Parliament at a press event – the first major action AGHA undertook. Through networking and outreach, we built a level of support and an advocacy platform which gave us the base from which to build our movement.

01
AGHA allies unite to support health workforce advocacy, one of several of AGHA's critical health rights campaigns.

<u>AGHA's advocacy campaigns – shaping ideals into action</u>

Once AGHA established itself as an organization, we began to organize concrete advocacy campaigns and targeted outreach programs to bring health rights to all Ugandans. This section will highlight three such programs to show the reach of AGHA and the kinds of advocacy possible by health professionals in a country grappling with multiple health rights challenges.

Health rights leadership building: Students for Equity in Health Care (SEHC)

Medical students represent the future of Uganda's health leadership. These students will shape Uganda's public health system and its responsiveness to human rights concerns. Our student outreach began small and spread quickly: AGHA invited four medical students to its first major conference in December 2004 to learn about our work, network with colleagues and get a sense of their role in health rights advocacy. Within four days, these four students had convened a task force of 13 to discuss how to start a health rights advocacy group on campus. Within a week, they had mobilized over

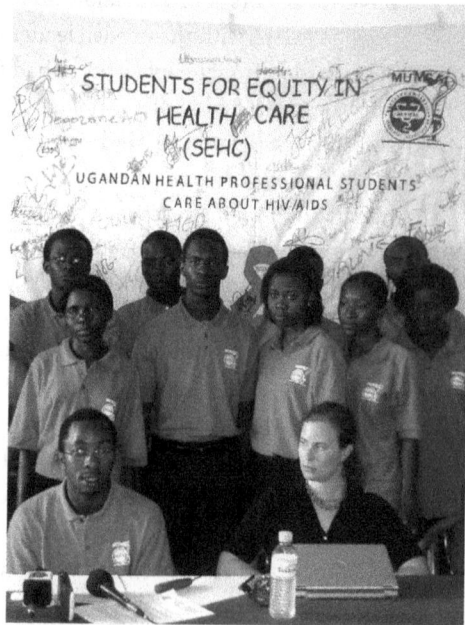

02
SEHC founder and Makerere University medical student Nixon Nyonzima speaks at an AGHA press conference on World Health Day 2006.

75 students for an advocacy training, and just three months later they held the first AIDS Week of Action ever at Makerere Medical School, which reached hundreds of students with health and human rights awareness and action messages.

SEHC has grown exponentially since its auspicious beginnings. There are now SEHC chapters at all three public medical schools: At the flagship Makerere branch, which has expanded to include nursing and paramedical students; at Mbarara Medical School, located in an area with high rates of HIV; and at Gulu University in war-torn Northern Uganda, where health indicators are appalling. In 2008, Makerere held its fourth annual AIDS Week of Action, Mbarara and Gulu their second, and all three schools came together to host the third National Student Conference on health rights advocacy – this time expanding to include students in the law, economics and social science faculties.

SEHC has been deeply involved in advocacy to promote equitable access to quality health care in Uganda and strengthen student leadership and empowerment. During the first AIDS Week of Action at Makerere, SEHC advocated for provision of a hepatitis B vaccine to medical students in Uganda, an action which led the Ministry of Health to promise the vaccine to all health workers country-wide. SEHC students have also written and disseminated their own Stigma Handbook to educate health students about the causes and consequences of HIV/AIDS-driven stigma and discrimination on patients and providers. They continue to hold health and human rights workshops to sensitize students to the importance of the human rights aspect of health care, and build national and international partnerships to improve health rights, including close ties with PHR's medical student chapters across the United States.

SEHC has not only made an impact on how health students view human rights, but has fundamentally changed the way many students look at their future. Nixon Niyonzima came to medical school ready to study surgery. After working with SEHC, he has become an impassioned human rights leader:

> "Before you join medical school, you have different perceptions of what
> medical school is and really what medicine is. Before I was in medical school,
> I thought that medicine was about prestige, about success. Not so. Medi-
> cine is sacrifice. Joining AGHA and starting SEHC gave me a very important

opportunity to learn what little extra we need to add to our profession to make it medicine. SEHC is a voice through which we advocate for our and patient's rights; above all, it provides an avenue to learn and teach fellow health workers the difference between human and inhumane, and the need to treat patients as human beings with human rights."

AGHA's health financing campaign: Innovative research for advocacy through a drug stock out survey

"Under-funding of the health sector is tantamount to deliberately giving an under-dose of medication to a patient and hoping that he will still get better. Government needs to commit to the 15 per cent (promised at the Abuja Summit in 2001) to help alleviate these issues."
Honourable Dr. Francis Epetait (Member of Parliament and Shadow Minister of Health for the Opposition Party at the Launch of AGHA's Drug Stock Out Survey)

In 2006, AGHA Uganda launched its health financing campaign, with the goal to improve the health and human rights of all Ugandans by advocating for increased health sector financing. Through concerted advocacy and outreach to civil society and the media, AGHA has increased awareness about the urgent need for higher health spending, and has gained allies in civil society, the Ministry of Health and Parliament.

AGHA realized it needed three things to make a real impact in this campaign. First, we needed better data on the realities in rural clinics to show the wide gaps between government policies and what is actually happening on the ground. Second, we wanted to connect better with our members, especially those in rural areas, and give them a way to participate more deeply in advocacy. Finally, we needed something splashy and sensational to capture the attention of policy makers and the media.

To meet all these needs, AGHA and PHR launched their innovative "Stock Out Survey" in late 2006. The survey, which took place in three new districts in rural Southwestern Uganda, collected data on the supply of essential malaria and antibiotic medicines and staffing levels at selected health facilities. This data was combined with informant interviews and community input from AGHA members and others to illuminate the key road blocks in supply-chain management, drug distribution, and staffing in Ugandan health facilities. The resulting report illuminated the consequences of inadequate

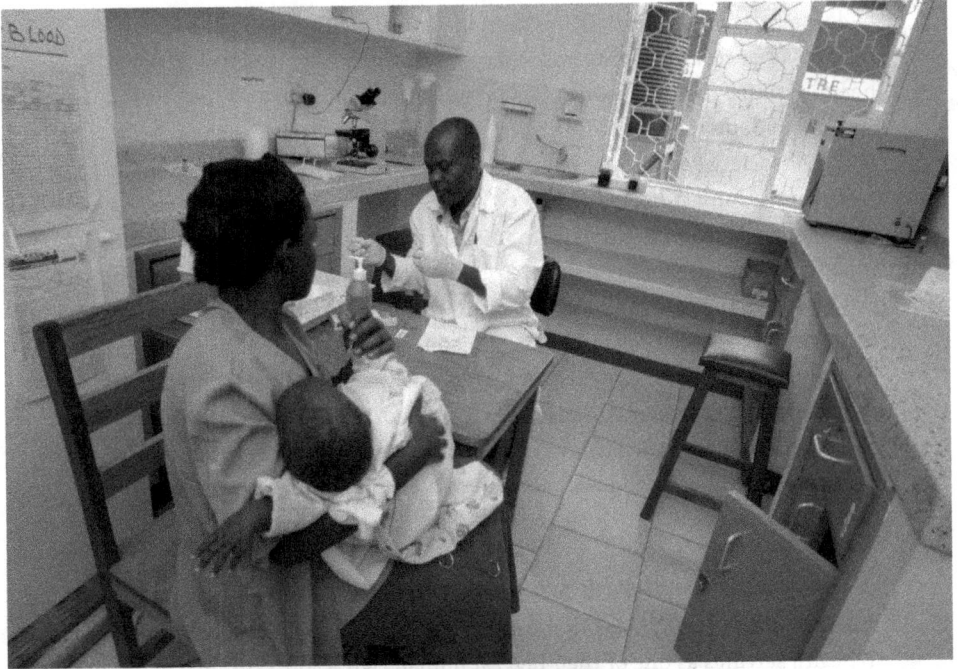

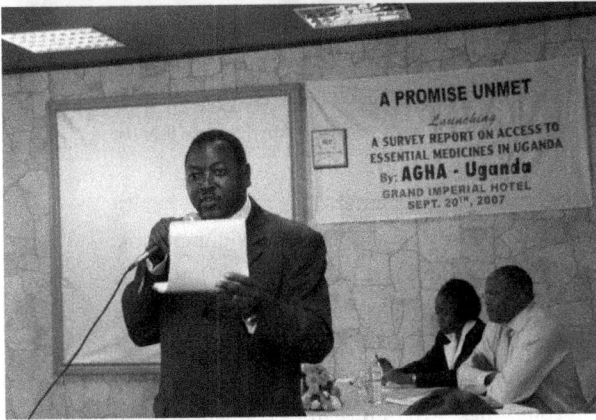

03
Patients receiving care at Lyantonde
Hospital, one of the clinics surveyed.
04
Honorable Dr. Emmanuel Otaala, Minister of State
for Health (Primary Care), addresses the participants
at AGHA's Drug Stock Out Survey Launch.

budget allocation on the health system in rural areas, and brought the critical voice of health workers to policy discussions on how to create responsive health systems that will protect and promote health for all.

On 20 September 2007 Members of Parliament, health professionals, and civil society representatives attended a meeting to launch the report "A Promise Unmet: Access to Essential Medicines in Three New Districts of Uganda". A diverse group of more than 50 stakeholders reviewed the findings of the research and discussed the implications of the findings on the health status of Ugandans. The event drew 13 Members of Parliament from various key committees. The Minister of State for Health (Primary Health Care), Dr. Emmanuel Otaala, who was the chief guest, stated that this workshop represented "the type of collaboration we at the Ministry of Health are always advocating for. When we work together as partners in health, we are able to address our common vision and overcome the barriers ahead of us."

Grassroots outreach and action: AGHA's anti-stigma campaign

From the start of AGHA's work, health professionals have identified stigma in health settings as one of their biggest human rights concerns. AGHA believes that stigma starts and stops in the hearts and minds of health workers, and thus we began our anti-stigma campaign with peer education and leadership building. This outreach provided an excellent entry point for organizing and engaging deeper with members, while training leaders to bring anti-stigma messages to the wider community.

AGHA held an initial stigma "training-for-trainers" for 25 AGHA health worker and Persons Living With AIDS (PLWA) members in November 2005. Participants at the training hailed from all four of AGHA's operational districts (Kampala, Tororo, Mbarara and Rakai) as well as from Makerere Medical School. Following the training, participants organized themselves into district based task forces and took the messages they had learned from AGHA to their peers and colleagues. AGHA has since trained 25 more leaders and the task forces have held more than ten member-led stigma trainings for health workers in the four districts, reaching over 200 health workers. AGHA is now working with district leadership in all four districts to integrate anti-stigma training into continuing medical education electives, thus institutionalizing this movement and creating a wider opportunity to promote health and human rights for people living with AIDS.

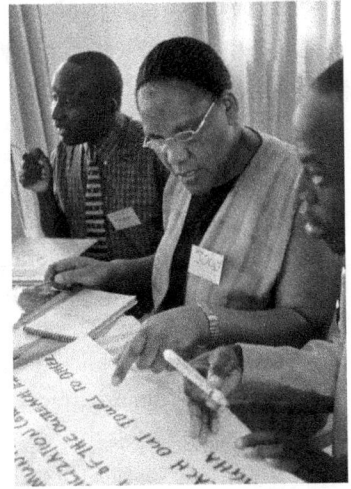

The critical importance of this work can best be shown through the work of the Mulago Anti-Stigma Task Force, made up primarily of nurses at Mulago Hospital, Uganda's national referral hospital. In April of 2006, the Foundation for Human Rights Initiative came out with a report, authored in part by TASO, which outlined high levels of stigma in the Mulago maternity ward against HIV-positive mothers – with nurses implicated in much of the discriminatory behaviour. The nurses AGHA had trained, immediately set up an anti-stigma training for their peers, to discuss the report, and to find ways to combat this stigma, and forge better relationships with patients. This kind of quick and compassionate response helped support both nurses and patients, during a trying time, and brought human rights to the fore at Mulago Hospital.

Successes, challenges and next steps

Five years ago, AGHA's founding members were meeting under the stars for tea at Fairview Hotel; today, AGHA is one of the leading health and human rights organizations in Uganda. The results of AGHA's work are inspiring and a testament to the power of health professionals in human rights advocacy:

—— **The paradigm of medicine is changing to accommodate and embrace human rights:** The Uganda Medical Association has started a human rights committee, which AGHA will chair. AGHA's health student leadership programme – Students for Equity in Health Care SEHC – now boasts over 600 members from chapters established in the medical school universities of Makerere, Mbarara and Gulu. The AGHA Stigma Task Force has trained over 200 health workers in four districts about stigma and what they can do to prevent it, and is working with district medical leaders to get this training integrated in continuing medical education classes – critical to stemming the tide of discrimination and promoting patient rights.

—— **The health budget in Uganda is increasing:** In April 2007, the parliament announced an 8 billion Uganda shilling increase in the health budget – small in the face of a shilling deficit of over 200 billion, but significant because the health budget was in fact set to be cut by billions until civil society, led by AGHA, was able to convince policy makers to reverse this harmful course and help support the right to health. Another budget increase came in 2008 – more proof of the power of health professionals to have a national impact.

—— **Health workers and their patients have better protection in health settings:** As a result of SEHC activism, Ministry of Health officials pledged to vaccinate all health workers against hepatitis B and to improve provision of post exposure prophylaxis for patients and providers at Mulago Hospital.

—— **Health rights activism is spreading across Uganda and Africa:** In Uganda, AGHA has spearheaded the establishment of a new Health and Human Rights Coalition called Voice for Health Rights, whose goal is to unite health and human rights civil society organizations in order to advocate for improved health service delivery. Approximately 20 organizations have subscribed to the coalition, which AGHA believes will strengthen the civil society response to critical health rights challenges in Uganda. AGHA is also spearheading the Uganda Health Workforce Advocacy Forum, a collaboration between key health professional leaders whose goal is to advocate for human rights-based health workforce development plans and programmes. This movement is spreading across the continent: Together with the International Federation of Health and Human Rights Organizations (IFHHRO), AGHA held a training and networking meeting for over 30 health rights activists from across Africa in February 2007, in order to create an African focal point for collaboration and information exchange.

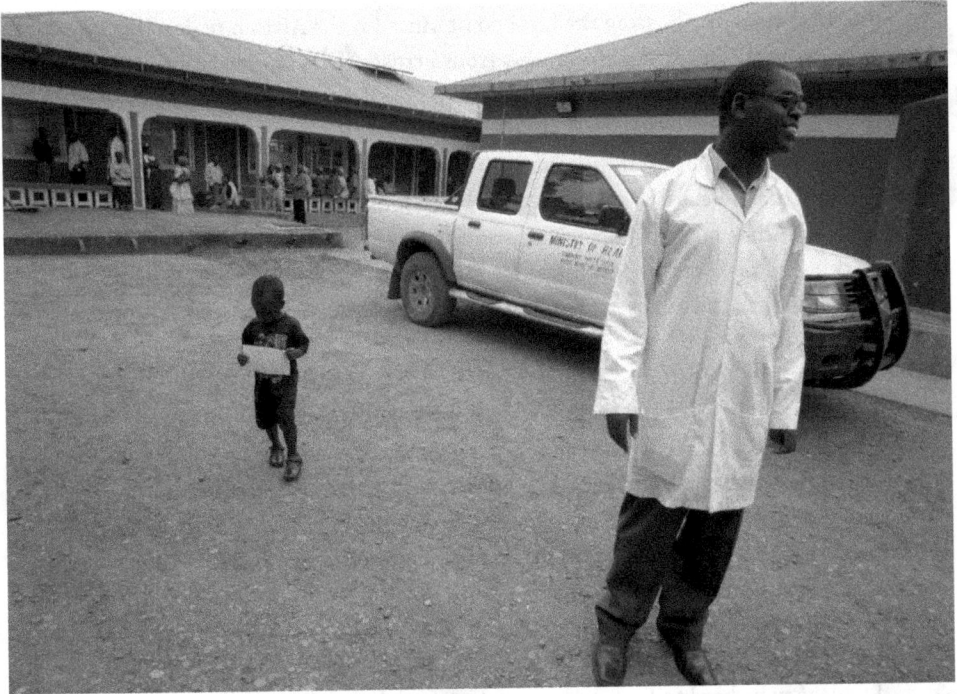

06

06
Dr. Katumba outside Lyantonde
Hospital in Southwestern Uganda.

AGHA is currently hosting the focal point office for the African region that aims to unite health rights groups from across Africa in education and monitoring the right to health.

This success has not been without deep challenges. The intricacy of building a rights-based health system in a resource-poor country can be daunting, but AGHA has focused its advocacy on the issues we think are both most critical and that we can best influence. While the community perception of human rights and advocacy remains guarded, AGHA is always looking for ways to deepen and broaden our member base and commitment, as well as opportunities for action. Keeping members involved and engaged, especially those who live in rural areas and do not have ready access to email, continues to be a challenge. Finally, finding funds and achieving long term sustainability remains difficult for AGHA. Many grants are small and for one year only, which makes it hard for a young organization to truly build programs that work, and to hire staff for long term progress and organizational development.

But health rights are being recognized in Uganda, and AGHA will remain a strong advocate as a result of the deep commitment of its members. Funds may be hard to find, and advocating for human rights will always be an uphill battle. But for AGHA it is no longer a dream, it is a goal. Health rights are attainable, and health workers from all cadres and from all areas of Uganda have risen to the challenge – and now encourage the world to do the same. Said Dr. Katumba Ssentongo, a long time AGHA member:

> "I have always believed that everyone is born with a purpose. My purpose is to make a change in the lives of the community I serve – that is my calling. AGHA helps me fulfill this purpose. I work at Lyantonde Hospital, a new hospital which lacks a lot of equipment. We have done advocacy to strategic groups who can help us equip our hospital so we have enough space, equipment, and materials, with the eventual goal to ensure our patients achieve their right to health. This is a new fight – we want people in the Philippines, in Chile, and around the world to join this movement. Together, we can succeed."

*   For more information about our work and how you can partner with us, please contact the AGHA secretariat at: AGHA Uganda, Mailing Address: P. O. Box 24667 Kampala, Office Location: Kamwokya, Plot 69 Kanjokya Street, phone: 041 348 491, email: info@aghauganda.org, website: http://www.aghauganda.org.

For having kindly permitted us the use of their photographs, we thank:
p. 395, 396, 399 (bottom): PHR
p. 399 (top), 401, 403: Vanessa Vick

08

STRENGTHEN-ING HEALTH CARE SYSTEMS

Drilling Down: Strengthening Local Health Systems to Address Global Health Crises

Lynn P. Freedman*

Introduction

Rock stars, movie stars, and business stars: Are they the canaries in the coal mine? – We stand at a pivotal moment in the global health field as large infusions of new money create great expectations of dramatic improvement in the trends of death and disability that plague the poorest regions of the world and threaten the rest. Certainly there have been some notable successes in public health over the past 50 years, including the eradication of smallpox and the introduction of oral rehydration therapy to substantially reduce death from diarrheal diseases. Yet the excitement and energy that have accompanied the splashy arrival of health onto the world's poverty-reduction agenda compete with a brooding sense of crisis, with an inchoate understanding that something is deeply wrong with the way things work in the field of global health.

For the moment, the canaries are singing an alluring melody and the resources are starting to roll in. But the miners working far below the surface, who are expected to produce results day after day, continue to slog away under desperate conditions. The air they breathe is still dangerously thin and their shouts can barely be heard. The products of their work, though sometimes glitteringly fabulous, are more often paltry, hard to process and burnish into value.

We must be careful not to mistake the canaries' music for oxygen itself. Unless there is profound change in how we understand, invest in, and act on global health problems, the risk of failure runs very high.

This paper argues that a rights-based approach, strategically constructed, plays a critical role in ensuring that the resources mobilized for global health have the kind of impact that will initiate the long-term processes of building social and political institutions essential for true change in global health.

The global health crisis

The crisis in global health has multiple dimensions:

—— Major diseases are decimating families and communities, causing suffering on a massive scale. HIV/AIDS, tuberculosis and malaria have recently attracted the most attention. But persistently high child mortality and maternal mortality, poor sexual and reproductive health, and epidemics of trauma and violence also have enormous implications for the quality of human life.

—— Deep and poisonous inequities characterize the global health scene. A woman in Niger has a 1 in 7 chance of dying in pregnancy or child birth over her lifetime, while a woman in Ireland has a 1 in 47 600 risk.[1] The disparities within countries, across class, race, gender and other lines of social disadvantage, may be less dramatic, but they are experienced more directly and destructively. Rarely documented or measured, less often addressed, these intra-country inequities regularly escape official notice altogether.

—— Health systems in poor, high-mortality countries are in serious disarray, sometimes in full collapse. In vast parts of the world, health facilities stand empty and deteriorating. In others they are overwhelmed and unable to cope. User fees and "informal" payments prevent the poorest from accessing what services exist, yet under-the-table payments are often the only way providers can earn a living wage. Drug shortages force patients into the streets to find life-saving supplies or to forego needed care altogether. A massive "brain drain" (see the chapters by Eric Friedman and Francis Omaswa, respectively, in this book) draws trained professionals out of countries, while policies of international financial institutions (IFIs) pressure for bans on government hiring to replace them. Existing medical and nursing schools do not even begin to meet the demand for health workers, yet donor funding is too unpredictable and short-term for poor-country governments to invest with confidence in new medical and nursing schools that will take years to build. Those professionals who remain in the system are often poorly trained and supervised, leaving even the best-intentioned providers without confidence or skills. Over-worked and demoralized, they can barely cope with their workloads, much less follow protocols for improved inter-personal relationships with clients. Indeed, in many places, shocking maltreatment of patients and their families is almost routine.

___ Poor health and health systems themselves are causing poverty, in both its economic and social dimensions and at both the individual and the population levels. WHO estimates that 100 million people each year are pushed below the poverty line by the costs of illness and/or obtaining health care. Poor health of the workforce is seen as a major obstacle to economic growth, while faltering growth renders countries unable to make the investments necessary to improve health – the so-called "medical-poverty trap".

One more dimension to the global health crisis should be added:

___ In many quarters there is a perception that increased money for the health sector does not yield improved health outcomes. A sense of "public health nihilism"[2] creeps into policy debates, bringing cynicism and paralysis with it.

What's wrong with "business as usual"?

Rock stars and movie stars have done much to open the rich world's eyes to the terrible toll that ill-health is taking on the world's poor, but it is the Millennium Development Goals (MDGs) that have facilitated health's arrival onto the formal poverty-reduction agenda of governments and international development agencies. Virtually every report about the health MDGs (including our own) begins and ends with the same conclusion: "Business as usual" will not be enough to reach any ambitious target for improving the health of populations. But the typical call to exceed "business as usual" is ultimately a call for more – lots more – of the same, with precious little analysis of why standard approaches have generally been so deficient.

Three aspects of "business as usual" need to be acknowledged and challenged. At the risk of over-simplification, they can be described as the established approaches set out below.

The epidemiological approach to public health

The dominant approach to the formulation of health policy and the distribution of health resources relies heavily on the evidence generated by epidemiologic research and cost-effectiveness analysis. It is a technocratic, largely top-down process, in which "business as usual" consists of a familiar sequence of steps:

1. Select priority diseases/conditions (usually according to burden of disease)
2. Document the proximate causes of death from those conditions
3. Identify technical interventions to address those causes
4. Do demonstration projects to prove effectiveness and cost-effectiveness of the interventions and to identify "best practices" in delivering them
5. Disseminate information about best practices
6. Call for "scale-up"
7. Advocate for "political will" to get the job done

The result is a collection of discrete, theoretically cost-effective interventions (often termed an "essential minimum package") focused on specific diseases. For most interventions, high-mortality, resource-poor countries are stranded at step 5 with levels of coverage dangerously low and inequitably distributed. Virtually all commentators working from within this paradigm agree that delivery at scale is the challenge.

But "scale up" is rarely conceptualized as anything beyond the multiplication of interventions to ever larger populations and ever wider geographic areas. The political obstacles to structural change are assumed to be surmountable through the determined exercise of national leadership, the familiar "political will". Until recently, the (crumbling) health systems on which equitable delivery of such interventions ultimately depends have been widely ignored, or intentionally avoided, by much of the health field, leaving their fate largely in the hands of economic policymakers and ideologues, as well as local powerbrokers.

Social and economic determinants of health

An important counter-weight to the epidemiologic approach is one that focuses on the social and economic determinants of health. A vast literature demonstrates that changes in key social and economic conditions – including education (particularly of girls and women), income, nutrition, water and sanitation – are associated with improvements (or deterioration) in health. The work of the WHO Commission on the Social Determinants of Health reinforces the importance of tackling these factors through intersectoral action.[3]

The problem with the "business as usual" versions of this approach is that they typically end with identifying these important correlations and calling for priority to be given to economic growth and to interventions outside the health sector, simply assuming that overall development will automatically have a positive impact on health. Little attention is paid to the "mechanisms of action", the processes by which economic development can ultimately improve population health equitably, and the conditions that are required for putting those processes into place in any particular setting.

This kind of economic determinism and its enduring currency in the health field owe much to the groundbreaking work of Thomas McKeown and his analysis of the steep mortality declines that followed the industrial revolution in 19th century Britain.[4] Writing in the 1970s, McKeown argued that, contrary to then-conventional wisdom, only a tiny proportion of mortality improvements prior to the 1930s could be attributed to the technical interventions of medical science. Instead, he argued, it was economic growth and the resulting improvements in living conditions – particularly in nutrition – that accounted for the leaps in life expectancy.

McKeown's implicit attack on the high-tech strategies of the day was certainly welcome in progressive circles where the turn toward community-based, locally appropriate interventions was crystallizing into the concept of Primary Health Care announced in the Alma-Ata Declaration of 1978. In the area of women's health, attention to social and economic determinants of health played a crucial role in the transition from demographically-driven contraceptive supply programs, to holistic, user-centered notions of reproductive health.

But as subsequent critics have pointed out, McKeown's thesis also proved highly convenient for the neoliberal economists and their rising influence over global development policy in the 1980s and 1990s.[5] Assured

that good health would automatically follow strong economic growth regardless of medical or public health interventions, the IFIs and donor countries pressed for structural adjustment programmes that slashed health
sector budgets, called for the withdrawal of the state from social services,
and put all faith (and, indeed, it was more faith than fact) in the magic of
the market to ultimately improve the health of all.

While McKeown was certainly correct that the medical profession
and medical technology made little contribution to the mortality declines
of the late 19th and early 20th century in Britain, his dismissal of the role
of the state, of the new public health movement (the "Sanitary Idea") and
of human agency, in favour of the invisible forces of economic growth,
have been largely discredited. Indeed, Simon Szreter's close analysis of
the same data from 19th century Britain comes to a significantly different
conclusion:

> "The most that can be said in favour of modern economic growth is that the
> wealth that it accumulates creates the longer-term potential for population
> health improvements. *But whether or not this potential is realized depends
> entirely on a set of quite distinct social and political negotiations and decisions
> on how exactly that wealth is to be used and distributed.*"[6]

In fact, Szreter demonstrates that, in the short-term, economic growth
causes intense social disruption which, unless carefully managed by an in-
terventionist state, leads to disruption, deprivation, disease and death (the
"4 Ds"). In the case of 19th century Britain, he points to the importance of
the politics of public health, the social and political movement initiated by
the "Sanitary Idea" (improved living conditions) and the crucial actions of
local (not central) government in building cross-class consensus for the investment of tax revenues in the health-related infrastructure, including water and sanitation systems.[7]

Arguably globalization is causing similar disruption, and the lessons
Szreter draws from the historical British experience (and from other European and East Asian cases) can inform the building of an effective rights-
based practice.

The standard human rights approach

Human rights now occupy an important place in global health discourse. The formal legal instruments of human rights – treaties and declarations – have generated exceptionally wide consensus in the international community. The human rights vision of individual dignity and equality, together with its language of social justice, has "crystallized the moral imagination" of many.[8] Use of a rights-based approach to programming has now become the official policy of UN agencies such as the United Nations Children's Fund (UNICEF) and the UN Population Fund (UNFPA), and of international NGOs such as CARE and Save the Children.

I would argue, however, that standard approaches to the use of human rights in health – "business as usual" – fail to fulfill its transformative potential.

The elaboration of formal law is, of course, an essential part of building a strong human rights system. Understanding of the right to health has benefited enormously from the excellent General Comment No. 14 of the UN Committee on Economic, Social and Cultural Rights, and from the important and creative work of the Special Rapporteur on the Right to Health (both dealt with at the beginning of this book). But methodologies for actually using human rights in practice in the health field are still wanting.

In global and national policy discussions, human rights often stay suspended at the rhetorical level, with broad assertions of entitlement that, generally lacking any formal mechanism for adjudicating specific cases or controversies, ultimately ring hollow. Health policymakers, schooled in the dominant paradigms sketched out above, and always searching for hard numbers to guide (or justify) their decisions, regularly express skepticism about the usefulness of human rights to answer the specific problems they face.

For many health managers and programmers, rights-based approaches have become synonymous with a programmatic requirement to service the poor and marginalized first – end of story. In practice this is often expressed as the juxtaposition of the (supposedly) rights-based approach of "pro-poor targeting" in contrast to the supposedly trickle-down approach of universal access.

For rights activists who turn their attention to health, human rights have often been neatly conflated with medical ethics and confined to promoting the dignity and autonomy of individual patients or they have focused on discrete incidents of abuse and wrongdoing. The traditional human rights methodologies of "name and shame" or "expose and denounce", so effective for a certain kind of civil and political rights, have had little traction. The heart of the challenge in global health is less about stopping abusive practices and more about building conditions necessary for the fulfillment of rights.

Why these approaches fail to transform the health situation in developing countries

So, what, ultimately, is wrong with these three established approaches? First, they only scratch the surface of the problem, certainly contributing essential ingredients to the ultimate solutions, but fundamentally failing to address the power dynamics that lie at the heart of the global health crisis. The rights-based approach that I advocate here keeps this understanding of health itself at the centre of the analysis and at the crux of strategic choices in terms of policies and programmes: Health, although it has physiological expressions and biological causes, is not just a technical issue. It is always also political. Health outcomes and their patterns within and across populations depend not just on genetic pre-disposition and physical environment, but fundamentally on access to, and distribution of, power and resources of many kinds including money, information, technology, social support networks and other forms of social capital.

Second, the established approaches fail to address the social and political institutions through which power ultimately operates. The epidemiologic approach gives us the "what" of effective interventions, but never the "how" needed for implementing them broadly and equitably. It also fails to address the need to invest in broader health systems, a complex construct that does not fit neatly into the menu of discrete cost-effective interventions.

The social and economic determinants approach certainly taps into the bigger social processes that influence health but it often ignores the actual institutions through which resources generated by economic growth and social development are converted into health-enhancing interventions and distributed across societies. Indeed, the operation of the inverse care law (those who need it least, get it first) in countries with weak health systems has been repeatedly confirmed by benefit-incidence studies showing that it is the rich and powerful who derive the most benefit from public spending in health.[9]

The standard human rights approach, floating at the rhetorical or formal legal levels, fails to capture the way in which health systems "are not only producers of health and health care, but they are also purveyors of a wider set of societal norms and values."[10] People's interaction with that system thus defines in critical ways their experience of the state and of their place in the broader society – matters at the core of the human rights idea.

Perhaps the most obvious way in which health systems communicate and enforce values and norms is in the way providers treat patients. In many parts of the world, poor people experience appalling abuse in health facilities.[11] As reported from the Voices of the Poor studies:

> "Rude, humiliating and inappropriate treatment are common complaints. A man from Tanzania says: 'We would rather treat ourselves than go to the hospital where an angry nurse might inject us with the wrong drug.' Elsewhere in Tanzania, men, women and young people say over and over again that they are treated 'worse than dogs'. Before they have a chance to describe their symptoms, they 'are yelled at, told they smell bad, and [that they are] lazy and good-for-nothing ...'"[12]

The ways in which health providers are themselves treated by the system sends equally powerful messages about societal norms and values, and no doubt influences their treatment of patients as well.[13] Sometimes those who struggle in the most challenging conditions to provide ethical, compassionate, high-quality care, find themselves unrewarded – or even punished – for taking initiative, while those who exploit a poorly functioning, ill-supervised system to shirk their responsibility or enrich themselves, do so with impunity. Yet in other settings, the system is organized to pay serious attention to accountability and to communicate the importance it places on responsible provider behaviour.[14]

Norms and values are also communicated by the choices that governments make (albeit often under pressure from international actors) in the actual structuring of their health systems. For example, a purely market-based approach in which access to health care depends on the ability to mobilize cash resources, explicitly legitimizes exclusion of the poor.[15]

Building a rights-based approach to health: The strategic place of health systems

But the solution to all of this cannot be a blueprint for the theoretically ideal health system imposed by fiat from the center or, worse, from donor countries. As Pritchett and Woolcock have convincingly shown, solutions favoured and imposed by the development community have regularly become the problem that the next generation of solutions must address.[16] Their analysis of "solutions" in social sectors in which key public services are both highly discretionary and transaction-intensive – services such as curative health care – finds a common structure to the repeated failure.

Starting with attempts by postcolonial states in poor countries to meet the needs of their people with a needs/supply/civil service model, Pritchett and Woolcock contend that the common structure of failed solutions is found in a kind of "bureaucratic high modernism",[17] a push to find simple, measurable, replicable, standardized, top-down solutions – solutions that attempt to replicate the end points of successful social sectors in high-income countries without going through the often contentious, painstaking, and lengthy social and political processes that preceded such successes.

A rights-based approach that focuses on the building of local health systems has the possibility of addressing each of these deficiencies in the "business-as-usual" scenarios. It begins by understanding health systems as core social institutions, as part of the very fabric of social and civil life. This fact often goes unnoticed in societies where basically health systems work. But where health systems have failed – and even more, where they have failed for poor and marginalized populations – that failure is experienced "as a core element of social exclusion ... Health care systems that do not offer care – that take a narrow or an abusive view of their duties – thereby contribute profoundly to people's experience of what it is to be poor."[18] Equally important is Mackintosh's insight that "the culture and operation of the health care system (as a whole, public and private) is the way in which claims are established, legitimated and denied or fulfilled by 'society.'"[19]

This has significant implications for the development of rights-based approaches to health, including mechanisms that will ensure constructive accountability. I use the phrase "constructive accountability" to make clear that accountability is not primarily about blame and punishment when things go wrong. Rather, it is about developing an effective dynamic of obligation and entitlement between people and their government, and within the complex system of relationships that form the wider health system, both public and private.[20]

A strategy built on ideas drawn from human rights transforms the health system from a static agglomeration of buildings, equipment, drugs and staff, into a dynamic entity through which citizens interact with their government and wider civil society. Mechanisms of constructive accountability give people the potential to effect change – from the micro level of interactions with local health workers, to the macro level of health sector reform in the context of international development policies.

A rights-based approach to strengthening health systems puts equity as a top priority. This is a far cry from the rather glib approach of "propoor targeting". Rather it is about identifying and creating the conditions under which redistribution – understood as "all social processes that create increasingly inclusive or egalitarian access to resources"[21] – can be initiated and sustained. The Millennium Project Task Force on Child Health and Maternal Health used this approach to identify and articulate several principles that can guide policy on basic issues such as private sector regulation, financing mechanisms, and hospital management structures, in ways that promote such redistribution.[22] The Commission on Social Determinants of Health's Knowledge Network on Health Systems provided additional elaboration on how health systems can be structured to prioritize equity.[23]

The human rights principle of progressive realization is also useful here. Although it surely will take a massive increase in resources to create health systems that are able to provide consistently the level of equitable, respectful care envisioned by human rights norms and spelled out in many countries' constitutions – far more than the 10 to 15 dollars per capita per year that the poorest countries now spend[24] – all states, no matter how poor, can take immediate, concrete, deliberate and targeted measures to advance the right to health. At the same time, allocations of budget and official development assistance are clearly relevant to the fulfillment of human rights. Discretionary, harmful cuts to the health budget as well as IFI policies that unreasonably constrain countries in addressing public health emergencies such as basic access to safe water arguably violate the right to health.[25]

In addition, the principle of progressive realization can be used to inform prioritization of interventions – a dilemma at the centre of health policymaking. Not all interventions are equally important for ensuring enjoyment of a right. When fundamental rights are at stake, particularly when the historical context points to a legacy of neglect, some interventions must take priority over others. This principle has been invoked in the HIV/AIDS field (*Minister of Health v. Treatment Action Campaign* 2002[26]) and we have argued elsewhere that it has important application in the field of maternal mortality as well.[27]

Finally, a rights-based approach focused on the strengthening of local health systems is a strategically effective way to build the kind of social movement that historically has been so critical for improvements in population health. Participatory approaches to health policy and programme have human rights value in and of themselves. Moreover, consciously political struggles coalescing around human rights principles have the potential to challenge the power structures that block equitable access to the range of resources that make good health possible. For example, making budgets and flows of funds transparent would assist communities in holding their governments accountable for timely and equitable disbursements.

The rights-based approach to strengthening local health systems that I have started to sketch out here is not meant to be a set of pre-formed policies that constitute rights-based solutions, or even a standardized technique for "doing human rights". It is instead a fluid practice that wrestles with very specific problems in the delivery of health services, analyzing them in historical and political context, using multiple forms of evidence to craft solutions, identifying the workings of power that have blocked progress, strategizing ways to mobilize those directly affected (as well as those directly and indirectly responsible) to use the values, norms, and vision of human rights to call for specific rearrangements of power and resources necessary for serious change. Examples of this approach are as specific as confronting the issue of who should be permitted and trained to deliver anesthesia for life-saving obstetric care,[28] or as general as the prioritization of different strategies for addressing big goals such as the reduction of maternal mortality.[29]

Last of all, let us be clear: this is not a fast or simple process. It is decidedly not a "quick fix". But without this kind of investment in the social and political institutions of poor, high-mortality countries, without the building of local people's movements to demand and enforce accountability for access to life-saving care under humane conditions, progress in global health will be as fleeting as the flap of a canary's wings.

*   A version of this paper was presented at a seminar on 'Tackling Global Challenges with the Tools of Human Rights: Assessing Progress, Mapping Future Directions' convened by Realizing Rights: The Ethical Globalization Initiative in 2006. The author thanks the participants in that seminar for their helpful comments on the earlier draft.

1   World Health Organization (WHO), United Nations Children's Fund (UNICEF) et al., *Maternal Mortality in 2005: Estimates Developed by WHO, UNICEF, UNFPA and The World Bank* (Geneva: World Health Organization, 2007).

2   A. Fairchild and G. Oppenheimer 'Public Health Nihilism vs. Pragmatism: History, Politics, and the Control of Tuberculosis' 88(7) *American Journal of Public Health* (1998), at 1105–1117.

3   Commission on Social Determinants of Health, *Closing the Gap in a Generation: Health Equity Through Action on the Social Determinants of Health: Final Report of the Commission on Social Determinants of Health* (Geneva: World Health Organization, 2008).

4   J. Colgrove, 'The McKeown Thesis: A Historical Controversy and Its Enduring Influence' 92(5) *American Journal of Public Health* (2002) 725–729.

5   S. Szreter, 'The Population Health Approach in Historical Perspective' 93(3) *American Journal of Public Health* (2003), at 421–431.

6   Ibid. (emphasis added).

7   S. Szreter, 'Economic Growth, Disruption, Deprivation, Disease and Death: On the Importance of the Politics of Public Health for Development' 23(4) *Population and Development Review* (1997), at 693–728.

8   P. Uvin, *Human Rights and Development* (Bloomfield, CT: Kumarian Press, 2004).

9   F. Castro-Leal, J. Dayton et al., 'Public Spending on Health Care in Africa: Do the Poor Benefit?' 78(1) *Bulletin of the World Health Organization* (2000) 66–74; D. R. Gwatkin, A. Bhuiya et al., 'Making Health Systems More Equitable' 364 *The Lancet* (2004), at 1273–1280.

10 L. Gilson, 'Trust and Development of Health Care as a Social Institution' 56 *Social Science and Medicine* (2003), at 1453–1468.

11 R. Jewkes, N. Abrahams et al., 'Why Do Nurses Abuse Patients? Reflections from South African Obstetric Services' 47(11) *Social Science and Medicine* (1998) 1781–1795; S. Miller, A. Tejada et al., *Strategic Assessment of Reproductive Health in the Dominican Republic* (New York: Population Council, 2002).

12 World Health Organization (WHO) and World Bank, *Dying for Change: Poor People's Experience of Health and Ill-health* (Geneva: WHO, 2002).

13 Z. Mumtaz, S. Salway et al., 'Gender-Based Barriers to Primary Health Care Provision in Pakistan: The Experience of Female Providers' 18(3) *Health Policy and Planning* (2003), at 261–269.

14 J. Tendler and S. Freedheim, 'Trust in a Rent-Seeking World: Health and Government Transformed in Northeast Brazil' 22(12) *World Development* (1994), at 1771–1791.

15 M. Mackintosh, 'Do Health Care Systems Contribute to Inequalities?' in D. A. Leon and G. Walt (eds.), *Poverty, Inequality and Health: An International Perspective* (Oxford: Oxford University Press, 2001).

16 L. H. Pritchett and M. Woolcock, 'Solutions When the Solution is the Problem: Arraying the Disarray in Development' 32(2) *World Development* (2004), at 191–212.

17 J. C. Scott, *Seeing Like a State: How Certain Schemes to Improve the Human Condition Have Failed* (New Haven, CT: Yale University Press, 1998).

18 Mackintosh, *supra* note 15, at 184.

19 Ibid., at 185.

20 See L. P. Freedman, 'Using Human Rights in Maternal Mortality Programs: From Analysis to Strategy' 75 *International Journal of Gynecology and Obstetrics* (2001) 51–60; L. P. Freedman, 'Human Rights, Constructive Accountability and Maternal Mortality in the Dominican Republic: A Commentary' 82 *International Journal of Gynecology and Obstetrics* (2003), at 111–114.

21 M. Mackintosh, M. and P. Tibandebage, 'Inequality and Redistribution in Healthcare: Analytical Issues for Developmental Social Policy' in T. Mkandawire (ed.) *Social Policy in a Development Context* (Palgrave: Basingstoke, 2004), at 144.

22 UN Millennium Project, *Who's Got the Power? Transforming Health Systems for Women and Children* (Task Force on Child Health and Maternal Health, 2005).

23 L. Gilson, J. Doherty et al., *Challenging inequity through health systems: Final Report, Knowledge Network on Health Systems* (Geneva: WHO Commission on the Social Determinants of Health, 2007).

24 The Commission on Macroeconomics and Health suggested that an annual per capita expenditure of USD 34 to USD 40 is necessary to provide a minimum acceptable level of health care.

25 NYU School of Law Center for Human Rights and Global Justice, Partners in Health, RFK Memorial Center for Human Rights, Zanmi Lasante, *Woch Nan Soley: The Denial of the Right to Water in Haiti* (2008), available at http://www.chrgj.org/projects/docs/wochnansoley.pdf.

26 *Minister of Health v Treatment Action Campaign* (TAC) (2002) 5 SA 721 (CC).

27 UN Millennium Project, *supra* note 22.

28 L. P. Freedman, 'Shifting Visions: "Delegation" Policies and the Building of a "Rights-Based" Approach to Maternal Mortality' 54(3) *Journal of the American Medical Women's Association* (2002), at 154–158.

29 UN Millennium Project, *supra* note 22.

Building Rights-Based Health Systems: A Focus on the Health Workforce

Eric A. Friedman

A boy suffering from rheumatic heart disease goes into cardiac arrest in Medical Ward 4C in Mulago Hospital, the national referral hospital in Kampala, Uganda. He apparently never received the antibiotics that could have prevented him from reaching this desperate moment. His family is poor, so he has ended up in this ward, devoid of equipment save the occasional IV line. He is not hooked up to a heart monitor. Nurses try to save him; they call doctors, but none come; there are too few. The nurses' heroic efforts are not enough. The fourteen-year-old is dead. It is but another typically traumatic day in a crippled health system.

New initiatives like the Africa Health Strategy 2007–2015, the International Health Partnership, and the Campaign for the Health Millennium Development Goals (MDGs), each launched in 2007, are too late for the boy whose short life ended three years earlier, but perhaps they will enable more people to exit Medical Ward 4C alive, or avoid entering it in the first place. Developing country governments and international partners alike are looking to reinforce the basic building blocks of the health systems, including the health workforce, as they recognize that dilapidated infrastructure and undersized and under-motivated health workforces obstruct progress towards global targets for health improvements.

Today, 57 developing countries collectively suffer a shortage of some 4.3 million health workers; African countries alone need to more than double the size of their health workforce.[1] Broken or without health workers trained in their use, half of the medical equipment in developing countries goes unused.[2] Weak health systems are the largest obstacle to ramping up

HIV services,[3] and most of the more than 500 000 annual maternal deaths, and the nearly 10 million annual child deaths, could be prevented with well-functioning health systems.[4]

Here lies an historic opportunity to advance the right to the highest attainable standard of health. As countries develop, revise, and implement national health sector and health workforce strategies, the health systems they create can – and must – become ones whose contours are defined by human rights principles.[5]

Seizing this opportunity will require a greater understanding of what it means to weave human rights into the fabric of redesigned and re-energized health systems. What principles drive a human rights approach to health systems, and how can countries operationalize them? This chapter focuses on accountability as the starting point of national health sector and health workforce strategies. It will describe how accountability and several other key right-to-health principles – participation, equity, and quality – inform health workforce challenges, and will briefly cover other aspects of the health system as well.[6]

A starting point: Accountability

Health strategies should be, in essence, right to health accountability road-maps – plans to achieve obligations for which the government must be accountable. And they need transparent monitoring systems to track and evaluate their implementation. Right to health obligations give shape to the nature of health services required and the outcomes that health systems must be designed to achieve.

Basic features of the right to health establish a general but important initial baseline: Universal access to health care. These features include the universal nature of the right itself; its requirement to take steps to create "conditions which would assure to all medical service and medical attention in the event of sickness;"[7] the right's "interrelated and essential elements" including available and accessible health facilities, goods, and services; the right's focus on "equality of access to health care and health services," and; the core obligation to provide "essential primary health care."[8] The central questions then become: What health care? And by when?

The key treaty guaranteeing the right to health obligates countries to commit the maximum of their available resources to fulfilling this and other human rights, and "to move as expeditiously and effectively as possible towards the full realization of" this right, thus providing guidance on how quickly this health care must be provided.[9] As elaborated upon in Article 12 of the International Covenant on Economic, Social and Cultural Rights (ICESCR) and in General Comment No. 14 of the Committee on Economic, Social and Cultural Rights, universally available health care must give priority to reproductive, maternal, and child care, immunizations, nutrition, safe water and adequate sanitation facilities, preventing and treating epidemic and endemic diseases, making available essential medications, and addressing other major health concerns of the whole population, based on epidemiological evidence.[10]

Other commitments give further shape to priorities and timelines. Among these are the MDGs, including three-quarter reductions in maternal mortality rates and two-third reductions in child mortality by 2015 compared to 1990, and reducing the incidence of malaria and other major diseases by 2015;[11] universal access to HIV treatment, prevention, care, and support by 2010;[12] universal access to reproductive health by 2015;[13] and, an African Union commitment to a package of essential health services by 2015.[14]

These commitments form the context for understanding the principles of progressive realization and maximum available resources, as well as the obligation of international assistance and cooperation.[15] Since these commitments represent a belief that these goals are achievable,[16] and given that the vast majority of countries have committed themselves under international law to realizing the right to the highest attainable standard of health,[17] health plans must be designed to achieve these commitments.

Unless these goals are the frame upon which countries build their health systems, even full implementation of existing health plans could leave a population's right to health unrealized. For example, in 2007 Uganda developed a human resource strategy designed to increase the number of health workers by 66% by 2020. Yet with the population expected to grow by 60% during this period, the ratio of health workers to population would improve only minimally.[18] Uganda would remain well short of the threshold below which, according to the World Health Organization (WHO), countries are "very unlikely" to achieve the MDGs.[19]

Encouragingly, recognizing the shortcomings of this strategy, Uganda's health ministry has since developed a draft supplement to the 2007 strategy. The supplement envisions a far more ambitious expansion of the health workforce. Its "Health for People" scenario would lead to "an equitably distributed workforce which is in size equal to the minimum number of health workers needed to adequately serve the people in Uganda" by 2020.[20] The supplement will still need to be turned into a plan of action and funded through considerably increased government and external resources.

Securing these funds will be a challenge. Uganda's 2007 strategy cites "sector budget ceilings, especially tight for the health sector."[21] In 2006/7 Uganda spent 9.6% of its budget on health,[22] even though in the 2001 Abuja Declaration, African leaders committed to spending at least 15% of their budgets on health.[23] The supplement recognizes the need for health to "become a higher political priority" and for the budget ceiling policy to be "tamed" or "abandoned."[24]

Even if they spend 15% of their budgets on health, many developing countries will still need significant donor support.[25] Wealthy countries, however, have yet to meaningfully commit to ensuring adequate funding for health plans designed to achieve the MDGs and other global targets. This missing commitment and low levels of foreign assistance point to a failure by many governments to fully comply with the obligation to provide international development aid.

An obligation to provide such assistance is rooted in major declarations and treaties, including the ICESCR responsibility to take steps "through international assistance and co-operation" towards full realization of economic, social, and cultural rights,[26] and through the UN Charter obligation "to take joint and separate action in co-operation with the [United Nations] for … purposes" including "universal respect for, and observance of, human rights."[27] To be genuinely aimed at progressively realizing the right to health, and to fully cooperate with the United Nations, such assistance and cooperation must support countries in moving "as expeditiously and effectively as possible" towards making health services universally available, and be sufficient to achieve such UN-endorsed goals as the MDGs and universal access to HIV services by 2010.[28]

Countries may be reluctant to develop true needs-based workforce strategies, fearing that if they expand their health workforce considerably or accept external assistance for health worker salaries, such expansions or foreign assistance would not be sustained. This is a legitimate human rights concern. The progressive realization requirement demands progress; improvements not sustained indicate retrogression. Yet, developing and sustaining a health workforce able to provide health services for all will prove unsustainable only if governments fail to spend the maximum available resources on human rights obligations,[29] wealthy nations fail to provide adequate assistance, or some combination thereof. Failure to sustain an adequate workforce would be evidence of human right violations. Countries can minimize the risk of unsustained funding by insisting on long-term commitments from donors, prioritizing health services that touch most directly on right to health requirements within national budgets, developing alternate budget scenarios,[30] and developing models of care that will reduce reliance on more expensive health worker cadres.

Health workforce: Accountability

To be accountable for the types of health commitments discussed above, health workforce strategies should aim to achieve the numbers, skills, and distribution of health workers required to meet specific health outcomes and service delivery goals. These estimates will help inform education policies (for example, how many new health workers need to be trained), remuneration and other incentives (for example, how effective retention policies need to be), and other aspects of the strategy.

These goal-driven estimates are part of the grounding of plans in epidemiological evidence that the right to health requires.[31] Without baseline estimates of what resources will be required to achieve goals, the odds of actually achieving them greatly diminish. These estimates will also highlight cases where innovative strategies are required, such as expanded use of community and mid-level health workers in places like Mozambique and Ethiopia, countries that have less than a fifth of the WHO-calculated minimum threshold level of doctors, nurses, and midwives needed to provide basic health services.[32]

Health workforce: Participation

Members of the general population have the right to participate in health-related decisions.[33] This entails their meaningful involvement in developing the health workforce strategy and evaluating its implementation. A combination of processes might be used to solicit input, such as including health civil society leaders in leadership teams spearheading the development of health workforce strategies and holding open public meetings and targeted consultations with community leaders and civil society representatives to seek input on the strategy.

Creating opportunities for participation in impoverished countries might seem to be an unaffordable luxury, and resource constraints may indeed affect the modalities and extent of participation. Yet far from a luxury, participation holds special importance to poorer and marginalized populations whose needs are most at risk of being under-valued or overlooked. Who better to insist that health strategies meet government responsibilities to marginalized populations, and to guide them, than rural dwellers, people with HIV/AIDS, people with disabilities, the elderly, refugees and internally displaced people, and other marginalized or socially disadvantaged populations themselves? Meanwhile, health advocates can hold the government accountable to obligations such as the MDGs.

Participation also has a two-way educational function. By creating space for health users to inform policymakers of their life experiences, the government may learn of problems – and solutions – of which officials might be unaware. Are certain segments of the population subject to discriminatory or ignorant health workers; for example, do health workers realize that people with disabilities can become infected with HIV? Are health providers unable to speak local languages, obstructing care?[34] Conversely, through their involvement in the planning process, people can become educated on how the health workforce strategy should function in their communities, enabling them to provide informed feedback on whether the plan's implementation is meeting its promise. They can also use political, media, legal, and other channels to insist on improved implementation where it falls short.

Health workers too must be involved in developing health workforce strategies. They have rights that these plans must address, such as the right to safe working conditions and to confidential health services, including HIV testing and treatment. Health workers are the surest advocates for such elements of the health workforce strategies.

Health worker participation is also central to developing effective strategies. Nurses, doctors, and pharmacists will have the most direct understanding of why their colleagues migrate, and what might encourage them to remain in-country or serve in rural areas. Furthermore, if they have a say in these policies and understand the rationales and trade-offs involved, health workers might be more willing to give them a chance.

In Ondo State, Nigeria, a new administration surveyed health workers in 2003 to determine their greatest needs. Some 62% prioritized having adequate equipment, supplies, and medicines. The government focused on meeting this expressed need. In combination with other development activities, this contributed to a dramatic increase in the proportion of nurses serving in rural areas, from 28% in 2003 to 66% by 2006.[35]

Health workforce: Equality and non-discrimination

Strengthening basic rural infrastructure is one element of a comprehensive approach to increasing the number of health workers in rural areas,[36] thus moving towards the equitable distribution of health services that the right to health demands.[37] Under a right to health approach, equality concerns infuse all aspects of a health workforce strategy. The Africa Health Strategy 2007–2015 recognizes two more approaches, incentives for serving in disadvantaged areas – the most common policy lever for increasing the number of health workers in rural areas – and community service requirements for new graduates.[38]

Community service, building basic rural infrastructure, and incentives are all important strategies for developing an equitably distributed workforce. For example, in an effort that has helped bring AIDS treatment to 5000 people, several dozen or more physicians in Zambia serve in rural areas on three-year contracts that include a package of incentives.[39]

A human rights-based plan will likely use other equity levers as well, including the education system. For instance, the mix of health worker cadres affects the rural/urban balance. Non-physician clinicians – health workers trained for three to four years with many of the competencies of a physician – are far more likely than physicians to serve in rural areas.[40] Certain types of nurses, such as community nurses, might be trained specifically for deployment in rural areas.[41]

Health professional training institutions have a critical role in promoting equality. Since health professional students from rural areas are more likely to return to serve in these areas,[42] recruitment and scholarship practices should be used to increase the number of students from underserved communities and marginalized populations. Curricula emphasizing primary health needs and programmes exposing students to these needs are also strategies to build equality into pre-service education.

Further, health training institutions should incorporate education on human rights – including on the right to health – into their curricula, and provide in-service human rights training to health professionals.[43] Such approaches will introduce health workers to their obligations to provide non-discriminatory care, necessary for equal access for marginalized populations. Beyond this, health workers may view their own roles and responsibilities in a new light, making them more likely to serve in rural areas. And since some health workers will become policymakers, ensuring that health workers are educated on human rights is one of the best ways to ground health strategies in human rights.[44]

Health workforce: Quality and the private sector

Another right to health requirement with implications for the health workforce is that health services should be of good quality.[45] As medical and nursing training institutions increase intake to overcome health workforce shortages, they should ensure that the resulting influx of students does not compromise the quality of education. Also, ensuring effective, supportive supervision of health workers must be a priority.

Providing quality health services requires regulating private sector health providers and ensuring that private health providers adhere to principles of equal treatment and non-discrimination.[46] Further, given the size of the private sector in many countries,[47] a health workforce strategy would be remiss if it failed to consider ways in which private health providers can contribute to national health goals. The obligation that states use the maximum available resources towards fulfilling the right to health covers not only financial but also human resources.[48] Strategies should consider ways in which partnerships with private health providers can expand access to health services and contribute towards achieving health commitments. This might include contracting with private sector personnel to provide certain services, regulating their training to cover priority health areas, or helping fill gaps in public facilities.[49]

Beyond the health workforce

Human rights principles that inform health workforce strategies also provide guidance to other aspects of health systems. For example, ordinary health service users, marginalized groups, health advocates, and health workers should all have opportunities to participate in developing an overall national health sector strategy and its various components. The strategy should include mechanisms to enable people to participate in health-related decisions at the community level,[50] such as through village health committees.

Equity concerns should inform decisions throughout the health system, such as where to locate new health facilities and where to direct funds to upgrade facilities (based on the requirement of equitable distribution and geographic accessibility for all),[51] for which level of the system to prioritize financing (with priority to primary level facilities),[52] what data health information systems should track (including disaggregated data to measure impact of health services on women, poor people, ethnic minorities, and the elderly),[53] and how to finance health systems.

Like the distribution of health workers, how health services are financed can dramatically impact the accessibility of health services. Overwhelming evidence demonstrates point-of-service payments (user fees) block access for the poor.[54] Outpatient health services utilization jumped 50–100% when Uganda removed user fees for government health facilities in 2001.[55] Exemptions for the poor routinely prove ineffective.[56] User fees should be removed, replaced by financing schemes that meet the requirement that health goods and services be affordable for everyone, including disadvantaged groups. It matters how an approach works – and can be expected to work – in practice. A social insurance scheme may provide subsidies to the poor and other marginalized groups, but if the subsidies are inadequate, or fail to reach all who need them, the scheme would fall short of right to health demands. Further, a health financing scheme should address transportation and other costs that are not direct health service charges, but may place health services beyond the reach of some segments of the population.

The job ahead: Incorporating the right to health into health systems

"We are suffering," admitted one of the nurses who tried in vain to save the boy in Mulago Hospital's Medical Ward 4C. If the right to health becomes a standard that informs the development and financing of health systems, her suffering might end, and millions of people otherwise headed towards death will live.

Everyone has a role to play toward realizing this goal. Schools, the media, health workers, and community leaders can educate people about the right to health, its importance, and its manifestations. The public can work within their countries' political, civil, and legal space to educate, pressure, or compel policymakers to adhere to their obligations under the right to health, including by instructing them on its practical benefits, such as the positive impact of strengthened health systems on health outcomes and the economic benefits of a healthy population.

Health workers themselves have a critical role in merging the right to health with health systems, both as informed policymakers and as forceful advocates, such as Uganda's Action Group for Health, Human Rights and HIV/AIDS (described elsewhere in this volume).[57]

The international community must stand behind the right to health, through political will and technical expertise. Voters in developed countries should insist that their political leaders prioritize human rights and global health – and remain faithful to their obligations – including by meeting international commitments and obligations on foreign assistance. International health and development agencies, including WHO, should adopt guidelines to assist countries in orienting their health systems towards human rights.

Perhaps one day human rights will be widely recognized as the proper underpinning for societal structures, including health systems. For now, though, we all have our work cut out for us.

1 World Health Organization (WHO), *World Health Report 2006* (2006), at 12–13, available at http://www.who.int/whr/2006/.

2 WHO, *Everybody's Business: Strengthening Health Systems to Improve Health Outcomes: A Framework for Action* (2007), at 9, available at http://www.who.int/healthsystems/strategy/everybodys_business.pdf.

3 See, for example, Michael Perry, 'Medical "brain drain" hindering AIDS battle' *Reuters*, 23 July 2007 (quoting Debrework Zewdie, World Bank, Director, Global HIV/AIDS Program, who stated "Our most difficult challenge is ... the limited health system capacity in countries with the highest disease burden"), available at http://www.reuters.com/article/healthNews/idUSSYD164580 20070723.

4 Lynn P. Freedman, Ronald J. Waldman, and Helen de Pinho, *Who's Got the Power? Transforming Health Systems for Women and Children* (2005), at 4–5, available at http://www.unmillenniumproject.org/documents/maternalchild-complete.pdf; UNICEF press release, *Releasing Declining Numbers for Child Mortality, UNICEF Calls for Increased Efforts to Save Children's Lives*, 12 September 2008, available at http://www.unicef.org/media/media_45607.html.

5 For a guide on developing a health workforce plan that is rooted in human rights, see Physicians for Human Rights, *The Right to Health and Health Workforce Planning: A Guide for Government Officials, NGOs, Health Workers and Development Partners* (2008), available at http://physiciansforhumanrights.org/library/documents/reports/health-workforce-planning-guide-2.pdf.

6 These are among the major human rights principles informing health system development, though it is not an exhaustive set. Others include, for example, issues of cultural acceptability and additional aspects of accountability including benchmarking. For a more comprehensive review, see, Paul Hunt, *Report of the Special Rapporteur on the right of everyone to the enjoyment of the highest attainable standard of physical and mental health to*

the *UN Human Rights Council*, 31 January 2008, UN Doc. A/HRC/7/11.

7 International Covenant on Economic, Social and Cultural Rights (1966) (ICESCR), at Article 12(d) (emphasis added).

8 Committee on Economic, Social and Cultural Rights (CESCR), *General Comment No. 14 on the right to the highest attainable standard of health*, 11 August 2000, UN Doc. E/C.12/2000/4, at paras. 12, 19, 43.

9 Parties to the ICESCR commit "to take steps, individually and through international assistance and co-operation, especially economic and technical, to the maximum of [their] available resources, with a view to achieving progressively the full realization of the rights recognized in the present Covenant ...": ICESCR, *supra* note 7, at Article 2(1). General Comment No. 14 further explains that "progressive realization means that States parties have a specific and continuing obligation to move as expeditiously and effectively as possible towards the full realization of" the right to health: *General Comment No. 14, supra* note 8, at para. 31.

10 ICESCR, *supra* note 7, at Article 12; *General Comment No.14, supra* note 8, at paras. 14–17, 21, 43–44. Effectively addressing major health concerns requires gathering epidemiological evidence, as well as information on the current health system and how it is addressing these health concerns.

11 United Nations Statistics Division, *Millennium Development Goals Indicators: The Official United Nations Site for the MDG Indicators*, http://unstats.un.org/unsd/mdg/Host.aspx?Content=Indicators/OfficialList.htm. A strong case can be made that most (if not all) of the MDGs, including those related to child and maternal mortality and major diseases, have achieved the status of customary international law. Philip Alston, *A Human Rights Perspective on the Millennium Development Goals* (2004), at paras. 40–42, available at http://www.hurilink.org/tools/HRsPerspectives_on_the_MDGs--Alston.pdf.

12 Political Declaration on HIV/AIDS, adopted by the UN General Assembly, 15 June 2006, UN Doc.

A/Res/60/262, at para. 20, available at http://data.unaids.org/pub/Report/2006/20060615_HLM_PoliticalDeclaration_ARES60262_en.pdf.

13 UN World Summit Outcome, 60th session, 2005, UN Doc. A/60/1, at para. 57(g), available at http://www.un.org/summit2005/documents.html.

14 "[We hereby] commit ourselves to the achievement of Universal Access to Prevention, Treatment and Care by 2015 through the development of an integrated health care delivery system based on essential health package delivery close-to-client …": Gaborone Declaration on a Roadmap Towards Universal Access to Prevention, Treatment and Care, Second Ordinary Session of the Conference of African Ministers of Health, Gaborone, Botswana, 10–14 October 2005, at para. 2, available at http://www.africa-union.org/root/au/Conferences/Past/2006/March/SA/Mar6/GABORONE_DECLARATION.pdf.

15 Specific targets such as those contained in the Millennium Development Goals do not obviate the existing treaty obligations such as the use of the maximum of available resources. If countries can exceed such targets through using the maximum of their available resources, they have an obligation to do so.

16 At present, certain goals in some countries may seem very difficult to achieve. This does not mean that the goals were unrealistic in the first place, but rather this is largely a result of inadequate action towards achieving them. With the consequent lack of progress as the goals' deadlines draw nearer, the challenge of achieving the goal by the target date grows, with large gaps to be filled in relatively little time.

17 Nearly all states are party to the Convention on the Rights of the Child, which recognizes the child's right to the highest attainable standard of health. Convention on the Rights of the Child (1989), at Article 24. About three-quarters of countries have ratified the ICESCR. Moreover, the World Conference on Human Rights, held in 1993 and with representatives from governments of 171 countries, affirmed that all states have a duty to promote and protect all human rights. Thus, even states that have not ratified relevant treaties or guaranteed the right to health under national law are expected to promote and protect the right to health: Judith Asher, *The Right to Health: A Resource Manual for NGOs* (London: Commonwealth Medical Trust, 2004), at 4, available at http://shr.aaas.org/pubs/rt_health/rt_health_manual.pdf; Office of the High Commissioner for Human Rights, *World Conference on Human Rights*, available at http://www.unhchr.ch/html/menu5/wchr.htm.

18 Uganda Ministry of Health, *Uganda Human Resources for Health Strategic Plan 2005–2020* (2007), at 21.

19 *World Health Report 2006, supra* note 1, at XVIII.

20 Uganda Ministry of Health, *Uganda Human Resources for Health Strategic Plan 2005–2020 Supplement 2008*, final working draft (October 2008), at 26.

21 *Uganda Human Resources for Health Strategic Plan 2005–2020, supra* note 18, at 14. Uganda's Health Sector Strategic Plan II raises similar concerns: "Attempts have been made to mobilize additional funds for the sector but these have been constrained by macroeconomic concerns and the rigid sector ceilings." Uganda Ministry of Health, *Health Sector Strategic Plan II: 2005/6-2009/10* (Volume 1), at 55. These constraints highlight the impact macroeconomic policies can have on fulfilling the right to health.

22 Uganda Ministry of Health, *Annual Health Sector Performance Report Financial Year 2006/2007* (October 2007).

23 Abuja Declaration on HIV/AIDS, Tuberculosis and Other Related Infectious Diseases, Organization of African Unity summit, adopted 27 April 2001, Abuja, Nigeria, at para. 26, available at http://www.uneca.org/adf2000/Abuja%20Declaration.htm.

24 *Uganda Human Resources for Health Strategic Plan 2005–2020 Supplement 2008*, final working draft, *supra* note 20, at 7.

25 In 2005, the Commission for Africa estimated that for African countries to provide a basic health package, they would need to increase health

spending to 15% of their budgets, and would still require donors to increase annual health assistance to Africa by USD 10 billion immediately, and by USD 20 billion annually by 2015 – plus HIV/AIDS assistance: Commission for Africa, *Our Common Interest* (2005), at 195, available at http://www.commissionforafrica.org/english/report/introduction.html.

26 ICESCR, *supra* note 7, at Article 2(1).

27 UN Charter, Articles 55–56.

28 Along with foreign assistance, the obligation to respect the right to health requires countries to develop their own health workforces in ways that do not rely on health workers from developing countries, which could harm the right to health elsewhere: Paul Hunt, *Report of the Special Rapporteur on the right of everyone to the highest attainable standard of physical and mental health*, 12 September 2005, UN Doc. A/60/348, at paras. 61–62 available at http://www2.essex.ac.uk/human_rights_centre/rth/docs/GA%202005.pdf.

29 Factors in determining whether governments are spending the maximum available resources on fulfilling their human rights, and in particular their right to health, obligations include: comparing government health spending (including total spending, spending as a proportion of the Gross National Income [GNI], and spending as a proportion of overall government spending) to comparable countries (for example, countries in the same region or with similar per capita income levels); comparing government health spending levels to relevant government commitments; measuring how spending has changed over time, how changes in health spending compare to changes in GNI, how health spending compares to other areas of the budget (and how these other areas relate to advancing human rights), and what the government actually spends on health (and other budget areas) compared to what it budgets; and, examining government revenue and opportunities to increase the resources available to it, including the proportion of GNI that tax revenue constitutes (how this compares to international standards and comparable countries) and to what

extent the government is actively seeking international assistance: Fundar – Centro de Análisis e Investigación, International Budget Project, and International Human Rights Internship Program, *Dignity Counts: A Guide to Using Budget Analysis to Advance Human Rights* (2004), at 35–39, available at http://www.iie.org/IHRIP/Dignity_Counts.pdf; Physicians for Human Rights, *Deadly Delays: Maternal Mortality in Peru* (2007), at 107–108, available at http://www.physiciansforhumanrights.org/library/documents/reports/maternal-mortality-in-peru.pdf.

30 The Africa Health Strategy 2007–2015 recommendation that countries should develop several budget scenarios, including one that is consistent with health targets, is well-considered given the present realities of insufficient and often unpredictable, short-term donor assistance: Africa Health Strategy 2007–2015, adopted at the Third Session of the African Union Conference of Ministers of Health, Johannesburg, South Africa, 9–13 April 2007, at para. 41, available at http://www.africa-union.org/root/UA/Conferences/2007/avril/SA/9-13%20avr/doc/en/SA/AFRICA_HEALTH_STRATEGY_FINAL.doc. However, the need to fall back to a lesser scenario, inconsistent with health targets and virtually guaranteeing some (likely high) number of preventable deaths, means that the national government or wealthy nations are failing in their legal obligations.

31 *General Comment No. 14, supra* note 8, at para. 43(f).

32 WHO has calculated that on average, countries need a total of at least 2.3 doctors, nurses, and midwives per 1 000 people to enable 80% of births to be covered by a skilled birth attendant, and has labelled those countries that are below this threshold and do not attain this level of coverage as having critical shortages. *World Health Report 2006, supra* note 1, at 11–13. Ethiopia had 0.25 doctors, nurses, and midwives per 1 000 population in 2003, and Mozambique had 0.35 doctors, nurses, and midwives per 1 000 population in 2004, based on the latest data available through

the WHO Global Health Atlas, available at http://www.who.int/globalatlas/.

33 *General Comment No. 14, supra* note 8, at paras. 11, 17, 43(f).

34 A Physicians for Human Rights report on maternal mortality in Peru found that the inability of health providers to speak an indigenous language is a contributing factor to maternal death in rural Peru: *Deadly Delays: Maternal Mortality in Peru, supra* note 29, at 69–75, 131.

35 PowerPoint presentation by the Commissioner for Health, Ondo State, Nigeria, and CHESTRAD International, *Ondo State, Nigeria: Evidence, Learning & Action for Human Resources for Health*, presented August 2006, in Akure, Ondo State, Nigeria, at slides 10, 30 (available on file with author).

36 Zambia will receive support from GAVI to bring clean water and power to rural health facilities as part of that country's effort to retain health workers in rural areas: Personal communication with Lisa Oldring, Special Advisor, Realizing Rights: The Ethical Globalization Initiative, 1 November 2007 (on file with author).

37 *General Comment No. 14, supra* note 8, at para. 43(e).

38 Africa Health Strategy 2007–2015, *supra* note 30, at para. 61.

39 'Rural doctors number soars – Chituwo' *Times of Zambia*, 28 July – 4 August 2005, available at http://www.times.co.zm/news/viewnews.cgi?category=4&id=1122582782; Office of the Global AIDS Coordinator, *The President's Emergency Plan for AIDS Relief Report on Work Force Capacity and HIV/AIDS* (July 2006), at 12, available at http://www.state.gov/documents/organization/69651.pdf; Jaap Koot et al., *Supplementation Programme Dutch Medical Doctors 1978–2003 Lessons Learned; Retention Scheme Zambian Medical Doctors 2003–2006 Suggestions: Final Report* (December 2003), at 27.

40 Twenty-five sub-Saharan African countries have non-physician clinicians, including nine of which have more non-physician clinicians than physicians, including Malawi, with twenty times more non-physician clinicians than physicians: Fit-

zhugh Mullan and Seble Frehywot, 'Non-physician clinicians in 47 sub-Saharan African countries' 370 *Lancet* (2007) 2158–2163, at 2161.

41 Personal communication with Isabella Mbai, Head, Department of Nursing Sciences, School of Medicine, Moi University, Eldoret, Kenya, 10 October 2006 (on file with author).

42 A study in South Africa found graduates from schools of medicine were three to eight times more likely to practice in rural areas if they were from rural areas: Elma de Vries and Steve Reid, 'Do South African medical students of rural origin return to rural practice?' 93 *South African Medical Journal* (2003), at 789–793.

43 General Comment No. 14 includes health personnel training "on health and human rights" among the "obligations of comparable priority" to the core obligations: *General Comment No. 14, supra* note 8, at para. 44(e).

44 See Paul Hunt, *Report of the Special Rapporteur on the right of everyone to the enjoyment of the highest attainable standard of physical and mental health*, 17 January 2007, UN Doc. A/HRC/4/28, at paras. 38–47 available at http://www2.essex.ac.uk/human_rights_centre/rth/docs/council.pdf.

45 *General Comment No. 14, supra* note 8, at para. 12(d).

46 Ibid. at paras. 18, 35, 43(a), 51.

47 In many developing countries, private sector health personnel provide a large portion of, and even the majority of, health services: Ndola Prata, Dominic Motagu, and Emma Jefferys, 'Private sector, human resources and health franchising in Africa' 83 *Bulletin of the World Health Organization* (2005) 274–279. Overall, the private sector (including for-profit and not-for-profit) is responsible for approximately half of health service provision in sub-Saharan Africa: International Finance Corporation, World Bank Group, *The Business of Health in Africa: Partnering with the Private Sector to Improve People's Lives* (2007), at VII, available at http://www.ifc.org/ifcext/healthinafrica.nsf/Content/FullReport. Approximately 75% of health provider contacts in Bangladesh occur outside the public

sector: *Everybody's Business: Strengthening Health Systems to Improve Health Outcomes*, supra note 2, at 9.

48 Robert E. Robertson, 'Measuring state compliance with the obligation to devote the "maximum available resources" to realizing economic, social and cultural rights' 16 *Human Rights Quarterly* (1994), at 693–714.

49 *The Business of Health in Africa*, supra note 47, at 26–28.

50 *General Comment No. 14*, supra note 8, at para. 11 ("A further important aspect is the participation of the population in all health-related decision-making at the community, national and international levels").

51 Ibid. at para. 12(b), 43(e).

52 Ibid. at para. 19.

53 Ibid. at para. 43(f): "a national public health strategy and plan of action ... shall include methods, such as right to health indicators and benchmarks, by which progress can be closely monitored."

54 See, for example, Margaret Whitehead, Göran Dahlgren, and Timothy Evans, 'Equity and health sector reforms: Can low-income countries escape the medical poverty trap?' 358 *Lancet* (2001) 833–836, at 834.

55 Rob Yates, *Should African Governments Scrap User Fees?* (2004), at 2. Fees were not abolished at private wings of some large hospitals.

56 See Joanne Carter and Rick Rowden, *User Fees on Primary Health and Education*, available at http://www.holycrossjustice.org/ResultsUSA.htm.

57 See further the chapter in this book on 'The Health Professionals' Voice in Achieving the Right to Health: Case Study from the Action Group for Health, Human Rights and HIV/AIDS Uganda' by Dr. Nelson Musoba and Sarah Kalloch.

Health Worker Migration: Perspectives from an African Health Worker

Francis Omaswa

The early African experience

My early experience with the international movement of health workers dates back to my school days in Uganda during the early sixties. One Sunday afternoon, a man came to the school to give us a talk following his triumphant return to Uganda after passing the final examination for the Fellowship of the Royal College of Surgeons. He was the very first indigenous person in East and Central Africa to achieve this feat. He returned home immediately, was received as a hero, and went on to render outstanding service to the country, to the African region, and the world, while all the time being based in Uganda.

A few years later, I joined Makerere Medical School myself, the only centre which trained doctors at the time for Kenya, Tanzania, Uganda and other neighbouring countries. There were undergraduate programmes for doctors and nurses at the teaching hospital at Mulago, but higher training could only be undertaken abroad, usually in the United Kingdom. There were waves of doctors, nurses, physiotherapists, radiographers etc. who left the country for higher training and all returned to Uganda after completing their training. The story told is that in the check-list for the preparations for the final examinations, an air ticket was included so that successful results were celebrated back at home. I witnessed this same experience in Kenya where we spent some time as guinea pig students for the new Medical School that was being developed there, and the same story can be told for Tanzania as well.

These health professionals came back home and found conducive and favourable working conditions. The salaries were adequate, perhaps even more than adequate, the hospitals and health facilities functioned well, with good material and human resources management. These professionals enjoyed job satisfaction and were recognized and appreciated by the society. They willingly accepted and served in postings in all corners of the countries. This applied equally to those health professionals who had not left the country to go for further studies. I completed my training and was recruited in 1970 into the civil service in Uganda, as a Medical Officer, and was sent to work in a recently built rural hospital. My seventeen Uganda classmates received similar postings. The hospital was well run, with running water, regular electricity, supplies were available and my salary was good enough for me to buy a car on hire purchase and to build a decent house for myself in the village. It is pertinent to mention that this high quality of health services was provided from the tax base of the Government of Uganda and there were no donors. Under these circumstances, the incentives to stay in the country overrode the benefits of migration. There were vacancies abroad, but these were not more attractive than the positive environment at home.

Problems in Africa

This favourable and positive environment started to change from around the mid-seventies, reaching different levels at different times in the countries. In essence, the economies in African countries began to decline with the collapse of commodity prices; governance deteriorated with military governments sprouting up all over; the cold war gave leeway for bad governments to thrive – as they could trade their votes at the UN and elsewhere for aid and patronage from either of the camps of the cold war. Bad governance led to conflicts, insecurity, sectarianism and hence to a slippery slope towards economic collapse, conflict and social insecurity. All these favoured the preponderance of the pull of migration over the incentives to stay at home. Health workers started to leave their countries.

Uganda typifies the situation. The government take-over by Idi Amin is generally credited with ushering in the onset of economic decline and poor governance, however, there is no doubt that, with or without Idi Amin, Uganda would still have joined other countries that felt the impact of the whole gamut of the decline era factors described above. In Zambia, copper prices fell; in Malawi, a dictatorship thrived; in Tanzania, a rigorous socialist doctrine exerted a demotivating influence on professionals. Ethiopia, Somalia and Sudan were all experiencing chronic conflicts, some of which persist to this day.

The Uganda case illustrates key core messages regarding the interplay between politics, human character, attitudes and behaviour in the face of the push and pull factors. Soon after the military take-over of government, the number of those who completed their studies and did not return went up sharply, others in the country who were members of certain ethnic groups did not feel secure and were leaving, initially in small numbers and reaching a peak in 1977 following the arrest and murder of Archbishop Janan Luwum. At this time, there was a massive migration of health workers, including the most senior, predominantly to Kenya and to other African countries such as Zambia, Botswana, and South Africa. Many also went to Europe, America, Australia and Canada. There were also health workers who stayed in the country in spite of the horrible security and economic conditions. The reasons that some stayed home varied, ranging from the need to take care of family, lack of tradable skills, apathy and, in some cases, the sorry situation provided opportunities for prosperity as caregivers and business associates of the rulers. There are also stories of heroes who persevered and stayed in their stations dutifully, faithful to the slogan "if I go away, what will happen to the people here and to the work that needs to be done here?"

The immediate post-Amin era produced another twist to the story of health workers. The factions that jostled for power at one point sought to discredit the incumbent by making the country appear ungovernable. One way to achieve this was to target doctors. A wave of politically motivated murders of top doctors took place during a period of several weeks, resulting in more migration and discouraging those who perceived the departure of Idi Amin as the signal to return home. This despicable political tactic has resurfaced in the stories currently emanating from the conflicts in Iraq and Afghanistan.

As Uganda started to settle down politically, a huge number of professionals, in health and other sectors, who had fled the country, returned home. At various times, there were even incentive packages through various agencies such as the United Nations High Commissioner for Refugees (UNHCR), the International Organization of Migration (IOM) (Tokten), and the government of Uganda. Two messages are worth sharing with respect to the phenomenon of return migration. The first is that we identified two categories of returning professionals. One type is those who want to come home, and any incentives given are of secondary relevance. They come back entirely on their own, settle down and quietly get on with their work. The second type is those who expect and demand incentives and support to return home. These people often fail to take root and tend to leave the country again, or even reap the incentives given and then leave. If they stay, they will grumble and complain until they have sufficient excuse to migrate again.

The second message is that tensions can develop between the returning professionals (returnees) and those who stayed in the country all along (stayees). Those who stayed may resent the arrival of those whom they feel were not loyal enough to the country and who then end up benefiting from both their exile as well as the incentives to return. These tensions needed to be managed. The lessons to be learnt from Uganda may be summarized as follows:

1. When local country conditions are positive, health workers stay and do not migrate.

2. The most powerful incentives to international migration are insecurity, injustice, poor working conditions and economic and social strife.

3. In spite of the most unfavourable environments, there are heroes who stick with their people and stay to provide essential services.

4. Sometimes targeted violence against health workers is used as a political tool.

5. When the conditions in the country revert from negative to positive, most health professionals return home, and their return needs to be managed without demoralizing those who did not migrate.

Creating a crisis

As conditions in African countries continued to remain challenging, the flux of health workers in and out of African countries resulted in a worrisome net outflow. Other external factors played their part too; in particular the aging of the population in developed countries that called for extra numbers of health workers, the dearth of young people joining training schemes and caps slapped on training places by some of the professionals in developed countries. In the Middle East, oil revenues helped to accelerate health care growth, and against a backdrop of cultural practices that discouraged local female trainees from joining the profession and a simultaneous insistence on certain services to be provided by females only. Quality of life concerns by health workers in developed countries is a factor not often given due prominence. Examples include reluctance to work in remote locations, so that these vacancies get filled by international migrant health workers; work-life-balance where working hours have been reduced; and the feminization of the profession, with the women in the predominantly female workforce taking time off to have families. All these factors add to an increased demand for health workers in developed countries.

In developing countries, on top of the push factors already described, a heavy disease burden of emergent and resurgent infectious diseases such as HIV and AIDS, tuberculosis, highland malaria (introduced and fanned by climate change), and new threats like SARS and avian flu, have increased demand for health workers. On top of this, the prevalence of non-communicable diseases such as diabetes, cardiovascular disease, hypertension and mental health problems compound the so-called double burden of disease afflicting developing countries and call for more health workers.

The Joint Learning Initiative, a two year study on the global health worker situation, whose report 'Human Resources for Health: Overcoming the Crisis' was published at the end of 2004, shone a light on what has come to be known as the Global Health Workforce Crisis.[1] It highlighted the shortages, poor working conditions, inadequate financing and health worker migration.

Governments wrangle

In the face of this health worker shortage, we have a straightforward market place where those with strong purchasing power outbid those with weaker purchasing power. There are governments that have chosen not to train, but to recruit those already trained by others, as this is cheaper. There are programmes in countries that do not train, but only recruit from poor competitors, and there are professions who limit the number of those who can train to maintain a premium on their own demand. There are communities who are left without health workers because they are too poor. There are poor countries whose meager resources train health workers who are pirated away by recruiters from rich countries who have set up recruitment camps in those countries. The migration of a few of the already depleted critical health workers from a community or a country can lead to a cata-strophic situation, where basic health care, such as attendance to deliveries of pregnant mothers, immunization of children or disease surveillance, can no longer be provided, resulting in increased illness and deaths.

This has sparked fierce arguments between governments. I have attend-ed several meetings of Ministers of Health at the World Health Assembly, and of the British Commonwealth, where the Ministers were furious with each other, hurling allegations such as "you are stealing our health work-ers", "you do not care about us". At three consecutive World Health Assem-blies, Ministers of Health from developing countries forced through three resolutions demanding a variety of responses by the global community and WHO to this problem. It is these resolutions that called for the 2006 World Health Report 'Working together for health'.[2] And it is this report, echo-ing the Joint Learning Initiative that called for the establishment of a glo-bal stakeholder alliance – the 'Global Health Workforce Alliance' hosted by WHO – of which I was privileged to become its first Executive Director.[3]

The Global Health Workforce Alliance

The Global Health Workforce Alliance (GHWA) is a partnership dedicated to identifying and implementing solutions to the global health workforce crisis. It is constituted by governments, multilateral agencies, civil society, academia and the private sector. The secretariat is provided by the World Health Organization in Geneva and was formally launched in May 2006, al-though preparatory work started already in April 2005.

GHWA envisages a ten-year life span, during which time it aims to support the development of evidence-based comprehensive and coherent country-level approaches to the health workforce crisis. Through the coor-dinated actions of its members, it works to scale-up significantly country, regional and global actions to ensure that every person in every village eve-rywhere has access to a skilled, motivated and supported health worker.

To achieve this, a dual strategy has been adopted, namely: First, acceler-ating country-led actions by strengthening national planning and manage-ment; and secondly, bringing stake holders together to tackle trans-nation-al constraints such as financing, priority research, knowledge sharing and migration. To achieve this, GHWA will ensure political visibility of the cri-sis, advocate for solutions, assemble and disseminate knowledge and best practice. Its methods of work include establishing time-bound and result-oriented task forces and working groups which bring together both technical know-how, as well as political and advocacy support. These methods generate knowledge and technical frameworks as public goods on human resources for health.

At present, the following Task Forces and Working Groups have been established; some have completed their work while others are in advanced stages, and yet others have recently been launched:

1. Task Force on Tools and Guidelines has created a planning framework for countries to use in making health workforce plans at country level.

2. Task Force on Scaling up Education and Training has issued a report with recommendations on skill mix, how to scale-up, and critical success factors gleaned from nine country studies.

3. Task Force on Health Workforce Financing is in advanced stages of generating recommendations and tools on how to plan for resources for health workforce plans and their implementation.

4. Working Group on Positive Practice Environments is a partnership between GHWA and the health professions, namely nursing and midwifery, physicians, dentists, pharmacists and physiotherapists. Guidelines have already been launched on "Positive Practice Environments" which will now be followed by a five year campaign to advocate and popularize them.

5. Task Force on Universal Access to HIV and AIDS will seek to support the achievement of universal access in a manner that integrates HIV and AIDS work with the rest of the health system.

6. Task Force on the Private Sector and Human Resources for Health will examine how the private sector can contribute to health worker development.

7. The Health Worker Advocacy Initiative is an independent partner of GHWA and is led by advocacy groups whose mission it is to bring the health workforce crisis to the attention of global and national leaders and call for commitment to pledges made.

8. The Health Worker Migration Policy Initiative addresses the key subject of health worker migration including developing principles for a global code on international recruitment of health workers. These principles have been handed over to the Director General of WHO and will subsequently be submitted to the World Health Assembly.

The health worker migration policy advisory council

The challenge of health worker migration poses unique dilemmas to policy makers from both developed and developing countries. Health workers have the right to emigrate in search of a better life, yet people have the right to health in countries hard hit by emigration. Addressing the imbalances resulting from health worker migration is thus complicated by the need to balance these two fundamental rights: The right of an individual to leave one's own country, and the right to health.

It is estimated that we now have a worldwide shortfall of almost 4.5 million health workers. Across the developing world, health workers face economic hardship, deteriorating infrastructure and social unrest, which has led to increased emigration. In many countries, HIV/AIDS has further decimated the health workforce. In Ghana, for example, in a recent year, 70 physicians were trained and 67 left the country immediately after graduation. This crisis, in turn, has been compounded by the ever-growing demand for health workers in developed countries due to aging populations and medical advances. Migration is a politically sensitive issue residing at the heart of a nation's sovereignty. What is certain is that the global shortage and asymmetrical migration of health workers cannot alone be solved by a single national policy response, but rather requires an international and coordinated response based on the principles of equity and fundamental human rights.

It was in response to this challenge that the Health Worker Migration Global Policy Advisory Council was formed as part of a larger Health Worker Migration Initiative of the GHWA, the WHO and the non-governmental organization Realizing Rights. Established in 2007, the Health Worker Migration Global Policy Advisory Council has as its mission to review, discuss and promote innovative global, regional and national policy action to support improved management of health worker migration globally. Composed of Ministers of Health and Development from source and destination countries and experts, the guiding principle of the Council is to forge solutions that respect the rights of migrants to seek a better life while also acknowledging the responsibilities of sending and receiving nations to minimize the negative impacts of health worker migration and to enhance its positive effects.

The Council, together with its technical partner, the Migration Technical Working Group, whose secretariat is the WHO, has provided a constructive forum for solutions-oriented debate regarding innovative policy action to address health worker migration. To date, the Council has been instrumental in mobilizing support and providing expert advice to the drafting of a new Global Code for the recruitment of health workers, which will come before the World Health Assembly in 2009; in compiling and analyzing current bilateral, regional and international codes for health worker migration; and in informing policymakers in both sending and receiving nations of promising practice they can pursue. The principle focus of these efforts has been to develop possible policy action that can be undertaken by countries that are global employers of health workers; to sensitize major destination countries to the effects of their recruitment and reliance on foreign health workers on source countries; and to promote a constructive global dialogue that recognizes roles and responsibilities on the part of both source and destination countries.

In my role as Co-Chair of this Council (with Mary Robinson), I have come to see the value of this platform in particular to health worker source countries, from Africa especially, who have not had opportunities to make their voices heard on this issue. In addition, the deliberations of the Council have allowed consensus ideas to emerge from both developed and developing countries as each listened to the concerns of the other. The Council and its partners, grounded in both the right to emigrate and the right to health as fundamental principles, have put forward pioneering and actionable solutions to the enormous challenge posed by health worker migration.

The Kampala Declaration and Agenda for Global Action (KD/AGA)

In March 2008, GHWA convened the first ever Global Forum on Human Resources for Health in Kampala, Uganda. This forum was a major milestone in health workforce development. It provided an opportunity for learning what works, and what does not and why, for fellowship by getting to know each other and galvanizing a global movement on human resources for health. It was addressed on video by His Excellency Ban Ki-Moon, the UN Secretary General, and was attended by Ministers of Health and global health leaders, civil society and academia. A Declaration and an Agenda for Global Action were adopted that now guide countries and the international community.[4] It was also included in the G8 Communiqué adopted in Hokkaido, Japan, last July 2008.

The KD/AGA addresses six interconnected strategic areas:

1. Building coherent national and global leadership for health workforce solutions
2. Ensuring capacity for an informed response based on evidence and joint learning
3. Scaling up health worker education and training
4. Retaining an effective, responsive and equitably distributed health workforce
5. Managing the pressures of the international health workforce market and its impact on migration
6. Securing additional and more productive investment in the health workforce.

The KD/AGA enjoins GHWA to monitor progress with its implementation, and to report on progress at the second global forum on Human Resources for Health that will take place in 2010. By that time, it is hoped that a number of countries will be on the way to implementing comprehensive health work force programmes that will contribute to the achievement of the MDGs and delivering better health to populations in need around the world and thus fulfilling a global aspiration for the right to health for all.

1   The Joint Learning Initiative, *Human Resources for Health: Overcoming the Crisis* (Cambridge: Harvard University Press, 2004).

2   World Health Organization (WHO), *World Health Report 2006: Working Together for Health* (Geneva: WHO, 2006).

3   See further, Global Health Workforce Alliance website at http://www.who.int/workforcealliance/en/.

4   GHWA, *The Kampala Declaration and an Agenda for Global Action,* adopted at the Global Forum on Human Resources for Health, available at http://www.who.int/entity/workforcealliance/Kampala%20Declaration%20and%20Agenda%20web%20file.%20FINAL.pdf.

Human Rights and Aid Effectiveness

Rahel Bösch

Introduction

The Paris Declaration on Aid Effectiveness constitutes a turning point in aid delivery. Endorsed in 2005, the Paris Declaration is a commitment by governments and organizations to strengthen efforts to achieve harmonization, alignment and better management of aid for results, with a set of actions and indicators which can be monitored over time.[1]

This chapter will provide a brief summary of the five pillars of the Paris Declaration and explore the role of human rights in implementing the commitments set out in the Paris Declaration. Efforts undertaken by the Human Rights Task Team of the Governance Network (GOVNET)[2] of the Development Assistance Directorate (DAC)[3] of the Organization for Economic Cooperation and Development (OECD) will be discussed, and a number of recommendations will be put forward on how a human rights perspective can contribute to enhanced aid effectiveness in development cooperation in the area of health.

Understanding the aid effectiveness agenda: The five pillars of the Paris Declaration

The Paris Declaration is more than yet another international statement of general principles. Evolving from the Monterrey Consensus[4] and Marrakesh Memorandum,[5] the Paris Declaration constitutes an action-orientated roadmap to improve the quality of aid and its impact on development. The partnership commitments set out in the Paris Declaration are organized around five key pillars: Ownership, alignment, harmonization, managing for results, and mutual accountability. Overall, and in particular for the pilot countries participating in the Paris Declaration survey, targets for the year 2010 have been set in order to encourage progress at the global level among the countries and organizations adhering to the Paris Declaration. In order to monitor progress, the targets were enriched by 12 indicators. Around 90 governments and 26 multilateral organizations have signed the Paris Declaration on Aid Effectiveness.

This comprehensive commitment to join efforts for increasing aid effectiveness constitutes a turning point in development cooperation for different reasons. First it challenges the traditional donor-recipient relationship by establishing national ownership as the core principle. Second, the Paris Declaration promotes a strong model of partnership, aimed at moving from an often one-sided approach to accountability, where only recipient countries are held responsible for results, to one in which donors are also accountable for fulfilling their commitments.

The first principle or key pillar, which promotes the ownership of national development plans, means that partner countries exercise strong and effective leadership over their own development policies and strategies. In other words, national development strategies and priority policy initiatives should be nationally driven by recipient countries rather than by donors. This concept is at the core of the Paris Declaration.

The above concept leads logically to the second key pillar – alignment. Through the Paris Declaration, donor countries have committed to aligning their development programmes and projects with priorities set out in the partner countries. In order to do so, donors have to harmonize their varied and diverse procedures in aid delivery amongst themselves. This third pillar on harmonization poses quite a challenge to donor governments and their national aid delivery procedures and protocols. It also requires a shift of paradigm from more donor-driven agendas to agendas owned and steered by the partner countries.

Overall, efforts towards ownership and alignment should be driven by common management for results, the fourth pillar of the Paris Declaration. Finally, this common approach should be led by mutual accountability. The OECD-DAC working party on Aid Effectiveness[6] highlights the importance of increased accountability:

"The Paris Declaration promotes a model of partnership that improves transparency and accountability in the use of development resources. It recognizes that for aid to become truly effective, stronger and more balanced, accountability mechanisms are required at different levels. At the international level, the Paris Declaration constitutes a mechanism to which donors and recipients of aid are held mutually accountable and compliance in meeting the commitments is to be publicly monitored. At the country level, the Paris Declaration encourages donors and partners to jointly assess mutual progress in implementing agreed commitments on aid effectiveness by making best use of local mechanisms."[7]

What are the links between development cooperation and human rights? The work of the Human Rights Task Team of the Development Assistance Directorates Governance Network (DAC/GOVNET)[8]

In parallel with the Paris Declaration process, efforts to promote good governance as an essential precondition for sustainable and effective development cooperation were evolving as well.

On the one hand, consensus was reached by the international community in the United Nations Millennium Declaration and reconfirmed in the Millennium Summit, around the importance of governance and human rights in reaching the Millennium Development Goals.[9] On the other hand, the donor community together with partner countries had elaborated a clear-cut commitment to increasing aid effectiveness with the Paris Declaration. In short, both processes are part of overall efforts by donor and recipient countries, including civil society and multilateral institutions, and in particular the OECD and the UN, to enhance the impact and quality of aid and development cooperation.

When it comes to implementing the Paris Declaration, crucial questions remain on the links between human rights and governance and the Paris Declaration agenda, which prioritizes increased quality and impact of development cooperation. Why should the implementation of the Paris Declaration on Aid Effectiveness be linked with the promotion of human rights? What would be the added value of bringing these two agendas together?

The role of human rights in poverty reduction

In 1997, the Development Assistance Directorate had already affirmed in the Final Report of the Working Group on Participatory Development and Good Governance that the promotion of human rights is part of promoting good governance. However, this was a rather limited approach focussing on civil and political rights and in particular on judicial reform. In the evolving debate on promoting good governance, human rights were no longer actively considered in the agenda of the Governance Network of the Development Assistance Directorate (DAC/GOVNET), which is a subsidiary body bringing together representatives from bilateral and multilateral donor agencies on governance related issues.

But over the last decade, human rights and development have been gradually converging. Today, poverty is increasingly understood in all its dimensions, not only the economic aspects, but also the social and cultural dimensions. This is reflected in the DAC Guidelines on Poverty Reduction. The guidelines resulted from a broad-based consultation process involving development practitioners, representatives from civil society and governments. The guidelines confirm the value added of rights-based approaches, as they "address the causes of poverty by identifying rights-holders and duty-bearers for the realization of all human rights – civil, cultural, political, social and economic. The emphasis on human rights shows that justice is a matter of rights, not charity."[10]

Bilateral and multilateral donors have increasingly looked to human rights as a means for improving the impact of aid on development. The evolving understanding of the role of human rights in development links closely with the promotion of gender equality and governance. UN agencies have played an essential role in defining a human rights-based approach to development.[11] This consensus was not reached easily but the experiences and good practices by UNICEF[12] and UNIFEM[13] in particular provided a sound base for common ground.

These developments provided the foundation for bringing human rights back to the working agenda of the DAC/GOVNET. Thanks to the individual commitment of the members of the Task Team representing various bilateral donor countries, as well as the interest of multilateral organizations and DAC/GOVNET's secretariat and the support of the then chair of the DAC/GOVNET, the Human Rights Task Team was challenged to prepare concrete suggestions in a policy paper which would include agreed actions.

Donor approaches, experiences and challenges in integrating human rights and development

Indeed, the paper was the first major challenge. The Task Team worked intensively to achieve more coherent understanding of human rights in development based on practical approaches. A study on donor approaches, experiences and challenges in integrating human rights into development was commissioned from the Overseas Development Institute.[14] The idea was to build common ground from disparate experiences. The Task Team did not want to add another study on the growing pile of lengthy documents but instead aimed to produce a synthesis of existing practices and lessons learned. The study looked at programming experiences at the project level, as well as country programmes and practices by global initiatives. It analysed more "traditional" governance interventions to promote civil and political rights, in particular through judicial reforms and access to justice projects and programmes.

Equally important, it examined human rights mainstreaming, with special focus on children's, women's and minority rights.

The study concluded that:

—— Human rights is the only internationally agreed framework which provides a coherent global normative and analytical framework. It puts the human being at the centre of the analysis, linked to state obligations and citizens' entitlement.

—— The human rights framework is broad enough to be adapted to different cultural and political environments.

—— Human rights principles can effectively be operationalized with human rights-based approaches (HRBA) building upon the UN common understanding.

—— Human rights promotion and protection is instrumental to improved development quality but has also an intrinsic value in itself.

—— Governance is an extremely broad concept which can be concretized by integrating a human rights perspective, because the latter clarifies roles and responsibilities of the state and its citizens. By (broadly) defining rights and duties, a human rights perspective in governance defines lines of accountability and hence legitimacy. It links non-discrimination and defines approaches to have a meaningful participation.

—— Human rights contribute to identifying the structural and root causes of poverty by starting with basic rights and duties in the analysis: "Instead of a needs based framework, human rights-based programming looks at states' ability to meet their obligations as well as their capacity and political will constraints."[15]

____ Human rights help to identify and prioritize excluded and marginalized groups as human rights-based programming directly tackles disparities.

____ A human rights perspective enhances aid effectiveness by helping donors and NGOs to understand the need to move away from direct delivery and to work at the level of the overall legal and policy framework, institutions and programmes – it contributes to a shift from service delivery to capacity development.

Bearing the five pillars of the Paris Declaration on Aid Effectiveness in mind – it is clear that these findings can and should enrich the understanding and realization of ownership, alignment and harmonization.

Enhancing aid effectiveness: The consensus reached in the Action Oriented Policy Paper on Human Rights and Development

The study was submitted to interested donors and partner countries and discussed by representatives of civil society and academia in October 2006 at a meeting convened in Paris. The response was extremely positive and paved the way for formulating the long expected Action Oriented Policy Paper on Human Rights and Development (AOPP).

The AOPP formulates ten principles for promoting and integrating human rights in development cooperation[16] (see Box on Ten Principles.) and identifies two new focus areas: Aid effectiveness and fragile states.

"Changes to the international development context, and an agenda of ambitious reforms in the international aid system, present new challenges and opportunities for addressing human rights. Donors and partner governments alike are increasingly focused on improving aid effectiveness, including in fragile states. This opens up opportunities for protecting and promoting human rights and integrating key human rights principles – such as participation, inclusion and accountability – into development processes in a more effective way."[17]

Ten principles for promoting and integrating human rights in development

The Action Oriented Policy Paper details the DAC's position on human rights and development and highlights new challenges in promoting and protecting human rights and integrating human rights in development.

The DAC has identified 10 principles intended to serve as basic orientation in key areas and activities where harmonized donor action is of particular importance:

1. Build a shared understanding of the links between human rights obligations and development priorities through dialogue.

2. Identify areas of support to partner governments on human rights.

3. Safeguard human rights in processes of state-building.

4. Support the demand side of human rights.

5. Promote non-discrimination as a basis for more inclusive and stable societies.

6. Consider human rights in decisions on alignment and aid instruments.

7. Consider mutual reinforcement between human rights and aid effectiveness principles.

8. Do no harm.

9. Take a harmonized and graduated approach to deteriorating human rights situations.

10. Ensure that the scaling-up of aid is conducive to human rights.

(See the DAC Action Oriented Policy Paper on Human Rights and Development, 2007)

Consider human rights in decisions on alignment and aid instruments

The ongoing work of the Human Rights Task Team aims at making use of the potential of linking the two agendas instead of moving ahead on disconnected tracks. Three of the ten principles set out in the AOPP are directly linked to aid effectiveness: Principle Six, concerning human rights in decisions on alignment and aid instruments; Principle Seven, on mutual reinforcement between human rights and aid effectiveness principles; and

Principle Ten, which calls for the scaling-up of aid which is conducive to human rights.

By adopting the AOPP, the DAC members[18] agreed to consider "the inclusiveness of government strategies, and their responsiveness to the perspectives of different interest groups and actors in a country – including the marginalized and most vulnerable – into consideration when assessing ownership and making decisions on alignment behind government strategies."[19] In addition, relying on the information and recommendations on a broad range of development issues, such as e.g. economic, social and cultural rights, (including the right to health) or discrimination against women or child protection provided by the corresponding human rights monitoring bodies, it is also important to take into account the country-specific human rights context – and based on that, to balance the support to state and non-state actors. In particular, human rights monitoring provides information on those groups who have difficulties in accessing services and exercising their rights.

DAC members are encouraged to "consider human rights principles, analysis and practice in the roll-out of the Paris Declaration's partnership commitments."[20] This can be approached by including the human rights principles of non-discrimination, inclusive participation and accountability in the 12 indicators for the Paris Declaration. Building in participation and non-discrimination will lead to questions on the process and on the set up of institutions, and how policies are established whose interests are taken into account and which priorities are set.

The third principle on ensuring that the scaling up of aid is conducive to human rights means that human rights performance and context should be taken into account by donors. Mainly, "efforts to increase aid should therefore move in tandem with the strengthening of human rights institutions, accountability mechanisms and related capacities."[21]

Starting from this consensus, the HR Task Team commissioned further studies in collaboration with the Overseas Development Institute (ODI) including on aid effectiveness and human rights, which explores each of the Paris Declaration's key principles and pays particular attention to areas in which human rights can make positive and practical contributions to the improvement of development quality and aid effectiveness. Some key messages are summarized in the box.

Aid effectiveness and human rights: Strengthening the implementation of the Paris Declaration

The Paris Declaration calls for country ownership of the development agenda. By taking on human rights obligations, countries have already gone some distance towards identifying national priorities. As well, human rights focus on the quality of the relationship between governments and citizens, and the processes and mechanisms of domestic accountability that are fundamental to ensuring meaningful and inclusive citizen-based ownership.

Under the principle of alignment, donors have committed to channelling support through countries' own institutions and procedures. Experience from human rights-based work to support budgeting processes can be drawn on to help ensure that financial and administrative mechanisms are responsive to a country's human rights obligations and to the views of rights holders themselves.

The fact that both donor and partner countries have ratified the international human rights treaties provides a uniquely valuable reference point for harmonization efforts. A mutually agreed, universal normative framework already exists, supported not only by political commitment, but also by the force of legal obligation. As well, at the operational level, there is growing convergence on the integration of human rights in development.

Human rights principles and standards can and should be used to define the results to be achieved and the strategies needed to achieve them. There is no inherent conflict between support for human rights implementation and managing for results.

The international legal regime established through the human rights treaties is a global accountability mechanism that is not the exclusive property of either donor or partner countries. It would be important to explore what use can be made of this global mechanism when devising approaches to mutual accountability for aid effectiveness, particularly since the Paris Declaration promotes a model of partnership that improves transparency and accountability on the use of development resources and that requires accountability mechanisms at different levels. From a human rights perspective, strengthening domestic accountability between governments and their own citizens is essential for ensuring effective use of aid to produce sustainable development outcomes.

Source: Human Rights and Aid Effectiveness – DAC Update – April 2007

Further steps towards reaching a common understanding

In parallel with the efforts of the HR task team of the DAC/GOVNET, two other subsidiary bodies of the DAC – on gender equality and environment – worked to further these issues as substantial development concerns in the Paris Declaration. These efforts were nourished by emerging experience and lessons learned in the field, illustrating that ownership of national strategies must be broad-based and inclusive, and that donors should not align with national priorities which leave out substantial issues, such as gender equality and social inclusion. In short, there is no increased aid effectiveness if quality and performance issues are left out.

The efforts to bring human rights, gender equality and the environment into a central position in the context of the Paris Declaration were furthered significantly by the Dublin Workshop on "Development Effectiveness in Practice" in 2007. Organized jointly by the DAC/GOVNET, the DAC Networks on Environment and Gender Equality, and the DAC Working Party on Aid Effectiveness, the workshop was to increase mutual knowledge and understanding of how practitioners are applying the Paris Declaration's overarching principles to advance gender equality, environmental sustainability and human rights. The long-term goal is to demonstrate how attention to these issues enhances development effectiveness.

Overall, the outcome of the workshop strongly re-emphasized the crucial role of human rights for development and aid effectiveness: "Human rights, gender equality and environmental sustainability are key goals of development. They are functionally essential to achieving the ultimate goal of the *Paris Declaration* – increasing the impact of aid on reducing poverty and inequality, increasing growth, building capacity and accelerating achievement of the MDGs."[22] The outcome of this very first meeting of representatives from GOVNET, Gender NET and the Working Party on Aid Effectiveness helped to further explore the value added of consciously integrating human rights along the five pillars of the Paris Declaration. Broadly summarizing the results of the Dublin Workshop, the following issues can be highlighted:

Ownership

Ownership goes beyond national governments; parliaments, civil society and decentralized government levels should own national development strategies. Only this broad ownership creates political leverage and links to the institutional and legal frameworks that promote and protect citizens' rights, and allow marginalized groups to participate in decision making processes that affect their lives. This links also to internal accountability. Broad participation and consultation opens doors for bringing in human rights, gender equality and environmental concerns and hence influencing priority setting in national development plans. This internal accountability also contributes to democratic ownership which is crucial for effective implementation of development and goes in tandem with monitoring progress in development.

Alignment

An essential lesson highlighted in Dublin was that "Alignment works best when environmental sustainability, human rights and gender equality are institutionalized in legal frameworks, national strategies and robust policies." Commitments undertaken by ratifying human rights conventions are in many countries translated in the national legal framework and provide therefore a common base for dialogues between donors and partner countries. In addition, public financial management is strengthened by participatory budgeting processes: "The practice of gender and equity responsive budgeting can strengthen national ownership by democratizing debates on national spending priorities and empowering society to participate meaningfully." In addition, it helps to direct discussions on budget allocations for equality issues and social inclusion, issues that are often tackled by national cross-cutting strategies without appropriate budget allocation.[23]

Harmonization

Increased donors' efforts with regard to harmonizing their agendas on human rights and gender equality will help to avoid fragmentation and lack of coherence and hence help to bring these agendas to the centre of the work on the Paris Declaration. Harmonizations needs trust, transparency and inclusiveness. Increased civil society participation being fundamental to ownership and alignment is also a precondition for harmonization. And overall: "Harmonization can bring gender equality, human rights and environment to the centre of Paris Declaration Implementation."

Managing for results

"Human rights, gender equality and environmental substainability are objectives in themselves – without results in these key policy areas, short term achievements in aid effectiveness will have little meaning."[24] Monitorable objectives on these issues are essential.

Mutual accountability

The Dublin findings also state:

> "A capable state needs a capable civil society. The *Paris Declaration* seeks to promote a model of partnership that improves transparency and provides stronger accountability mechanisms for the use of development resources. Strengthened domestic accountability through engagement with civil society is essential to democratic ownership, as is support for representative government, an independent judiciary and independent media. ... Mutual accountability, however, is one of the least developed of the Paris Declaration principles. There will be no accountability without accurate and reliable data, yet results-frameworks and indicators for gender, environmental sustainability and human rights are not widely used. Experience gained from work in these areas can add value and insights to its further development. Accountability is neither a technical exercise nor an end in itself but a dynamic socio-political process that is critical to achieving key development objectives and results. It is not just provided by states to citizens but also has to be demanded by citizens."[25]

Recommendations on human rights and aid effectiveness in the health sector

A recent study looks at the inter-linkages and synergies for improving development outcomes in the health sector.[26] Reviewing practice in various countries, this study is providing substantial recommendations for partner countries, donors and civil society organization on how utilizing the human rights framework can strengthen aid effectiveness and improve development outcomes in the health sector.

Selected recommendations for partner countries on how to do this cover the fields of legislation and resources.[27] For example, the study recommends that partner countries build health sector legislation, regulations and policies using international human rights standards, regional human rights charters and rights identified in the constitution. They should use the rights identified in constitutions, legislation and policies as a basis for identifying and communicating citizens' entitlements to health care through, for example, a charter of patients' rights drawn up on the basis of civil society consultation. When taking the lead on national debate about critical issues such as maternal mortality, the governments should use the human rights framework, including international human rights reporting mechanisms.

With regard to civil society participation, the study recommends to partner countries that they should support the engagement of civil society in national policy processes, including sectoral working groups, and ensure adequate allocation of resources in health sector budgets for enabling meaningful local level participation in decision-making processes. In order to enable civil society engagement in monitoring allocations timely information on health sector budget processes should be provided.

In order to ensure the equality and the prioritization of primary health-care services, health sector budgets should make reallocations on the basis of principles of equality. A further recommendation in the study includes parliament. It is recommended to establish parliamentary committees to review donor programmes as well as government's use of aid.

The study also draws important recommendations on how donors can integrate human rights in health sector development cooperation.

When engaging with partner countries on development policy, donors should recognize the importance of partner countries' international human rights commitments and constitutional commitments. And, based on that, support the capacities of the Ministry of Health at national, regional and local levels to address human rights issues, including gender equality and other forms of non-discrimination. When it comes to new aid modalities, donors should make sure that Sector Wide Approaches (SWAPs) or other forms of cooperation do not result in less attention to, and funding for, difficult agendas, such as reproductive and sexual health rights. In particular, they should ensure that channeling aid through budget support and SWAPs does not lead to a decrease in support to civil society organizations (CSOs) or to a reduction in the range of CSOs that are supported.

It is also recommended to use human rights analysis tools in joint planning and review missions to ensure that donor-supported programmes, at the very least, do no harm to the human rights of people in partner countries and consequently, to support the development of monitoring systems that can collect disaggregated data. With regard to monitoring, the support to the capacity of national human rights institutions to monitor and report on economic, social and cultural rights is recommended.

When including human rights in development cooperation in the health sector, the study highlights the importance of donor's respect of the use of international human rights mechanisms, including the UN Treaty Monitoring Bodies and Special Rapporteurs, to report on donor and partner country commitments and action.

Last but not least, donors could take an active role when it comes to strengthening donor accountability to partner country governments and their people through the provision of public information on programmes and enabling partner country parliamentary committees and national human rights institutions to review donor programmes.

For local, national and international human rights organizations the study points out that the inclusion of the Paris Declaration principles can help to inform understanding of some of the most effective ways of building strategies to promote human rights. Key issues identified include the importance of: Linking different accountability processes to enable, for example, broad-based participation in the monitoring processes of national human rights institutions and developing clear, prioritized operational solutions to context-specific health challenges.

Civil society organizations should focus on the translation of human rights principles of equality and non-discrimination into budget allocations through, for example, the development of needs-based allocation formulae and analysis of the equity impacts of resource allocations for universal versus targeted budget allocations.

Conclusions

Overall, it can be concluded that the mutual integration of aid effectiveness and human rights has moved ahead considerably in the last three years. This is also reflected in the third high level forum on the implementation of the Paris Declaration in Accra in September 2008.[28] Human rights are increasingly finding their proper place on the Paris Declaration implementation agenda. More work must be done, but the intensive efforts to ensure that human rights are central to aid effectiveness, including in the health sector, have made an impact.

1   For more information, see OECD/DAC, *The Paris Declaration*, available at http://www.oecd.org/document/18/0,3343,en_2649_3236398_35401554_1_1_1_1,00.html.

2   OECD/DAC, Paris, "The GOVNET's work covers some governance issues including governance assessments and capacity development, the fight against corruption, taxation and accountability, human rights and development, transparency in support of these elements of democratic governance." See further http://www.oecd.org/department/0,3355,en_2649_34565_1_1_1_1_1,00.html.

3   "The Development Assistance Committee (DAC, www.oecd.org/dac) is the principal body through which the OECD deals with issues related to co-operation with developing countries": See further http://www.oecd.org/dac.

4   The Conference on Financing for Development, held in Monterrey, Mexico in 2002 highlighted the importance of building partnerships among donors and developing countries as a means of making more effective progress towards the MDGs. More information available at http://www.un.org/esa/ffd/monterrey/MonterreyConsensus.pdf.

5   The Joint Marrakesh Memorandum was the result of the Conference on Managing for Development Results in 2004. The Memorandum called on international funding institutions to enhance their organizational focus on results, drawing from lessons learnt of different countries. The need for alignment with desired country development results and for relying on, and strengthening, country monitoring systems was recognized. More information available at http://www.escwa.un.org/divisions/sd_editor/Download.asp?table_name=Documents&field_name=ID&FileID=607.

6   The Development Assistance Directorate (DAC) Working Party on Aid Effectiveness (www.oecd.org/dac/effectiveness) was set up in May 2003 in the context of the international consensus reached at Monterrey on the actions needed to promote a global partnership for development and accelerate progress towards the Millennium Development Goals.

7   OECD/DAC, Paris, 'Three reasons why the Paris Declaration will make a difference significantly increasing the impact of aid', available at http://www.oecd.org/document/18/0,2340,en_2649_3236398_35401554_1_1_1_1,00.html.

8   The Human Rights Task Team of the Governance Network of the Development Assistance Directorate at the OECD (GOVNET) is the international network on human rights within bilateral and multilateral development agencies. It is working to enhance understanding and consensus on why and how donors should work more strategically and coherently on the integration of human rights and development. In pursuing this objective, the Task Team provides a framework for sharing of information and experience and for collective learning; promotes dialogue and collaboration between human rights practitioners and other development practitioners; develops policy guidance on how to integrate human rights more consistently into donor policies and practice; and acts as a resource to the DAC and its subsidiary bodies on human rights and development. More information available at http://www.oecd.org/document/21/0,2340,fr_2649_34565_35901653_1_1_1_1,00.html.

9   See further http://www.un.org/millenniumgoals/.

10 DAC Guidelines on Poverty Reduction, Paris, 2001, available at http://www.oecd.org/dataoecd/47/14/2672735.pdf.

11 The UN Common Understanding on a Human Rights-Based Approach, available at http://www.undp.org/governance/docs/HR_Guides_Common Understanding.pdf.

12 See further http://www.unicef.org/.

13 See further http://www.unifem.org/.

14 The draft of this study was completed by Laure-Hélène Piron, Overseas Development Institute (I).

15 OECD/DAC, *Integrating Human Rights in Development: Donors' Approaches, Experiences, Challenges* (Paris, 2006) at 63.

16 OECD/DAC, *Action Oriented Policy Paper on Human Rights and Development* (Paris, 2007) available at http://www.oecd.org/dataoecd/50/7/39350774.pdf.

17 Ibid.

18 An overview on DAC member states is available at http://www.oecd.org/linklist/0,3435,en_2649_33721_1797105_1_1_1_1,00.html.

19 OECD/DAC, Action Oriented Policy Paper on Human Rights and Development (Paris, 2007), Principle 6, available at http://www.oecd.org/dataoecd/50/7/39350774.pdf.

20 Ibid., Principle 7.

21 Ibid., Principle 10.

22 'Key Messages and Summary Record', Workshop on Development Effectiveness in Practice: Applying the Paris Declaration to advancing gender equality, environmental sustainability and human rights, Dublin, Ireland, April 2007, hosted by Irish Aid, organized jointly by the Development Assistance Committee's Networks on Environment and Development, Governance, and Gender Equality and the Working Party on Aid Effectiveness, funded by the Governments of Ireland and Denmark, 'Introduction' available at http://www.oecd.org/dataoecd/30/20/38933324.pdf.

23 Ibid., para. 15.

24 Ibid.

25 Ibid., paras. 18 and 19.

26 Clare Ferguson, *Draft Report for OECD/DAC GOV-NET, Human Rights Task Team: Human Rights and Aid Effectiveness: Inter-linkages and Synergies to Improve Development Outcomes in the Health Sector*, 5 April 2008.

27 Ibid., at 5–6.

28 The Third High Level Forum on Aid Effectiveness took place in Accra, in September 2008. The High Level Forum identified and agreed upon a programme of action, the Accra Action Agenda, to address the main challenges that have arisen, and map out a strategy for action to 2010.

09

CASE STUDIES ON THE ROLE OF GOVERNMENT AND CIVIL SOCIETY

The Democratization of Health in Mexico: Extending the Right to Health Care

Julio Frenk and Octavio Gómez-Dantés*

Health is moving steadily up the list of priority issues on the global agenda. During the past few years, health has been recognized as a key element of global security, sustainable economic growth, and effective governance. In foreign policy terms, global health has moved from the realm of "low politics" to that of "high politics".[1]

Recent reforms in Mexico illustrate the importance of health for governance. The main message of this chapter is that these reforms, by extending the right to health care to all the population, have strengthened the procedures and institutions of democracy. Undoubtedly, the democratization of health can contribute to the health of democracy.

Democracy and health

Huntington has spoken of "the third wave of democracy", which started in the 1970s in Southern Europe, then spread to Latin America and some Asian and African countries, and finally reached Central and Eastern Europe.[2] There are reasons to believe that this new wave is generating stable governments. However, the danger of stagnation haunts some younger democracies.

Huntington documented the existence of "reversions" in the two previous waves of democratization. Even though there are no signs of the development of a "third reverse wave",[3] the existence of trends that hinder the consolidation of newly established democracies has generated a search for means to further encourage democratic progress.

Salient among the conditions known to favour the consolidation of democracy are economic success or growth; the existence of a political culture that promotes tolerance and allows minorities to compete for power; the existence of cultural traditions that accept the separation of religion and politics; and the fair distribution of the benefits of economic growth.

In a recent United Nations Development Programme (UNDP) report on democracy in Latin America, the extension of the right to healthcare to all the population was recommended as a way to increase the effectiveness of democracies in the region.[4] The exercise of social rights, including education and health care, is intrinsically positive. However, the UNDP report highlights the efforts needed to incorporate these rights into legislation and ensure their implementation in ways which offer tangible benefits to all citizens. Doing so can contribute to establishing "full" democracies in those countries involved in the new democratic wave.

The Mexican health reform

In 2003, a legislative reform approved by a large majority of the Congress established a system of social protection for health in Mexico. This system will increase public funding by a full percentage point of gross domestic product (GDP) over a period of seven years to provide universal health insurance, which will benefit the 50 million Mexicans who have been excluded until now from formal social insurance schemes because they are self-employed, are out of the labour market, or work in the informal sector of the economy. Poor families can now enrol in a new public insurance scheme called Seguro Popular. Affiliation with this insurance scheme guarantees access to a comprehensive set of benefits. By the end of 2007, the number of persons enrolled in the Seguro Popular had reached 20 million.

This financial reform is being complemented by a micro-level management reform, which is strengthening delivery capacity through a series of specific interventions, including long-term planning of new facilities, better schemes for drug supply, human resource development, outcome-oriented information systems, facility accreditation, provider certification, quality improvement in the technical and the interpersonal dimensions of care, and performance benchmarking among states and organizations.

An external evaluation of the initial results of this reform showed, among other things, higher service utilization rates among those affiliated to the Seguro Popular than among the uninsured population; major improvements in the supply of drugs in health facilities that are offering services to these affiliates; and significant improvements in financial protection indicators among families affiliated to the new insurance scheme, including out-of-pocket expenditures and impoverishing and catastrophic health expenditures.[5] The researchers responsible for the quasi-experimental component of this evaluation concluded that most of these changes could be reasonably attributed to the implementation of the Seguro Popular.[6]

The democratization of health in Mexico

The guiding concept underlying the Mexican reform of 2003 was the "democratization of health", which involves the expansion of democracy to the realm of social rights.

The term "democratization", according to O'Donnell and Schmitter, implies the application of the norms and procedures of citizenship to those institutions that have been governed by other principles, such as coercive control, social tradition, judgment of specialists or bureaucratic processes.[7] Democratization also implies applying these norms and procedures to individuals who did not always enjoy the benefits and duties of citizenship, such as women, young people and children, ethnic minorities or workers in the informal sector of the economy.

Aristotle, in his "Politics", states that what defines a citizen is the possibility of holding office.[8] In other sources, the term citizen is associated with a range of rights and duties, of a diverse nature, not only political, as defined within a constitution.[9] In his seminal work, "Class, Citizenship and Social Development", Marshall recognizes three types of rights involved in the idea of citizenship: Civil, political, and social.[10]

Civil rights are those that define individual liberty: Freedom of thought and expression, the right to own property, and the right to an impartial trial. The institutions more directly related to civil rights are the courts. Political rights include the right to participate in the government of one's own country. The procedures through which these rights are exercised include voting, free political competition, and access to public information. Finally, social rights include those rights that guarantee the participation in the social heritage, including the right to adequate housing, health, education, and culture. Marshall states that citizenship culminates with the implementation of social rights, which are delivered through institutions such as the educational and health systems.

As a result of its democratization process, Mexico made important progress in the exercise of civil and political rights. It was clear, however, that the next great challenge was to bridge social gaps by assuring the universal exercise of social rights, including the right to healthcare.

This right was incorporated in the Mexican Constitution in the early 1980s. In practice, however, not all individuals had been equally able to exercise it. Half the population, by virtue of their occupational status, enjoyed the protection of social insurance. The other half was left without access to any form of health insurance. This portion of the population received health care at units of the Ministry of Health (MoH) through various forms of assistance, with huge variations of benefits: From a relatively large package of services in the big cities of the wealthy states, to a minimal set of preventive interventions for the rural poor of the southern states of the country.

So the legal recognition of health care as a social right was already there when the debate around the reform started, but its actual implementation was only benefiting certain sectors of the population. What was lacking was the definition of the explicit entitlements that ensued from such a claim, and the financial and organizational instruments to translate them into effective health services for all.

According to Brachet, the transformation of health care into a real social right requires, above everything, two things: A defined set of health benefits that all citizens, regardless of their labour or socio-economic status, should receive and can legally demand, and established mechanisms through which the costs of these benefits will be distributed to guarantee their financial viability.[11]

It is interesting to note that the point of departure of the Seguro Popular was the definition and costing of the specific entitlements that would give operational meaning to the right to health care enshrined in the Mexican Constitution. Thus, the law now stipulates a budgetary obligation for the federal and state governments in order to meet the expected demand from each family that enrols in the Seguro Popular. The government contributions are complemented by family contributions that are a function of the income level of affiliated households. Families in the first and second income deciles are exempted from these contributions.

More specifically, the guaranteed entitlements comprise two sets of benefits: First, a package of 255 preventive and curative essential interventions which account for the vast majority of demand for services in public institutions; second, a package of 18 high-cost interventions with potentially catastrophic consequences for families, including HIV/AIDS, critical neonatal conditions, and cancer in children, among others.

What are the implications of the use of a package of essential interventions, traditionally an instrument of technocratic approaches to healthcare, in a reform process that emphasizes equity and social justice?

These essential health services have been devised mostly as a priority-setting tool. In contexts of limited resources, cost-effectiveness analyses are used to identify those interventions that can generate the largest amount of benefits for the available resources. These interventions are usually targeted for the poor.

The Mexican reform packages responded to concerns over priority setting through three innovations: The incorporation of selection criteria covering more than cost and effectiveness; their use as a planning and quality assurance tool; and their extension to a universalistic conception of coverage based on the explicit definition of entitlements. We will now discuss each of these innovations.

First, interventions were selected using a broad set of criteria. Cost-effectiveness analyses were used as were social acceptability criteria, especially in the selection of benefits for the package of high-cost interventions. The intention is to ensure this package conforms with the norms of behaviour of the health professions and to broader social preferences, and to select the interventions through a fair and transparent process.[12] In this respect, a key component of the Mexican reform has been the creation of the National Bioethics Commission, which serves as an independent and credible deliberative body.

Second, the package of interventions provides the blueprint to estimate the resources required in order to strengthen the health system through three master plans for long-term investments in infrastructure, medical equipment, and health personnel, as well as a national programme to improve the availability of essential drugs. The package has also been used as a quality assurance tool, designed to guarantee that all necessary services are offered in accordance with standardized protocols. For the first time, the new law requires that every facility be accredited in order to participate in the insurance scheme. Accreditation is based partially on having the required resources to provide the stipulated interventions.

Finally, and this is what will be stressed in the remaining part of this chapter, the package has been used as an instrument for empowering people by making them aware of their entitlements. The new Mexican Health Law clearly states that Seguro Popular affiliates will have access to all health interventions included in both packages and to the respective drugs. In fact, at the moment of affiliation, all families receive a Charter of Rights and Duties that explicitly lists the health interventions to which they are entitled and the health facilities to which they can go to demand them.

The law also stipulates that the packages must be progressively expanded and updated annually on the basis of changes in the epidemiological profile, technological developments, and the availability of resources, which means that benefit coverage expands over time, not only as new technologies and money become available, but also as new diseases and risk factors are identified.

So the Mexican model may be seen as an option to reconcile two extremes: The selective, technocratic approach to the distribution of healthcare, which provides practical alternatives, but is usually morally neutral, and the rights-based approach, which has a strong value foundation but has lacked operational support.

The other prerequisite for turning health care into a social right has also been met. As mentioned previously, the financial mechanisms that will guarantee the sustainability of the Seguro Popular have been established by law, with the federal and state governments covering the vast majority of the costs through the general taxation system, complemented by a modest proportion of means-tested, progressive, and affordable contributions from families, with total exemption for those in the bottom 20% of the income distribution.[13]

In order to meet the resource requirements of the new scheme, between 2002 and 2006 the budget of the Ministry of Health increased, in real terms, by 72 percent, thanks mostly to the resources devoted to the Seguro Popular. If the expected trends in the mobilization of additional public resources continue to materialize, by 2010, the objective of increasing public funding for health by a full percentage point of GDP will have been met and the financial viability of the new public insurance scheme will be guaranteed. In this way, health care in Mexico will begin to be predominantly financed with public resources, as recommended by the Organization for Economic Co-operation and Development (OECD).[14]

Brachet identifies two other elements that also help to turn health care into a real social right: Mechanisms to guarantee that providers will be able to meet their responsibilities and monitoring and evaluation procedures that strengthen transparency and accountability.

As discussed in previous sections of this chapter, the health reform comes with a special initiative for strengthening the supply of public health services that includes: Three master plans for long-term investments in infrastructure, medical equipment, and health personnel; a programme to improve the availability of essential drugs, which includes periodic external surveys on the availability of drugs in ambulatory and hospital settings; and the compulsory accreditation of all health units providing services to the Seguro Popular.

On the evaluation side, an external assessment for the Seguro Popular was implemented between 2004 and 2006. This evaluation includes a quasi-experimental community trial measuring changes in service utilization, responsiveness, effective coverage, financial protection, and health conditions. For the system as a whole, a comprehensive evaluation model that includes the comparative monitoring of state and institutional health systems performance was designed. This involves external evaluations of the main policies and programs and monitoring and evaluation of personal and public health services. Part of the results of these monitoring and evaluation procedures are published in an annual report, *Salud: México*, that has attracted extensive attention from the federal and state governments, multilateral agencies, non-governmental organizations, the media, and the general public. Technical reports are also available in printed and electronic formats.

Conclusion

The effective exercise of social rights is a key component of citizenship and should be considered an intrinsic objective of all democracies. As illustrated by the recent health reform in Mexico, the universal exercise of social rights can also contribute to the consolidation of democracy.

Universal access to health care reduces poverty, improves educational outcomes, enhances productivity, and prompts economic growth. Prosperity and a fair distribution of its benefits contribute to democratic stability.[15]

In the case of Mexico, the extension of the right to health care is mostly benefiting the poor and it is taking place as part of a broad process of democratization. The message Mexican society is receiving is that the transition towards democratic institutions is paying off in terms of effective programmes with tangible benefits.

Equally important, recognition of health as a universal value favours the establishment of political agreements. These agreements, in turn, help to build social cohesion which nourishes democratic societies. In the Mexican case, the establishment of the Seguro Popular was the result of a broad political consensus.

Finally, the implementation of the right to health implies the use of democratic procedures, which also favours the consolidation of democracy. Salient among them are public deliberation, definition of entitlements, transparency, and accountability. The approval of the legal reforms that created the Seguro Popular required broad public discussion involving all the main actors: Health authorities, political parties, academic institutions, and NGOs. Clearly defined benefits have ensured that those who avail themselves of the public insurance scheme know the services and treatments to which they are entitled. At the same time, the implementation of the reform has fostered other important procedures including access to public information, open evaluation and dissemination of report cards, all of which are contributing to the consolidation of a democratic culture in Mexico.

* Some of the ideas included in this chapter were originally discussed in the following two papers: Julio Frenk and Octavio Gómez-Dantés, 'La democratización de la salud: Una visión para el futuro del sistema de salud en México' 137(3) *Gaceta Médica de México* (2001) at 281–287, and Julio Frenk and Octavio Gómez-Dantés, 'Ideas and Ideals: Ethical Basis of Health Reform in Mexico', *Lancet* (forthcoming).

1 D. Fidler, 'Health as foreign policy: between principle and power' VI *Whitehead Journal of Diplomacy and International Law* (2005) at 179–194.

2 Samuel Huntington, *The Third Wave: Democratization in the Late Twentieth Century* (Oklahoma: University of Oklahoma Press, 1991).

3 L. J. Diamond, 'Is Pakistan the (Reversal) Wave of the Future?' 11(3) *Journal of Democracy* (2000) at 91–106.

4 Programa de las acciones unidas para el desarrollo, *La democracia en América Latina: Hacia una democracia de ciudadanas y ciudadanos* (Lima, Perú: PNUD, 2004).

5 E. Gakidou, R. Lozano, E. González-Pier et al. 'Assessing the effect of the 2001–2006 Mexican Health Reform: An Interim Reportcard' 368 *Lancet* (2006) 1920–35; F. M. Knaul, H. Arreola-Ornelas, O. Méndez-Carniado et al. 'Evidence is Good for Your Health System: Policy Reform to Remedy Catastrophic and Impoverishing Health Spending in Mexico' 368 *Lancet* (2006) 1828–41.

6 Secretaría de Salud, 'Sistema de Protección Social en Salud: Evaluación de efectos', (Mexico City: Secretaría de Salud, 2007).

7 G. O'Donnell and P. Schmitter, 'Transiciones desde un gobierno autoritario' Paidos (1991) at 22–23.

8 Aristotle, *The Politics* (Chicago: The University of Chicago Press, 1984) at 87.

9 R. Scruton, *A Dictionary of Political Thought* (London: Macmillan, 1996) at 71–72.

10 T. H. Marshall, *Class, Citizenship and Social Development* (New York: Doubleday Anchor Books, 1965).

11 V. Brachet-Márquez, 'Ciudadanía para la salud: Una propuesta' In M. Uribe, López-Cervantes (eds.) *Reflexiones acerca de la salud en México* (México, D. F.: Médica Sur, Editorial Panamericana, 2001) at 43–47.

12 N. Daniels and J. Sabin, 'Limits to Health Care: Fair Procedures, Democratic Deliberation, and the Legitimacy Problem for Insurers' 26(4) *Philosophy and Public Affairs* (1997) at 303–350.

13 Secretaría de Salud, *Salud: México, 2006: Información para la rendición de cuentas* (México, D. F.: Secretaría de Salud, 2007).

14 Secretaría de Salud, *Sistema de Protección Social en Salud: Evaluación financiera* (México, D.F.: Secretaría de Salud, 2007).

15 T. Karl, '¿Cuánta democracia acepta la desigualdad?' 69 *Este País* (1996) at 46–51.

Health Care in Canada: Does a Health Care System Based on Shared Values Ensure Respect for the Right to Health?

Virginia A. Leary*

The Canadian publicly-funded, single-payer health system, while often praised, has not been free from recent stresses and strains. While few Canadians wish to change fundamentally their health care system, many see the necessity for substantial improvements.

Two recent developments are reflective of the concerns that many Canadians share regarding their health care system, in particular with regard to waiting times for non-emergency health services, the shortage of doctors and other health professionals, and the rising costs of pharmaceuticals. In 2002 the Royal Commission on the Future of Health Care in Canada published its final report, "Building on Values: The Future of Health Care".[1] Referred to as the Romanow Report after the Chief Commissioner, Roy Romanow, the report reaffirmed the basic values underpinning the universal, single-payer health care system in Canada, while outlining some 47 detailed and costed recommendations for substantial improvements in the system.

In a decision concerning waiting times for health services in Quebec's public health system, in 2005 the Canadian Supreme Court in *Chaoulli v. Quebec*[2] declared that provincial restrictions on purchase of private insurance for healthcare services covered by the government plan in Quebec violated the right to security of the person under the Quebec Charter of Human Rights and Freedoms. The Court held that where the publicly funded system does not provide timely access to health care, individuals should not be prevented from accessing the same services through private insurance, arguing that "access to waiting lists is not access to health care". While the decision was applicable only in Quebec, it nonetheless had the potential for wide repercussions since nearly all Canadian provinces had similar private health insurance provisions.

The Romanow Report and the *Chaoulli* decision could suggest an erosion of some of the fundamental aspects of the Canadian health system. Have the basic elements of the Canadian public health system survived despite these recent developments? To answer this question, it is first necessary to examine the history of the Canadian health system, and the fundamental values on which it is based. We will then turn to the Romanow Report and the *Chaoulli* judgment.

Canada's value-based health care system

Canada has long been party to key international human rights treaties which include the human right to the highest attainable standard of health. For many observers, the Canadian health care system appears to be grounded in core elements of the right to health including the availability, accessibility, and acceptability of quality health goods, services and facilities,[3] with due attention to underlying determinants of health related to lifestyle and the environment.[4] Yet the phrase "right to health" is not used in the Canadian Charter of Rights and Freedoms and to date there has been an apparent reluctance to give legal recognition to health as a human right in Canada. While most Canadians consider access to health care to be a human right, the terms "right to health" or "right to health care" are not mentioned explicitly in any of the documents establishing the Canadian health care system.

"Values" rather than "rights" is the term used in the founding documents to describe the ideological basis of the Canadian health system. Grounded in notions of equity, fairness and solidarity, these values have often been reiterated and were reaffirmed in the Romanow Report: Universality, portability, comprehensiveness, accessibility and public administration. For Canadians, according to the Romanow Report, these values are linked to their understanding of citizenship: "Canadians consider equal and timely access to medically necessary health care services on the basis of need as a right of citizenship, not a privilege of status or wealth."

The Canadian system of health insurance is a government programme, referred to as a universal single-payer system. The programme is financed both by provincial taxes, imposed directly on those who can afford to pay, and by federal contributions. Canadians freely choose their own physician, but the physician is reimbursed by the Government. Medical associations negotiate with the Government on the amount of reimbursement. Under the Canada Health Act, extra-billing and user fees for insured services are prohibited, and the federal government withholds contributions to any provincial plan which permits the purchase of private insurance for the same benefits covered under the government plan.

When receiving health care, or a stay in a hospital, patients show a healthcare card and are not required to make a direct payment. The system is universal, since all Canadians are required to belong to the system. Persons with low income are provided with care even if they are unable to contribute to the system. Portability is ensured; they may freely move to different provinces and the national system and the new provincial system remain fundamentally the same, with certain provincial variations.

Canadians may also freely choose their hospitals for treatment. The same facilities, however, are not available in all hospitals. Only a limited number of MRIs (magnetic resonance imaging machines), for example, will be available in a particular geographic area.

As the *Chaoulli* decision is directly applicable only in Quebec, the ultimate influence of the decision outside of the province is not yet clear. Within Quebec, some 100 doctors have opted out of the public system altogether. A Quebec proposal would allow hospitals to sub-contract to private clinics for hip and knee replacements as well as cataract surgery, in the event that the public system is not able to provide the care within six months. In 2006, Ralph Klein, then Premier of Alberta, proposed an Alberta Government plan permitting doctors to work in the public system and offer private services at the same time, while admitting that it may violate the Canada Health Act.[5]

Origins of the Canadian health care system: The role of the province of Saskatchewan

The province of Saskatchewan, a western Canadian province with a scattered, relatively small population, has played an extraordinary role in the development of the present Canadian health care system. The basic aspects of the Canadian federal health care system were adopted in 1965 following extensive hearings throughout the country led by a federal Royal Commission on the Delivery of Health Services, headed by Justice Emmett Hall of Saskatchewan. Roy Romanow, the head of the most recent Commission studying the Canadian health care system, was a former Premier of Saskatchewan. It is not surprising that the two most important Royal Commissions on health care have been led by citizens of Saskatchewan.

What explains the central role played by this sparsely populated province on the development of the Canadian health care system? Credit is usually given to Tommy Douglas, Premier of Saskatchewan from 1944 to 1960, whose influence led to the adoption in 1962 of the Saskatchewan Medical Care Act, a precursor of and major influence on the modern Canadian system. But what influenced Tommy Douglas? In 1944, the Co-operative Commonwealth Federation (the CCF), a socialist party, won the provincial election in Saskatchewan and formed official opposition in the three provinces of British Columbia, Manitoba and Ontario. The CCF led to the creation of the New Democratic Party (NDP), as it is known today. The CCF philosophy was more similar to the thinking of the Fabian Society in England than to the Communist Parties of Europe. It was a unique product of the situation of the prairie provinces. One of its early manifestos emphasized that citizens were entitled to a properly organized public health system.

As Tommy Douglas, a Baptist Minister, became a leader of the Party and the Premier of Saskatchewan, social ideas had begun to take hold in the Province. Following his own experience with health problems in childhood, Douglas had developed a firm belief in universal access to public health care, a belief he maintained throughout his tenure as both Minister of Health and Premier.[6] By the end of Douglas's period as Premier, Saskatchewan had established a progressive, public, universal health care system – a controversial development at the time – and Saskatchewan had become established, in Canadian minds, as a leader in health care. The progressive influence of Saskatchewan on health care developments in Canada continued through the Royal Commission reports of Emmett Hall, who recommended a joint federal/provincial system that would cover the costs of preventive health care services, including preventive, and hospital care for all Canadians, and of Roy Romanow.

Challenges to the Canadian health care system
The Romanow Report

The 2002 Report of the Royal Commission on the Future of Health Care in Canada, headed by Roy Romanow, was a significant development in the recent history of the Canadian health care system. While pointedly re-affirming the basic values of the Canadian system – universality, portabil-ity, comprehensiveness, accessibility and public administration – it made such extensive criticisms of the system and suggestions for improvement that it seemed to some to implicitly question the fundamental aspects of the system. Yet the Commission's mandate was not to question the ba-sis of the Canadian system but rather to engage Canadians in a national dialogue on the future of health care and make recommendations "to en-sure the long-term sustainability of a universally accessible, publicly fund-ed health system."

Not all reactions to the Romanow Report were positive. The 2003 *Sas-katchewan Law Review,*[7] which ran ten articles analyzing the Romanow Re-port, stated in its introduction that:

> "Despite the general approval of the Romanow Report, the underlying cur-rent of these articles is one of dissatisfaction: The authors recognize that in trying to review such a broad topic as Canada's health care system, the Report, not unexpectedly, comes up short on many issues."[8]

In general, however, Canadians welcomed the Romanow Report's conclu-sions and supported its recommendations for improvement. With atten-tion to improving equitable access to and quality of health care, addressing the social determinants of health, enhancing transparency and accountabi-lity, and focusing on the health needs of marginalized populations, many of the report's recommendations are consistent with promotion of the right to health.

The report recommended the establishment of a Canadian health cov-enant which would outline Canada's collective vision for health care and update the Canada Health Act, notably to add a sixth principle of "ac-countability" to address concerns that citizens lack sufficient information to hold duty-bearers accountable for delivering on health care. It recom-mended revisions to the relationship between the provinces and the fed-eral government in relation to health care financing, an increase in federal funding and the creation of five new targeted funds to address immedi-ate priorities until the minimum federal funding threshold is met. It ad-dressed the need to make the health system more comprehensive by in-tegrating priority home care services within the Canada Health Act and improving prescription drug coverage, improving timely access to quality care through special initiatives to improve wait list management, and fostering a national personal electronic health record system. It suggested the establishment of a Health Council of Canada to analyze and assess the national health system.

The report also contained detailed recommendations to address disparities in health and access to health care for rural and remote populations, and outlined a "new approach to Aboriginal health", including the establishment of Aboriginal Health Partnerships responsible for developing policies and providing services towards improving the health of Aboriginal peoples. While Canada's health care system is considered a model, albeit with weaknesses, the serious and persistent disparities in the health status of Aboriginal peoples as compared with other population groups merits particular attention from a human rights perspective.

The health status of aboriginal peoples in Canada

Canada appears to have a relatively good system of health care – generally comprehensive, universally accessible and of good quality. But the health status of important Canadian populations, in particular Canada's Aboriginal peoples, continues to differ considerably from that of the general population. In recent years the gap in life expectancy of registered First Nations people as compared with other Canadians has been estimated at 7.4 years for men and 5.2 years for women. In many places Aboriginal people are more likely to be exposed to substance abuse and other lifestyle-related illness, and the suicide rate among Aboriginal Canadians is reportedly three times that of the general Canadian population.[9]

Together with the National Aboriginal Health Organization, the Romanow Commission co-hosted a national forum on Aboriginal health which brought together people from First Nations, Metis, Inuit and urban Aboriginal communities to exchange experiences and views on the future of health care. From the outcome of these discussions, the Commission concluded that there is a need for an entirely new approach, "one that tackles the root causes of health problems for Aboriginal peoples, cuts across administrative and jurisdictional barriers, and focuses squarely on improving the health of Aboriginal peoples".[10] The report stressed that partnerships between the government and Aboriginal peoples should look beyond

narrow health issues and consider "broader conditions that help build capacity and good health in individuals and communities, such as nutrition,
housing, education, employment and so on."[11]

Recognizing health as a human right can help to underscore the importance of human health as more than access to health care, to include socio-
economic determinants such as the environment, access to clean drinking
water and food, and adequate housing, as well as health promotion. The
right to health also helps to shift the focus beyond national averages, highlight the disparate health status of marginalized populations and ultimately ensure that health systems are designed and implemented to meet the
health needs of all.

Chaoulli v. Quebec

In this decision, the Canadian Supreme Court effectively struck down provi-
sions in the Quebec health care system that prevented insurers from cover-
ing the same benefits as are covered by the public system. Section 15 of the
Health Insurance Act of Quebec and section 11 of the Hospital Insurance
Act prohibited the purchase of private insurance which, the appellants ar-
gued, violated their rights under section 1 of the Quebec Charter of Human
Rights and Freedoms and section 7 of the Canadian Charter of Rights and
Freedoms.[12]

The majority of the Court reasoned that wait times for certain procedures under the government health programme "increase the patient's risk
of mortality or the risk that his or her injuries will become irreparable" and
that "many patients on non-urgent waiting lists are in pain and cannot fully enjoy any real quality of life". The majority held that these amounted to
a violation of the right to life and personal inviolability under the Quebec
Charter, and that the violation was not justifiable under section 9.1 of the
Charter. The majority held that while the prohibition on private insurance
has a rational connection with the objective of preserving the public health
plan, such a prohibition is not strictly necessary to protect the integrity of
the public plan as other less intrusive measures could be taken to achieve
the same objective.

The Chaoulli case is considered highly controversial: The narrow 4–3
split decision apparently caught many in the health policy community by
surprise and has since been widely criticized by legal and health policy commentators.[13] It presented a potentially threatening legal intrusion into

health policy in that it suggested there are legal or constitutional limits on the permissible length of wait times, without necessarily providing any direction as to the definition of those limits. According to one commentator, the decision left healthcare administrators and policy experts concerned that it foreshadowed "fundamental change in the ground rules governing Canada's publicly funded healthcare system without any clear road map of what direction such change could or would take." In practical terms, however the decision appears to have had very little impact on the foundations of medicare in Canada, other than perhaps to have spurred much-needed attention to issues of wait-list reductions and the shortage of human resources for health in Canada.

Conclusion

The Romanow Report and the Supreme Court decision in *Chaoulli* each addressed major criticisms of the Canadian health care system, including lengthy wait times for non-life threatening medical procedures. But do these criticisms amount to an attack on the fundamental characteristics of the Canadian system? It is doubtful: While there is demand for major improvement, in particular to address the shortage of human resources, reduce wait times and address the rising costs of pharmaceuticals, most Canadians apparently are basically happy with their system compared with other health systems, particularly the system in the neighbouring United States.[14] The Romanow Report and the *Chaoulli* decision both reiterate the importance of the values on which the Canadian health system are based. There will continue to be calls for improvement to the system, but probably not many demands for the adoption of a system vastly different to the present single-payer universal health care system.

In relation to Canada's foreign and domestic health policy, the Romanow Report notes that "Canadians believe that access to health care is a fundamental human right" and that Canada should "move from merely talking about health as a human right to taking more concrete action to assist in improving the health of people beyond Canada's borders".[15] Looking to the future, a move beyond a restatement of values towards an explicit recognition of health as a human right, both in health policy documents and through the court system, would help to align the Canadian health system more closely with Canada's international human rights obligations.

* The author would like to acknowledge with gratitude Lisa Oldring for her contribution to this chapter.

1 Roy J. Romanow, *Building on Values: The Future of Health Care in Canada*, Final Report of the Commission on the Future of Health Care in Canada (Ottowa: Government of Canada, 2002).

2 *Chaoulli v. Quebec* (Attorney General), 2005 SCC 35 (Canada 2005).

3 Canada is party, inter alia, to the International Covenant on Economic, Social and Cultural Rights, the Convention on the Rights of the Child, the Convention on the Elimination of All Forms of Discrimination Against Women, the Convention on the Elimination of Racial Discrimination. A detailed definition of the right to health is contained in Committee on Economic, Social and Cultural Rights (CESCR), *General Comment No. 14 on the right to the highest attainable standard of health*, 11 August 2000, UN Doc. E/C.12/2000/4.

4 Canada hosted the First International Conference on Health Promotion, which led to the adoption of the Ottawa Charter for Health Promotion in November 1986, WHO/HPR/HEP/95.1, available at www.who.int/hpr/NPH/docs/ottawa_charter_hp.pdf.

5 See 'Alberta's Health Care Proposals Cause Alarm', *Prairie Messenger*, 8 March 2006, at 1 and 7; 'Alberta Policies Could Affect Whole Country', *Prairie Messenger*, 15 March 2006, at 3 and 7; 'Private Health Care will not save Canadian Medicine', *Prairie Messenger*, 12 September 2007, at 7.

6 Thomas H. McLeod and Ian McLeod, *Tommy Douglas: The Road to Jerusalem* (Toronto: Fifth House Publishers, 2004).

7 See *Saskatchewan Law Review*, Volume 66 (2003) which contains ten articles on various aspects of the Romanow Report.

8 Ibid.

9 According to the Royal Commission on Aboriginal Peoples (1995).

10 Romanow, *supra* note 1, at 212.

11 Ibid., at 227.

12 The Committee on Economic, Social and Cultural Rights referred to the *Chaoulli* decision in its concluding observations on Canada's periodic report in 2006, noting that "courts should take account of Covenant rights where this is necessary to ensure that the State Party's conduct is consistent with its obligations under the Covenant": UN Doc. E/C.12/CAN/CO/4, para. 36.

13 For a summary of reactions to the decision, see P Monahan, *Chaoulli v Quebec and the Future of Canadian Health Care: Patient Accountability as the "Sixth Principle" of the Canada Health Act*, C.D. Howe Institute Benefactors Lecture, Toronto, 29 November 2006, available at http://www.cdhowe.org/pdf/benefactors_lecture_2006.pdf.

14 For an interesting recent comment, see Sara Robinson, '10 Myths About Canadian Health Care, Busted, *AlterNet: Health and Wellness* (February 15, 2008), available at http://www.alternet.org/healthwellness/76032. See also Virginia Leary, 'So Close and Yet So Different: The Right to Health Care in the United States and Canada', in Rhonda E. Howard-Hassmann and Claude E. Welsh, Jr (eds.), *Economic Rights in Canada and the United States* (Philadelphia: University of Pennsylvania Press, 2006).

15 Romanow, *supra* note 1, at 240 and 242. See also Donna Greschner, 'A Colloquy on the Romanow Report: Public Law in the Romanow Report', 66 *Saskatchewan Law Review* 565, at 566 (2003): "Indeed, in the [Romanow] Report the word 'right' rarely appears. As a related consequence of this omission, there is almost no mention of the courts, which are the primary rights-enforcement bodies. It is as if the health care system operates on one plane and the judicial system on another."

Towards a Just and Equitable Society for Realizing the Right to Health: Case Study of Health Action International Asia-Pacific

Kumariah Balasubramaniam

HAIAP upholds health as a fundamental human right and aspires to build a just and equitable society in which there will be, among others, regular access to essential medicines to all who need them irrespective of their ability to pay for them. HAIAP actively promotes the concept of essential drugs, their rational and economic use through advocacy, research, education and action campaigns. (HAIAP Mission Statement)

Health Action International Asia-Pacific (HAIAP), established in 1986, is an independent and dynamic network of public health and public interest advocates, consumer groups and individuals from 18 countries in the Asia-Pacific region extending from Egypt to China, and including Australia and New Zealand. It is the Asia-Pacific arm of the global coalition Health Action International (HAI),[1] which was launched following a three-day non-governmental organization (NGO) Seminar on Pharmaceuticals held in Geneva from 27–29 May 1981.

In April 1987, HAIAP convened its first planning meeting in Bangkok, Thailand. The main agenda item was a two-day brainstorming session among the participants to identify and develop strategies and immediate and long term action plans to protect and promote the realization of the right to health, and to build a just and equitable society in which there will be, inter alia, regular access to essential medicines at affordable prices to all who need them. HAIAP's vision or ultimate goal is "Health for All" as outlined in the Alma-Ata Declaration.[2]

The realization of the right to health

The first step to formulate a strategy and develop action plans to protect and promote the right to health was to identify suitable ways in which the right to health could be made operational. One useful way to make it operational is to view the right to health as having three essential components.

1. The right to timely and appropriate healthcare;
2. The rights to the underlying determinants of health, such as access to an adequate, regular supply of safe food, nutrition and housing; healthy occupational and environmental conditions; access to safe and potable water; adequate sanitation; access to health related information and education; peace and security; and
3. The right of the population to participate in all health related decision-making at community, national and international levels.

Viewing the right to health as having different components enabled HAIAP to identify and develop immediate advocacy campaigns to protect and promote the right to timely and appropriate healthcare. It also allowed for a long term campaign to pursue the realization of the right of the population to participate in all health related decision making at community, national and international levels. HAIAP, assessing its resources, decided to focus on the first and third components of the right to health (as outlined above).

The right to timely and appropriate healthcare

A healthcare system has a number of identifiable characteristics. Central to HAIAP's work has been the process of identifying which characteristics are most important to protect the right to timely and appropriate healthcare. Based on our own findings in countries in the Asia-Pacific region, and the relevant literature, including the General Comment No. 14 on the right to the highest standard of health issued by the UN Committee on Economic Social and Cultural Rights, and World Health Reports, HAIAP determined that in order to provide timely and appropriate healthcare, the healthcare system in a country should ensure:

___ Universal and equitable access to essential medicines for all those who need them;
___ The quality, safety and efficacy of all medicines used;
___ That the prices of medicines are affordable to consumers and the government; and
___ That all medicines are used rationally.

Healthcare systems in developing countries

Although literature review, and our own findings in countries in the Asia-Pacific region, reveal that healthcare systems in the vast majority of developing countries do contain some of these aspects identified as essential to the provision of timely and appropriate healthcare, there is clear evidence of gross inequity and social injustice, as shown in reports that have been regularly appearing in the public domain since the 1970s. The following provide some examples.

Availability, quality and rational use

___ "By the 1970s effective medicines – though not always ideal – existed for nearly every major illness we know. Yet for half the world's population, it was as if they were still living in the 1880s. For them, modern medicines were unavailable, unaffordable, of poor quality or ineffectively used."[3]
___ In 2004 almost two billion people – one third of the global population – did not have regular access to essential medicines. In some of the lowest income countries in Africa and South Asia, more than half the people have no regular access to essential medicines.[4]
___ "The last decade has seen inequities in healthcare increase with reduced public budgets and increased reliance on the private sector. There is now a global cry for equitable access to essential medicines."[5]
___ Irrational use of medicines is a major problem worldwide. It is estimated that half of all medicines are inappropriately prescribed, dispensed or sold, and that half of all patients fail to take their medicines properly.[6]
___ Evidence suggests that more than half of all medicines in developing countries and those with economies in transition, and a substantial portion of medicines (particularly antibiotics) in developed countries, are

used inappropriately, thus wasting scarce resources. In addition, irrational use of medicines results in poor patient outcomes and can cause harm to patients.[7]

—— According to the World Health Organization about 70 percent of all drugs given to children may have little or no value.[8]

—— In many countries drug quality assurance systems are inadequate because they lack the necessary components. These components include adequate legislation and regulation and a functioning drug regulatory authority with adequate resources.[9]

Drug prices, access to medicines and the World Trade Organization's (WTO's) Trade-Related Aspects of Intellectual Property Rights (TRIPS) Agreements

—— "New international agreements, including WTO/TRIPS Agreement and the WTO Agreement on Technical Barriers to Trade (TBT) will undoubtedly affect access to medicines in developing countries."[10]

—— In developing countries, manufacturers of mainly generic drugs are likely to be adversely affected by the introduction of patent protection, as are consumers and governments who will need to pay more for drugs.[11]

—— In India, 32.5 million people fell below the national poverty line by making out-of-pocket payment for healthcare.[12]

HAIAP's advocacy campaigns

Achieving advocacy goals through partnerships

As stated in its mission statement, HAIAP works to achieve its objectives through advocacy, research, education and action campaigns. It does so through: Organizing regional and national meetings; presenting research papers on invitation by organizers of international and regional meetings; maintaining and updating the HAIAP website; and editing and publishing HAI News.

The success of HAIAP's campaigning for ensuring timely and appropriate healthcare depends on support from three important stakeholders. Medical and pharmacy educators (the academia) train future prescribers and dispensers; health ministry officials are responsible for healthcare systems and budget allocations. The media play a crucial role in increasing awareness among the general public. These important partnerships did not always come easily. At first, the academia believed that civil society campaigns and rhetoric are based on ideology; health ministry officials looked at civil society as anti-establishment which had nothing to offer them. The media told us that the information on health provided by civil society was not news-worthy. When we presented the empirical data we collected, critically analyzed them and provided appropriate recommendations and pragmatic conclusions, academia and the health ministry officials changed their views and agreed to collaborate with HAIAP. When we presented articles on the socio-economic determinants of health inequity, poverty, and hunger with empirical data and analysis, the media found them news-worthy and began collaborating with us and giving wide publicity to our campaigns. We were thus able to forge a new level of partnership between health activists, academia, officials from health ministries and the media in countries of the Asia-Pacific region.

Regional and national meetings and publications

HAIAP convenes regional and national consultations/seminars and workshops on selected themes and topics. Approximately 40–60 participants attend regional events and 20–25 attend national events. At these meetings, resource persons from academia, international NGOs and research institutes present research papers. Officials from ministries of health participate in some of the regional meetings. All regional and national events convened by HAIAP from 1987–2006 are listed in one of HAIAP's publications.[13] Press releases on meetings convened by HAIAP are distributed to newspapers in the region. HAIAP also publishes research papers and a regular newsletter, available on its website.

HAIAP's advocacy role

Based on a critical analysis of the problems facing developing countries, HAIAP initiated and carried out a number of advocacy campaigns aimed at strengthening national healthcare systems to enable them to pursue the realization of the right to timely and appropriate healthcare. These campaigns addressed issues such as:

1. Formulation, development and implementation of national drug policies;
2. Promotion of rational prescribing practices; and
3. Providing guidelines to develop public-health-sensitive national patent laws, in conformity with the WTO/TRIPS Agreement, to enable developing

countries to enact national patent laws to give public health interests precedence over private commercial interests.

HAIAP seeks to increase awareness among the various stakeholders including the public, health ministry officials responsible for national drug policies and drug regulation, academia and the media, on the need to formulate, develop and implement national drug policies which provide an adequate framework within which essential drugs of acceptable quality, efficacy and safety will be made available to all those who need them, at prices consumers and the governments can afford.

HAIAP's achievements

HAIAP is pleased that all countries in the South and South East Asia have developed their national medicines policies.[14] HAIAP has network partners and carried out campaigns in these countries (excluding Singapore).

The Sri Lankan Ministry of Health convened two-day workshops in February 2005 and again in July 2005 to develop a draft National Medicinal Drug Policy (NMDP). All stakeholders, including HAIAP, were invited to the two workshops. After extensive deliberations and discussions, the draft NMDP was accepted by consensus. It has now been adopted by the Government. The NMDP is posted on the WHO website.[15] A feature in the NMDP is that medicines should be registered on the criteria of quality, safety, efficacy, need and cost effectiveness. HAIAP has been campaigning for the inclusion of the last two criteria – need and cost effectiveness. This is a unique feature of the Sri Lankan NMDP.

Promoting access to affordable medicines:
Patents and prices

The effect of patents on prices of and access to medicines has become one of the major controversies of our time. HAIAP has focused on this issue since its inception in 1987 and it has worked hard on a campaign to increase awareness in the public and with policy makers in developing countries on the adverse impact of pharmaceutical patents on drug prices and the need for public sensitive national patent laws which will give precedence to public health interests.

Between 1990 and 2000, HAIAP carried out three global surveys of retail drug prices for a select number of commonly used drugs. A critical analysis of the empirical data obtained showed wide and indiscriminate variations in the retail prices of patent protected brand name drugs among developed and developing countries with retail prices even higher for some drugs in least developed countries than in OECD countries. For example, the retail prices of 10 out of 13 commonly used drugs for which comparable data were available in a 1998 study[16] were more expensive in Tanzania than in Canada. In India, 100 tablets of an anti-ulcer drug cost USD 2, while in Chile, 100 units of the same drug, manufactured by the same company, cost as much as USD 196. In all developing countries surveyed by HAIAP, the proprietary innovative brands were several times more expensive compared to their generic equivalents.

This research provided the basis for HAIAP's campaign for policy measures to make low-priced generic drugs available in all countries. We believe this will be possible only when developing countries can use the compulsory licensing and parallel importing provisions available in the TRIPS Agreement. However, the multinational drug industry opposes these provisions. When South Africa introduced parallel imports in its national legislation on patent laws in 1997, 39 pharmaceutical companies took the Government to court and obtained an order preventing the import of cheaper generic anti-retroviral drugs from India.[17] Several thousands of people living with AIDS were deprived of the life-saving drugs. There was universal condemnation, spearheaded by civil society, and the case was withdrawn in early 2000.

HAIAP, together with other civil society organizations including Third World Network, Médecins Sans Frontières (MSF) and Consumer Project on Technology, continued their campaign. Victory was achieved in 2001 when the WTO Ministerial Conference adopted the DOHA Declaration on the TRIPS Agreement and Public Health.[18]

The Doha Declaration specifically recognized concerns about the negative impact of patents on drug prices. The Doha Declaration states that each member has the right to grant compulsory licences and the freedom to determine the grounds upon which such licences are granted. Since many patented products are sold at different prices in different markets, the rationale for parallel importation is to enable the import of lower-priced patented products. The DOHA Declaration has reaffirmed that WTO members have the right to parallel importation.

HAIAP's campaign continues, with our members in the countries of the region lobbying their governments to amend their respective national laws on patents to include provisions for compulsory licensing and parallel importation.

The right of the population to participate in all health-related decision-making at community, national and international levels
People's health after the Alma-Ata Declaration

Primary Health Care (PHC) as outlined in the Alma-Ata Declaration failed for several reasons including:

—— The refusal of experts and politicians in developed countries to accept the principle that communities should plan and implement their own healthcare services.

—— Changes in economic philosophy led to the replacement of PHC by "Health Sector Reforms" based on market forces and the economic benefits of better health.[19]

From evidence available in the public domain, it is clear that governments and inter-governmental agencies have ignored their commitment made at Alma-Ata in 1978. HAIAP saw the need for a new approach to mobilize the interests, commitments and resources of a broader constituency for the poor, since it was clear that the current approaches have failed to reduce poverty and improve the health and living conditions of the poor.

A new and interesting development has been taking place all over the world. Socially conscious people from different walks of life, disillusioned with the apathy of their governments in tackling the urgent problems facing the poor, have been organizing at the grass-roots level to plan and implement development strategies to improve health and living standards of the poor. Literally thousands of socially oriented civil society organizations exist in the Third World. Social and political activism is not new but it can be put to new use at local, national, regional and international levels.

Peoples' Health Assembly

It was also evident that the annual World Health Assemblies, as a world forum of health policy makers, have not succeeded in changing health care policies in ways that focus on the poor and underprivileged. And so, HAIAP thought of an alternative, a Peoples' Health Assembly to provide a forum for socially conscious people from developing and developed worlds and hundreds of socially oriented indigenous groups from Africa, Asia, and Latin America to share their experiences and plan future strategies. In close collaboration with NGOs, including International Peoples' Health Council, Asian Community Health Action Network, Gonoshasthaya Kendra, Third World Network, and supported by the Dag Hammarskjold Foundation, HAIAP convened five planning meetings between 1998 and 2000 to convene a People's Health Assembly and its dream was realized when the first People's Health Assembly was hosted by Gonoshasthaya Kendra in Savar, Bangladesh in December 2000.

The 1500 people from 90 countries – activists, academics, professionals, health workers, and midwives – who participated spoke with one voice, demanding that they be heard in the global health decision-making processes. The outcomes of the Assembly were the Peoples' Health Movement (PHM)[20] and the Peoples' Health Charter,[21] now a worldwide movement, making the voices of the voiceless heard in the global health decision-making processes. HAIAP has been a member of the Steering Group of the Peoples' Health Movement since its inception. The Peoples' Health Charter is an advocacy tool used by health activists all over the world in their campaigns for the achievement of the right to health.

PHM has more than 60 country circles which are in constant contact with the PHM Global Secretariat in Cairo and perceptions, problems and solutions to their health or lack of it are shared in a two way process, highlighted and eventually brought for consideration at the WHO. Advocacy is undertaken at several levels and targets various categories of decision-makers. Direct advocacy is undertaken at the World Health Assemblies (WHA). Themes are identified and PHM country circles lobby country delegates to the WHA.

For the past six years beginning in May 2003, PHM delegates have been successful in lobbying, in partnership with a few civil society organizations including OXFAM, MSF and HAIAP.

PHM's strong challenge to the WHO has been to turn back to the letter and spirit of Alma-Ata and to act to promote primary healthcare (PHC), WHO's response has been to set up the task force on PHC. This will hopefully ensure WHO's commitment to the cause.

Conclusion

HAIAP's goal is to protect and promote the realization of the right to health. The first planning meeting in 1987 was a brainstorming session among the participants to identify and develop strategies and immediate and long term action plans to protect and promote the realization of the right to health and to build a just and equitable society. In retrospect it is clear that the strategy formulated enabled HAIAP to achieve its goals. This strategy was to identify suitable ways in which the right to health could be made operational. In doing so, it was determined that the right to health has three essential components (explained earlier).

Assessing its resources, HAIAP decided to focus on two of these three essential components:

—— The right to timely and appropriate healthcare; and
—— The right of the population to participate in all health-related decision-making at the community, national and international events.

In relation to HAIAP's work on promoting the right to timely and appropriate healthcare, HAIAP's advocacy goals are being achieved through partnerships with three other stakeholders in the health and pharmaceutical sectors, namely medical and pharmacy educators, policy makers in ministries of health and the media. Despite the apparently different agendas of these stakeholders, HAIAP was able to convince them that there were several commonalities in our agendas and that we could work together on particular issues. One of HAIAP's initial successes in achieving its goals was to forge a new level of cooperation between the health activities, academia, health ministry officials and the media.

This partnership enabled HAIAP to carry out a number of successful campaigns which addressed specific issues. HAIAP's achievements following these campaigns are described below.

Information on the successful campaigns along with the research and education and regional and national consultations, seminars and workshops related to these campaigns are posted on HAIAP website. The HAIAP website has several visitors ranging from grass-roots health activists to university students who look for intern places to carry out specific research studies in part fulfilment to complete their degrees. To date, three foreign students, one each from universities in France, India, and the US, have carried out elective periods of training in HAIAP.

In relation to the right of the population to participate in all health-related decision-making at community, national and international events, HAIAP quickly realized there are literally thousands of socially-oriented civil organizations in the Third World. These were working in isolation with minimal outputs. By collaboration with like-minded NGO's, HAIAP was able to bring all these civil society organizations under a global umbrella organization – the Peoples Health Movement (PHM). Now PHM makes the voices of the voiceless heard in the global health decision-making processes, with the aim of promoting equity and social justice.

This demonstrates how a small NGO, networking with motivated partners in 18 countries in the Asia-Pacific region, was able to achieve success in protecting and promoting the right to health.

1 http://www.haiweb.org.

2 WHO, Declaration of Alma-Ata, *Health for All*, Series No. 1 (Geneva: WHO, 1978).

3 'Essential Medicines: Access to Essential Medicines as a Global Necessity', speech by Dr. Gro Harlem Brundtland, Director General, World Health Organization, 25th Anniversary of the WHO Model List of Essential Medicines, Geneva, Switzerland, 21 October 2002, available at http://www.cfwshops.org/who_speech.html.

4 WHO, 'WHO Medicines Strategy: Countries at the Core 2004–2007' (Geneva: WHO, 2004) at 3.

5 Brundland, *supra* note 3.

6 WHO, *The World Medicines Situation* (Geneva: WHO, 2004) at 75.

7 WHO, *Progress in the Rational Use of Medicines*, Report by the Secretariat to the Sixtieth World Health Assembly, 22 March 2007.

8 G. Rylance (ed.), *Drugs for Children* (Copenhagen: WHO, 1987) at 11.

9 WHO, *How to Develop and Implement a National Drug Policy* (Second Edition, Geneva: WHO, 2001) at 3.

10 Brundtland, *supra* note 3.

11 Commission on Intellectual Property Rights, *Integrating Intellectual Property Rights and Development Policy* (London, Commission on Intellectual Property Rights, 2002) at 37–38.

12 C. Charn, Anup Garg, and K. Karan, *Health Millennium Development Goal 1: Reducing out-of-pocket expenditures to reduce income poverty: Evidence from India*, EQUITAP Project Working Paper No. 5, available at http://www.dfidhealthrc.org/meta/do cuments%5cMeta%20equity%20meet%20Oct%20 07%5CEquitap%20WP15_2005.06.28.pdf.

13 Radha Holla and Lakshmi Menon, '*Fast, Flexible and Furious': The Story of Health Action International (HAI) 1981–2006 with special focus on Health Action International Asia-Pacific (HAIAP)* (Colombo: Health Action International Asia-Pacific, 2006) at 59–63, available at http://haiap.org/up load/fandf.pdf

14 WHO, *The World Medicines Situation*, (Geneva: WHO, 2004) at 55.

15 http://www.who.int/medicines/areas/policy/NM DP_SriLanka.pdf.

16 K. Bala, I. Lanza, S. R. Kaur, 'Retail Drug Prices:

The Law of the Jungle', *HAI News*, April 1998, at 1–16.

17 http://www.cptech.org/ip/health/sa/pharma-v-sa.html.

18 http://www.who.int/medicines/areas/policy/doha_declaration/en/print.html.

19 John J. Hall and Richard Tailor, 'Health for All Beyond 2000: The Demise of the Alma-Ata Declaration and Primary Healthcare in Developing Countries' 178(1) *Medical Journal of Australia* (2003) at 17–20.

20 http://phmovement.org.

21 http://www.phmovement.org/cms/en/resources/charters/peopleshealth.

Health and Wellness for All: Mamelani Projects' Wellness Programme

Carly Tanur and Manmeet K. Bindra

It is estimated that in South Africa, nearly 600 people die per day of HIV and AIDS related causes.[1] Though efforts to curb transmission of the HI virus have been numerous, the number of people infected continues to rise at an alarming rate. In order to help reduce transmission rates, and improve quality of life for those living with the virus, there is a pressing need for effective health education to support care and treatment efforts. Mamelani Projects, a Cape Town-based public health non-governmental organization (NGO), runs a Wellness Programme that empowers individuals to take greater control over their bodies and health through self-care health education and psychosocial support. It aims to strengthen effectiveness of existing health care systems by helping people make better-informed decisions about how to access services and how to stay healthy, while emphasizing local resourcefulness among low-income communities.

Situation on the ground

The public health challenges facing South Africa, a country grappling with the legacy of apartheid and staggering inequality, are vast. It has an HIV prevalence rate of 18.8% and 5.54 million were estimated to be living with the virus in 2005.[2] Most prominently, the HIV health crisis is characterized by a public health system that is thin on the ground; high levels of food insecurity; limited access to treatment and care; lack of information about prevention and management of symptoms; and finally, mixed messaging around HIV/AIDS treatment options,[3] accompanied by stigma and social inequality. Consequentially, low-income communities are faced with the double burden of illness and poverty. Since most poor communities receive care from overcrowded clinics and emergency rooms, health education and psychosocial support are luxuries the health care system cannot afford.

Mamelani Projects' Wellness Programme: Supporting health care systems

While health education was traditionally the role of staff at public clinics, pressures on the resource-strained medical establishment prevent people from getting sufficient information to help prevent illness and maintain good health and, additionally, pose barriers to early testing. Nurses who are meant to see 35 patients per day are being forced to see up to 90.[4] Scores of cases of illness go unnoticed. A study in a community of high HIV prevalence in Cape Town estimated that 63% of community adult cases with pulmonary tuberculosis remained unrecognized by the health services.[5] Thus, the inaccessibility of health care facilities contributes to low levels of testing and a delayed response time to symptoms.

Mamelani Projects' Wellness Programme attempts to fill this gap by educating people about wellness and available health services in order to get the most effective care possible. It provides low-cost, practical information about how to boost the immune system and nutrition security; how to identify a range of illnesses; on correct usage of medication and treatments; and on the medicinal and nutritional value of locally available foods and home remedies. Facilitators educate groups on all available treatment options for commonly experienced illnesses and ailments, covering medical, traditional, as well as home-based care options.[6] Importantly, it encourages people who are unaware of their HIV status to get tested as soon as possible, while emphasizing that HIV is not a death sentence. Reducing the incidence of both opportunistic infections and HIV-associated morbidity and mortality requires both early testing and improved access to prevention and care services. Thus, improving nutritional status, increasing response time to infections and avoiding unhealthy activities may strengthen the immune system and delay disease progression.

Health education for all

Mamelani believes that every human being has the right and responsibility to have a basic understanding of how their body works and what steps can be taken to stay healthy. The workshops are tailored to the needs of low-income families and are taught in Xhosa. They stress the importance of wellness to the general population, without isolating HIV services or people infected by the virus. HIV education is integrated with wellness information in an attempt to reduce stigma associated with the disease, and to emphasize that it is everyone's responsibility – whether they are HIV positive or not – to be aware of how to prevent infection and how to stay healthy.

The following comment made by a participant demonstrates the power of health education to transform the way people view their role in managing their bodies and improving their health:

> "I always thought that these things about our bodies were only for the doctors to understand. I never thought I could understand these things. But now, after the workshops, I am curious, because I can see that I can also understand these things. This knowledge is really powerful to me because now I can make the right decisions."

By teaching people about their bodies, ways of staying healthy and their various options in responding to illness, people are able to view their bodies and their relationship to illness in a more positive light. Mamelani shows people that they can take control of their health by first understanding that they have the right and responsibility to gain insight into information that is traditionally perceived to be within the domain of the medical establishment. Mamelani facilitates this learning process by providing information and guiding people through the difficult challenges that they face in implementing this knowledge into their daily lives.

Importance of nutrition education for health care

Due to the high level of poverty and unhealthy consumption patterns, many South Africans have low levels of immunity, making them more susceptible to the symptoms associated with the virus. Nutrition should be integrated into care because it strengthens the body's ability to ward off diseases and symptoms that are commonly associated with the HI virus.[7] People living with HIV experience increased physical energy expenditure,[8] drops in food intake,[9] nutrient mal-absorption and loss, and altered metabolism that bring about weight loss and wasting, a common symptom of AIDS.[10] Further, anti-retroviral treatment (ARV) reduces the rate of viral replication, while nutrition "provides the body with what it needs to create new immune cells, and thus do its part in fighting infections."[11] Thus, limited access to proper nutrition and financial constraints affect an individual's adherence to the medication.[12] Good nutrition helps the body achieve the full benefits of ARVs; nutrition and ARVs work in tandem to sustain the immune system in different, though complementary ways. Supporting nutrition security of people living with HIV, especially when they are asymptomatic, may prolong the period of time before HIV develops into full-blown AIDS.

Another indication of the need for health education and nutrition-based responses to high rates of HIV, AIDS, tuberculosis (TB) and other illnesses is the rate of re-treatment for people. According to a study by the Human Sciences Research Council on major infectious diseases in the Western Cape, it was found that in areas with poor access to health facilities, re-treatment cases are the result of increased susceptibility brought on by advanced immuno-suppression. This is due in part because HIV creates an environment where the risk of reactivation of latent TB disease is exacerbated by a compromised immune system. Thus, the nutritional implications of HIV and TB are also critical due to the high co-infection rate. There is a greater risk of infection progressing straight to primary disease in instances of immune deficiency.[13]

The wellness workshop addresses how the immune system works, how different illnesses affect the body, how to respond to the symptoms of opportunistic infections, and how improved nutrition can strengthen the immune response at every stage of disease progression, including enhanced drug effectiveness. This information makes the workshop most useful for people who test positive but have not developed full-blown AIDS because a strong immune system prolongs the time before ARVs become necessary.

The component of the workshops which focuses on nutrition guides participants through a number of activities to demonstrate the importance of eating balanced meals using nutritious, locally available foods without incurring excess cost. For example, the Mamelani Wellness Programme promotes increased consumption of selenium, which is widely known to be vital for immune functioning. Selenium is found in beef, chicken liver, sunflower seeds, Brazil nuts and aloe (an indigenous South African succulent).

Facilitators demonstrate how to make aloe juice, which is locally grown and easily accessible. Mamelani also provides Brazil nuts at a subsidized rate to participants in order to provide an alternative, low-cost source of selenium. In addition, they discuss practical strategies for maintaining a healthy body weight, while fighting misconceptions that lead to poor health. Finally, the workshops discuss cooking methods that ensure maximum nutritional intake.

The workshops place extra emphasis on food-based responses that can strengthen the immune system and help the body cope with symptoms. One HIV-positive participant claimed that she frequently suffered from mouth sores, which forced her to take excessive periods of leave from work to access health services from the clinics. She could not afford to spend time waiting in clinics each time she experienced a mouth sore, and would normally postpone accessing treatment until the pain was so unbearable that she was unable to eat. After attending the wellness workshops, she began chewing sour fig leaves to halt the progression of the mouth sores. Responding promptly saved valuable time and her immune system sustained less harm.

Supporting people beyond information

Disproportionate numbers of people affected by disease in South Africa come from impoverished backgrounds. Staying healthy and preventing illness is further challenged by the fact that many live in crowded, unhygienic living environments and often come from socially marginalized communities. To negotiate and cope with the multiple impacts of illness and poverty, such as stigma, isolation and loss of employment, Mamelani provides psychosocial support and care so that participants can focus on their health to the best of their abilities. Support takes the form of one-on-one counselling, referrals to other NGOs and by serving as patient advocates. An important feature of the organization is that all of the facilitators come from the communities they serve, and conduct the workshops in a manner that encourages respect and dialogue, as opposed to providing information in a top-down manner.

Health education is an ongoing need, especially for people suffering from a chronic illness, and a virus for which there is no cure. Normally health professionals inform patients about wellness information under incredibly stressful circumstances (e.g. after getting tested), resulting in critical information about what to eat, and how to prolong the period before treatment is required, often being compromised. Thus, wellness workshops are conducted once a week for six weeks in order to give participants enough time to become comfortable with the facilitators, build trust with the group, and to absorb the information fully. One participant expressed her level of comfort in the workshop in the following way: "You always feel free to ask anything when you attend the workshop, about your health and even about the fears you have about the community." This climate of respect is necessary in order for participants to feel comfortable to discuss complicated and sensitive issues.

While the wellness workshops aim to empower people to take their health and lives into their own hands, Mamelani understands that many people live in situations where they are not fully in control of their decisions, irrespective of how much they know about their responsibilities to their health. One client, who was on ARVs, was struggling to follow her treatment regimen because she lived with relatives who pressured her to share her food with the family, thus compromising her ability to meet her special dietary needs. She often arrived home to find that the groceries she had purchased had already been consumed. The facilitator suggested that she eat smaller meals outside of the home and offered her emotional support until she was ready to speak with the family, in order to make them sensitive to the importance of her dietary needs. After speaking to the family, it was suggested that she would share certain staples, but that specific food items would not be shared. The deeply engrained Xhosa cultural norm of sharing all resources equally made separating this individual's food from the rest of the family's a difficult adjustment. However, after some time, the family became more accommodating, despite the extra financial burden and the break from traditional consumption patterns in the home.

In certain cases, facilitators take a more proactive role by serving as patient advocates. One participant approached Mamelani because her child's clinic card was burnt in a shack fire. Though the child was on treatment, the hospital refused to dispense the child's ARVs without the clinic card and instead sent her back to her local clinic, where she would need to start the application process for accessing ARVs all over again. By the time the Mamelani facilitator came to know about the case, the child had not been able to access treatment for two weeks. The facilitator responded immediately by reporting the child's situation to the management at the clinic, to bypass the tedious reapplication process, so that the child could resume his treatment regimen as soon as possible. To respond to more specialized needs, Mamelani actively refers individuals to partner NGOs that deal with a host of issues, ranging from domestic violence, family conflict, food security, skills training and employment.

Conclusion

Mamelani's Wellness Programme responds to a range of needs faced by people struggling to cope with chronic illness. It understands that care for chronic ailments, such as HIV and TB, cannot be treated effectively through short-term inputs, but rather by empowering individuals to become informed about their health, and by supporting them through the various impacts of illness on their lives. One facilitator observed the following:

> "Some people still cry when they are diagnosed with HIV. Some of our clients start drinking a lot and sleeping around because of anger. They feel angry towards their partners and blame them for their status. They do not talk about it and start to feel hatred and anger towards others. They experience fear – fear of dying, of losing their partners, of losing their jobs. They also experience confusion, not knowing what to do or what steps to take. Some people are still in denial, pretending as if nothing is wrong even if they are dying inside. They also experience stigma, feeling isolated from the family and friends. This is where Mamelani is helping – offering support and information. Knowledge is power. To know what steps can be taken and what the right thing to do is in order to stay healthy, shows people that they can stay strong and live positively for as long as possible before they progress to full blown AIDS. Even if someone is already on treatment, knowing what to eat and how to prepare healthy food can help with managing symptoms and adherence to treatment."

Though South Africa has a strong commitment to human rights, it has a long way to go in order to ensure that people have access to essential services to protect the right to health. Mamelani understands that in order to help people effectively improve their health and seek needed services, the health care system must be supported by interventions that provide basic health education to ensure that people are able to take control over their lives. Thus, the Mamelani Wellness Programme highlights the importance of health education as an entry point, in helping people at risk of illness and poverty live a better life by learning about their bodies, their rights in accessing health care, and their responsibilities to themselves and their communities.

1 'South Africa: AIDS Treatment Action' in *Africa Policy E-Journal*, 24 March 2003, available at http://www.africaaction.org/docs03/taco303.htm.

2 South African Department of Health, 'Broad Framework for HIV & AIDS and STI Strategic Plan for South Africa, 2007–2011' (Pretoria: Department of Health, 2006).

3 Key figures in the government have been denying the scale of the HIV epidemic and Dr. Mantombazana Edmie Tshabalala-Msimang, the former health minister, played a particularly damaging role in promulgating fallacious messages about how to respond to AIDS. The health minister persistently emphasized that AIDS should be treated with vegetables and good nutrition, while pointing out the high toxicity levels in anti-retroviral drugs. On the other hand, the Treatment Action Campaign (TAC) and health experts from around the world have rigorously been fighting the government to provide access to anti-retrovirals to people through the public health sector. Due to the confusing messaging and polarization around the debate between the government and the activists regarding the role of treatment and nutrition, many South Africans have been left with uncertainty about who to trust. As HIV and AIDS weaken the immune system, nutrition must be integrated into care and treatment for people who test positive. Thus, Mamelani Projects emphasizes the importance of testing, while educating people on what steps to take before they require treatment in order to prolong the period before treatment becomes necessary.

4 Aziz Hartley, 'Overworked Nurses Feel the Brunt', *Cape Times*, 15 April 2005.

5 Beverly Draper, Beverly, David Pienaar, Warren Parker and Thomas Rehle, 'Recommendations for Policy in the Western Cape Province for the Prevention of Major Infectious Diseases, including HIV/AIDS and Tuberculosis' (Western Cape: Human Sciences Research Council, 2007), at 27.

6 WHO, 'Traditional Medicine: Fact Sheet No. 134' (Revised May 2003), available at http://www.who.int/mediacentre/factsheets/fs134/en/. (In South Africa, 75% of people living with HIV/AIDS use

traditional medicine/complementary or alternative medicine (TM/CAM).)

7 HIV belongs to a group of retroviruses that affects the body by weakening the immune system, thereby making it more vulnerable to a host of different diseases and illnesses, such as TB, thrush, pneumonia, oral thrush, anaemia, as well as malnutrition. It is a slow acting virus and can remain in the body undetected for years; thus, it carries major long-term impacts that may not be detected early on. AIDS results when an HIV positive person contracts opportunistic infections (OIs) or when their CD4 count (a measure of the strength of the immune system) drops below 200 cells/mm. The length of time between HIV infection and AIDS depends on the strain of the virus, genetic factors, age, co-infections and the general health of the individual before and after infection.

8 "Asymptomatic HIV-positive individuals require 10% more energy, and symptomatic HIV-positive individuals require 20%–30% more energy than HIV-negative individuals of the same age, sex, and physical activity level.": E. Piwoz, *Nutrition and HIV/AIDS: Evidence, Gaps and Priority Actions* (Washington, D. C.: Academy for Educational Development, 2004). Additionally, for HIV-infected children experiencing weight loss, energy needs are increased by 50–100%.

9 Reduced food intake may be due to painful sores in the mouth or digestive track; depression, fatigue or other psychosocial problems; or lack of access to food or economic resources. The WHO recommends that effective ways of improving dietary intakes need development and documentation.

10 Food and Nutrition Technical Assistance (FANTA) Project, *HIV/AIDS: A Guide for Nutritional Care and Support* (Second Edition, Washington, DC: Academy for Educational Development, 2004) at 14; E. Piwoz, *supra* note 8.

11 David Patient and Nail Orr 'ART and Nutrition in HIV and AIDS', 5 *The Third Voice* (2006).

12 People on ART who do not correctly follow drug regimens may experience more opportunistic infections and faster progression of the virus. Non-adherence may also produce drug-resistant strains of the virus, increasing the transmission of the virus to those who cannot be treated by existing medications. T. Castleman, E. Seumo-Fosso and B. Cogill. 'Food and Nutrition Implications of Antiretroviral Therapy in Resource Limited Settings' in Food and Nutritional Technical Assistance (FANTA) Project, *Technical Note No. 7*, (Washington, DC: Academy for Educational Development, 2004) at 11.

13 Draper, *supra* note 5, at 22–26.

The Right to Health:
A People's Health Movement
Perspective and Case Study

Claudio Schuftan, Laura Turiano and Abhay Shukla

The progressive weakening of public health systems, the growing privatization of health care and the erosion of universal access to health care are worldwide phenomena. The health sector globally is still dominated by vertical and technocentric approaches, often supported by "public-private partnerships" active at several levels. There is thus an urgent need to replace this dominant discourse by a process aimed at universally achieving the "right to health and to health care" as the main objective. In this way, we can hope to achieve more equitable health care systems in both developing and developed countries. To counter and reverse the tide promoting "health care as a commodity", there is a need to establish a global consensus on "health care as a right".

Human rights violations are not accidents; they are not random in distribution or effect; they are linked to social conditions. It is the socio-political forces at work that determine the risk of most forms of human rights violations. Our understanding of human rights violations is thus based on the broader analyses of power and social inequality and their social, economic and political determinants. The promotion of equity is the central ingredient for respecting human rights in health.

It is mostly the poor who are the victims and they have too little voice and no influence, let alone rights. It is inequities of power that prevent the poor from accessing the opportunities they need to move out of poverty. Structures and not just individuals must be changed if this state of affairs is to change.

Since laws designed to protect human rights and the right to health are mostly not applied, what additional measures have to be taken? This is what the People's Health Movement's "Right to Health and Health Care Campaign" (called RTHHC Campaign for short) sets out to explore.

It is not enough to improve the situation of the poor within the existing social relationships. Rights are claimed through social action and the latter depends on how power is distributed and used to address health issues.

Human rights legislation alone – without enforcement mechanisms – is not up to the task of relieving the suffering already at hand. Rights are not equal to laws – they are realized through social action and by changing the prevailing power relations. Rights cannot be advanced but through the organized efforts of the state and of organized civil society. To work on behalf of the victims of violations of the right to health invariably means becoming deeply involved in pressing for social and economic rights.

Public health must be linked to a return to social justice. Denial of care to those who do not pay is simply legitimized in the free-market system. The commodification of health care changes people from citizens with rights to consumers with (or without) purchasing power. This leaves those who are economically marginalized also marginalized from accessing comprehensive health care.

The global campaign proposed by the People's Health Movement (PHM) is a step in the direction outlined above, i.e., it seeks the social transformations indispensable to resolve the inequities found in health.

The right to health: A holistic overview of its components and tasks for the global health movement

The right to health has been defined as the "right to the enjoyment of a variety of facilities, goods, services and conditions necessary for the realization of the highest attainable standard of health".[1]

This right includes both the right to all the underlying determinants of health besides health care (such as water, food security, housing, sanitation, education, a safe and healthy working and living environment, etc.), and the right to health care (i.e. the right to the entire spectrum of preventive, curative and rehabilitative services plus health education and promotive activities).

The following diagram shows the main components of the right to health and some of its interrelationships.

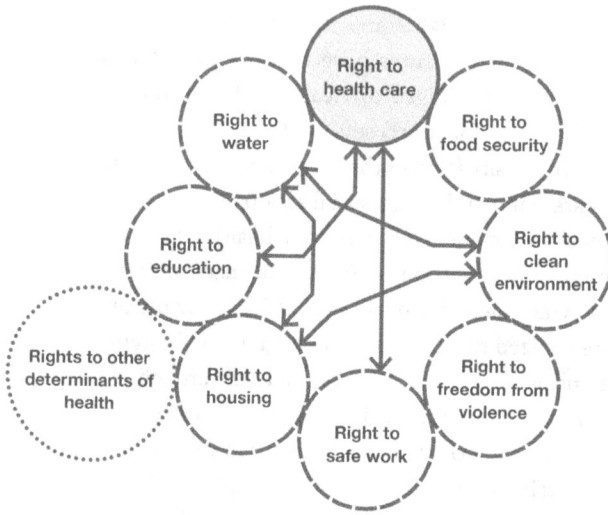

In practice, this suggests two types of tasks for the global health movement: Tackling the right to all the underlying determinants of health, and strengthening the right to health care.

Tackling the right to the underlying determinants of health

Supporting and even co-initiating, campaigns or initiatives addressing key health determinants (for example campaigns for water, for food security, or for housing) is important and justified by itself. There are initiatives already working on behalf of these rights, not necessarily spearheaded by health activists. We contend that the focal points for each of these initiatives should be the organizations with the most experience and commitment to that particular issue (e.g. water, food security, housing, the environment). This recognition places an obligation on health activists to actively support and strengthen such initiatives though not necessarily to take up the responsibility of primary leadership of such groups. When liaising with these groups, PHM will bring the health perspective into their campaigns.

An additional important role that has to be played by health activists is to help document violations of the right to the underlying determinants of health, for example, showing how denial of food security leads to worsening malnutrition, increased morbidity and mortality. Health-based arguments can indeed significantly strengthen the demands of claim-holders to tackle these determinants from a right to health perspective.

Strengthening the right to health care

The global health movement has a primary and unquestionable responsibility to take the lead on this. The urgent need for action within the health care sector has already been pointed out. We are all witnesses to the often catastrophic consequences of the lack of economic access to adequate health care and the poverty trap that leads to avoidable morbidity and mortality.

What does the right to health imply and what is the added value of the human rights-based approach?

In every development process, there are three types of actors: Claim-holders, duty bearers and agents of accountability. When the state does not respect human rights, claim-holders have to demand their rights directly from the duty bearers in government plus interact with agents of accountability (e.g., human rights commissions, ombudsmen, human-rights-oriented NGOs) who oversee the procedures being put in place by government and make sure duty bearers fulfill their obligations (including remedies and restitutions). If claim-holders do not do it, it is in part their fault. One can thus say that it is also the duty of those of us who are aware of human rights to generate awareness about the bases of these rights, in partnership with the marginalized and underserved groups we work with.

The right to health is thus violated, when the poor, the marginalized and the discriminated, as claim-holders, do not have the capacity to effectively demand (claim) their rights; rights are also violated because duty bearers do not have the capacity or the will to fulfil their obligations (technically called "correlative duties").

Therefore, in the human rights-based approach one has to carry out three types of analyses:

1.   Situation analyses in which one determines the causes of the problems placing them in a hierarchical causality chain of immediate, underlying and basic causes or determinants;

2. capacity analyses in which one determines who are the individuals/institutions that bear the duty to do something about the above causes calling them then to fulfil their duties as per their country's obligations as signatories of the UN human rights conventions; and

3. analysis of and liaison with accountability agents.

Herein lies the call for human rights activists to carry out rights awareness work, for instance to educate and inform the broader society about what these rights mean and what accountability mechanisms should be put in place and made to work. These three types of analyses have to be carried out with the representatives of the local community and the beneficiaries of the health system so that the rights being violated can be identified jointly and those responsible also be jointly confronted – for them to do something about the problems identified.

Note that the rights activists' ultimate goal is not to look for health policies that favour the poor ... What is sought is significant poverty reduction policies that directly address the social determinants of health.

As rights activists, we are no longer going to go and beg for changes to be implemented; we are now going to demand them based on existing international law already in force in most of the countries where we work. Disseminating this concept is in itself empowering. We should note that people in countries that have not ratified these covenants do have the same rights. Their problem is that their governments have not made a commitment to honour them.

PHM seeks to overcome the culture of silence and apathy about the human rights violations in health that we all know are happening. This, because human rights and the right to health will never be given to poor, marginalized, discriminated and indigenous persons. Rights are never given, they have to be fought for! And this is what PHM's Global RTHHC Campaign is attempting to do.

As regards the added value of adopting a human rights-based framework, several advantages come to mind:

1. A RTHHC Campaign has a big social mobilization potential – and this is an indispensable part of any campaign;

2. as said, the human rights approach is backed by international law;

3. the right to health approach demands – from a position of strength – that decision-makers take responsibility;

4.   human rights imply correlative duties that are universal and indivisible; and

5.   the human rights approach is focused on processes that lead to outcomes (just setting goals, like the Millennium Development Goals (MDGs),[2] is thus not sufficient in the human rights-based framework).

What may be realistically achieved through the proposed process?

PHM has no illusion that systematically raising the issue of the "right to health" will, by itself, lead to an actual, complete implementation of this right in countries across the globe. The universal provision of even basic health care services involves major budgetary, operational and systemic changes; in addition to shifting to a rights-based framework, major political and legal reorientations are thus needed – and such major changes cannot be expected to happen in full in the near future, given the political economy of health care in most countries of the world today.

However, PHM expects to and can work on a number of more achievable objectives that can take us towards the larger human rights goal. Some of these "achievables" to be considered are: (a) The explicit recognition of the right to health care at country level; (b) the formation, in some countries, of health rights monitoring bodies (accountability agents) with PHM and civil society participation; (c) a clearer delineation of health rights at both global and country levels; (d) the shifting of the focus of the World Health Organization (WHO) towards health rights/universal access systems and the strengthening of groups within WHO that will work along these lines; (e) the bringing of the right to health care more into the global agenda thus making it a central reference point in the global health discourse; and (f) the strengthening of the human rights activists' network in as many countries as possible so that all its members work around a common and broad rallying point, along with building partnerships with other networks.

Why the global RTHHC Campaign?

Nearly 150 countries around the world are parties to the International Covenant on Economic, Social and Cultural Rights. General Comment No. 14 of the Committee on Economic, Social and Cultural Rights (CESCR), adopted in 2000, elaborates on and clarifies the right to health by defining the content, the methods of operationalization, the violations and the suggested means to monitor the implementation of this right. There is now a need to launch a global process of mobilization to actually implement the provisions of General Comment No. 14 in all ratifying countries. This clearly calls for measures to operationalize the right to health and to review and recast all global and national health sector reform initiatives in the light of the framework of health as a right (such as, for instance, recasting the reforms that are now being pursued to achieve the Millennium Development Goals).

There are a host of reasons to adopt the right to health approach. Among them is the fact that the basic human needs approach (has) never delivered. Other valid justifications are: (a) The human rights-based framework is now UN policy, and (b) PHM is founded on the principles of the right to health and to equitable access to health care services at all levels with no discrimination.

While PHM continues to struggle for the right to health as a basic human right at various levels, there is now growing recognition of the need for a global initiative to address health system issues in a rights-based framework.

There is also a growing worldwide need for solidarity in, and mutual learning from, our struggles, so as to strengthen our efforts in the various countries and regions. There is a related need to challenge the dominant global discourse of "safety nets for those left outside the existing packages of benefits" that results from health services being increasingly commodified and from governments retreating from funding the provision of universal health care, limiting their role to supporting said "safety nets" or other kinds of reduced public health services "for the poor". We need to counter this with a strong "health care as a human right" strategy that unequivocally asserts the central role of the state and public health systems – and their responsibility to provide health services for all.

Given the above, the following overall strategy has been adopted by PHM: PHM country circles will continue to strengthen and expand their involvement in various concerned initiatives within their countries and regions. They will, at the same time, analyse the interrelatedness between various health determinants so as to enable PHM and its circles to develop integrated and holistic strategies.

PHM is focusing on its Global Right to Health and Health Care Campaign. The RTHHC Campaign will concentrate on strengthening the right

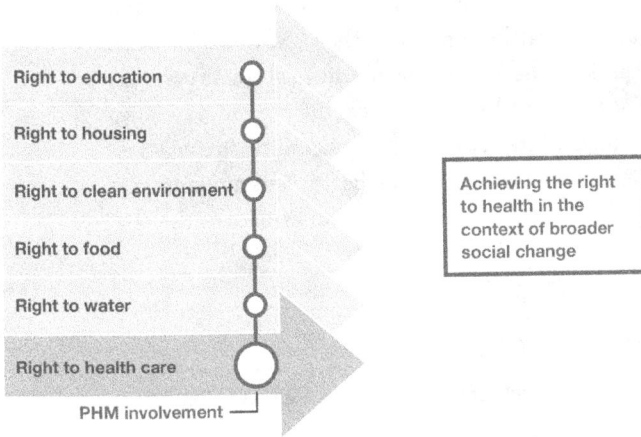

The diagram shows, from top to bottom, a vertical sequence of points:

- Right to education
- Right to housing
- Right to clean environment
- Right to food
- Right to water
- Right to health care

with "PHM involvement" indicated at the bottom, and a box to the right reading "Achieving the right to health in the context of broader social change".

to health care since we argue that PHM has a primary responsibility regarding this issue. The RTHHC Campaign will focus on tasks in which PHM (along with partners in the global health movement) can take the lead and primary responsibility.

The overall perspective about how the global health movement should approach the right to health is depicted in the diagram above.

Focus of the RTHHC Campaign

The RTHHC Campaign is, in its first phase, focused on the issue of access to quality health care which can be acted-upon from within the health sector. This is being broadened by PHM's vision of health care that, as in the Alma-Ata Declaration, includes preventive, curative and rehabilitative health services, as well as health promotion services, e.g., nutrition, quality drinking water and sanitation, health education, health information systems. Specific important aspects of this right such as women's and children's right to health care, mental health rights, HIV and AIDS-affected persons' health care rights, workers' health rights, and the right to essential drugs, are all being woven into the RTHHC Campaign, bringing diverse branches of the global health movement into a broad coalition that strengthens universal access to health care.

At the same time, PHM is denouncing and acting upon adverse existing and new policies that are having negative impacts on the right to health (such as the privatization of services, the weakening of universal access systems, vertical programmes that fragment health systems, the current 90/10 gap in research funding, the unjust international trade regimes – to name just but a few). These policies, and violations of key health determinants, are being identified at the country level and are taken up as part of the proposed RTHHC Campaign.

The three phases of the RTHHC Campaign

In moving towards the full implementation of the RTHCC Campaign, phases have been designed as follows:

Preparatory phase (3rd quarter of 2006 to fourth quarter of 2007)
This involved:

—— Creation of a broad consensus on the RTHHC Campaign concept. In each country, identified groups were invited to become part of the RTH-HC Campaign. At the global level, a "Core Campaign Steering Group" was formed. This team actively supports a host of regional and local organizers and leads the international network, plus the up-front fund-raising and advocacy work for the Campaign.
—— Identification of existing PHM or newly associated groups that will take regional and local responsibilities.
—— Identification of short and long-term sources of funding for the various aspects of the RTHHC Campaign, at the regional and global levels, plus the development of a budget.
—— Completion of a multilingual "Assessment Guide" for the preparation of papers depicting "The State of the Right to Health" in each country. (This was finalized in November 2006 and is now available in four languages.[3])
—— Contribution to the discussion and planning of the 2008 edition of the "Global Health Watch II" (the alternative world health report).

Documentation and analysis phase (late 2007 to late 2008)
During this period, country and regional reports are prepared. Over 25 countries are now engaged, are studying and implementing the ad-hoc Assessment Guide and are at different stages of organization.

PHM does not see these (or any) reports as an end; rather, the real end is the process launched to mobilize civil society to produce these reports.

The phase culminates with: (a) The holding of national workshops to discuss the results of the assessment of the right to health and to prepare a commensurate action plan for the PHM circle and associates; and (b) the concrete planning of Regional Assemblies on the Right to Health in all five or six regions of the world.

Regional assemblies and subsequent action phase (following the World Health Assembly of May 2008)

___ One assembly in each region where the campaign is ongoing will be held, one after the other. These assemblies will be convened by PHM, with the involvement of the UN Special Rapporteur on the Right to Health and the WHO, and will be attended by national health officials, national human rights committees and PHM, as well as other health and human rights activists. Plans will be made to have health workers and beneficiaries represented in these meetings as well. Country reports on the right to health will be presented and discussed. This will be complemented by a regional analysis paper in each region, dealing with how international macro and structural factors and global agencies are affecting the right to health in the region. Action plans to implement the right to health will be drawn up, discussed, and presented in the second half of the assemblies.

___ This series of regional assemblies may culminate in a resolution being proposed for adoption at, say, the World Health Assembly in Geneva in 2009 or 2010. Such a resolution will call for time-bound, progressive implementation of the right to health.

___ Preparation of a "Global Action Plan on the Right to Health Care". Such a document will, with facts and figures, convincingly show how quality essential health care services could be made available now to every human being on earth, provided certain key reallocation of priorities and resources are enacted. These global recommendations will be accompanied by practical recommendations for the countries in each region.

___ Governments will be lobbied to accept the major points suggested during the regional assemblies and the 2009 or 2010 World Health Assembly will be asked to adopt a "Declaration on the Right to Health for All" for implementation by member countries. The same will have time-bound, specific and monitorable benchmarks. The aim will be to foster more effective community involvement and monitoring in health to operationalize the right to health. Universal access to comprehensive health care will be endorsed as an overarching principle, together with a related call for definitive changes in the global trade and patents regime as they affect health.

Expected outcomes of the RTHHC Campaign

In its work, the RTHHC Campaign will use four broad approaches:

—— Documenting violations and facilitating redress for those violations.
—— Policy advocacy (denunciation of existing policies and formulation of new ones) at the national and international levels.
—— Raising awareness and education.
—— Establishing alliances and embarking on civil society mobilization.

There is a need for a shift in the focus of the WHO towards the human rights-based framework to health; a shift that puts universal access to public services at the centre of WHO's work, and that strengthens a group inside WHO that will continue to work and provide leadership on this work.

The strengthening and broadening of the PHM network in various countries across the globe will be both an outcome, and also an imperative to take PHM forward around the common, broad rallying point of the RTHHC Campaign.

A clarification on the implementation of the RTHHC Campaign

The RTHHC Campaign uses a participatory process to inform people about their right to health and actually involves them in preparing the assessment of the right to health care in their country – at the same time that it builds and mobilizes a sustainable PHM network.

Collecting the data that bring out the evidence of the violations of the RTHHC does not, by itself, spur the victims of such violations into action. Victims must be present when the assessment is carried out and when data are analysed. By going through this process, victims will learn about what the right to health and health care is all about and may thus meaningfully contribute to its operationalization.

Country-level activities are the heart of the campaign. How the RTHHC Campaign is organized in Country X is up to the campaign committee in that country. PHM's overall concerns are that the process involves as many people from different sectors and tendencies as possible, and that the final assessment report covers the different parameters described in the campaign's RTHHC Assessment Guide as closely as possible. As written, the Guide provides a step-by-step, user-friendly explanation of the reasoning process to be followed to identify violations of the right to health. Therefore, regardless of how country circles end up using this tool, it is recommended they consider its five main steps in reporting their findings so as to make country reports comparable.

The most important goal of this campaign is to empower and involve ordinary people in representing their own interests in a political process/movement that has the power to influence both the national and the international levels of decision-making. PHM wants to bring people's claims for their health rights to a level that cannot be ignored.

As already stated, the point of this campaign is not to produce RTHHC Campaign reports. The reporting process is a process to find evidence, to educate people about their rights and about key principles of public health, as well as to bring them together behind shared, common, goals. This is what is needed to make effective demands on governments.

For the above reasons, before engaging in the actual assessment, it is crucial to set up a credible network of strategic allies. Country focal points for the campaign should therefore contact such allies (including individuals and institutions). Establishing such a network is key. To arrive at a point when the time is right to launch the assessment, PHM circles ought to take as many weeks or months as are needed to assure success. Consequently, the criteria for proof of social mobilization preceding the launching of the first phase of the campaign are as follows:

___ Organizing at least two national level (or regional in bigger countries) meetings to discuss the campaign, involving participants from various organizational backgrounds, preferably including some from different regions of the country.

___ Formation of a first campaign coordination group which will take collective responsibility for expanding and developing the campaign.

___ A formal agreement on the provisional decision-making mechanisms for the development of the campaign in the country.

___ Existence of a functional e-group/list-server or other means of communication among the participating organizations/individuals to facilitate campaign communications.

Each country will decide for itself how to use the assessment process as a tool for additional mobilization.

Countries do not have to do their assessments all at the same time, nor finish all at the same time. But there does have to be a certain critical mass of countries in a region that have gone through the assessment process and the national strategic action planning before it makes sense to have a regional meeting (the second phase). Each of the regional meetings should nevertheless happen within a reasonable period of time so that international momentum can be generated.

To summarize, each new or strengthened national PHM circle needs to create the critical mass of popular support/power so as to be able to follow-through with the relevant action plan.

If the campaign does not succeed in mobilizing claim holders and their organizations to be ready for, and to actively participate in, the assessment, there is the risk that the campaign may backfire. We have to be careful not to build expectations only to then let down the people whose right to health is being violated (as well as those persons who contributed to the assessment process).

The local political context has to be analysed by the PHM circle so that committed strategic allies can be aligned and given concrete responsibilities, as part of an ad-hoc plan for the whole campaign as duly agreed with them. The question also has to be asked, then, whether the timing for launching the campaign is right, given the concrete local political realities.

Putting pressure on duty bearers by using the results of the assessment, therefore, has to go hand-in-hand with mobilizing the participating claim-holders for actions at different levels: The process is as important as the outcome!

The assessment process is not a technical "desk exercise" that only analyses data, but it should preferably include documentation of testimonies of denial of health care, and participatory case studies of health care facilities or health-related services being successfully carried out by participating organizations. Such activities simultaneously build evidence and generate involvement. Holding of dialogues between groups of health activists and health authorities, public hearings, workshops on the right to health, and/or carrying out symbolic protest actions of various types will be important features of the campaign.

Only starting the mobilization drive after the assessment, when all the evidence is in, would be considered to be too late – although the mobilization will gain momentum after the assessment results are presented and constitute an incontrovertible "evidence base" of violations of the right to health care.

As part of the mobilization effort, country PHM circles can choose from the beginning to hold public hearings on the right to health (as PHM India and PHM South Africa successfully did), or other community-based action.

The campaign will greatly depend on proactive country-level organizers that are willing to commit quality time, not only to do a desk job or carry out a mere assessment project: This is not the essence of the campaign. An assessment report so produced will be of limited use; it will gather dust in duty bearers' in-boxes – and has never been the intention of the campaign.

Some countries may centre their mobilization around already strongly felt needs in the population and, as an entry point to the campaign, address these strongly felt needs as they relate to the right to health. Connecting the campaign to ongoing national popular struggles is essential.

The campaign will not attempt to be confrontational, unless needed. The lobbying strategies outlined in the Assessment Guide discuss ways to work with duty bearers in a constructive manner.

Finally, the campaign highly encourages the early involvement of health workers and their unions. They are, at the same time, claim-holders (i.e. claim-holders of decisions made at higher levels), and duty bearers. Their involvement will give the campaign access to valuable information, as well as greater depth and additional credibility. The endorsement of the campaign by well-known personalities and prestigious institutions is also invaluable.

1 Committee on Economic, Social and Cultural Rights (CESCR), *General Comment No. 14 on the right to the highest attainable standard of health*, 11 August 2000, UN Doc. E/C.12/2000/4.

2 Millennium Development Goals, available at http://www.un.org/millenniumgoals/.

3 See www.phmovement.org and follow the leads to the Right to Health Campaign.

10

STRATEGIES FOR REALIZING THE RIGHT TO HEALTH

Global Health Diplomacy: The New Recognition of Health in Foreign Policy

Ilona Kickbusch and Christian Erk

Health is a valuable resource, both for the individual as well as for society. The protection and improvement of individual and public health can be argued to be a major rationale and goal of the nation state.[1] However, securing the health of the public goes beyond focusing on the health status of individuals.

There is solid evidence that many determinants of individual and population health extend beyond the control of what is commonly understood as health sector activities and are to a large extent determined by other societal and economic factors. A variety of policies influence and shape the conditions in which we live and work, and these conditions may have positive or negative consequences for the health of a given population and its individuals. This interconnectedness is not only acknowledged by the World Health Organization (WHO) which states that "health is a state of complete physical, social and mental well-being, and not merely the absence of disease or infirmity",[2] but also developed in academic writing.[3] Most of the models of health determinants see health influenced by macro level (e.g. social, economic, cultural, and environmental) and middle level conditions and policies (working conditions, education, sanitation, health care services, unemployment, food production, housing, neighbourhood and communities). These determinants are complemented by micro level individual factors (lifestyle, behaviour, constitution) which, in return, heavily depend on the availability of, and support for, healthy choices in everyday environments on the macro and middle levels.

Given this network of health determinants, health is often best influenced by policies and actions outside the health sector, such as, inter alia, transport, housing, regional and environment policy, education, fiscal, tax and economic policies.[4] Actions, decisions and policies in these sectors can have positive or negative impacts on the above-mentioned health determinants which are reflected in health outcomes and the health status of the population – though some of these influences are direct and self-evident while others are indirect and difficult to predict. In return, health has important effects on the realization of goals in other sectors, such as economic wealth. There is an increasing body of evidence that better health contributes to higher levels of education and economic growth, while countries with weak conditions for health have a hard time achieving sustained growth due to a reduction in labour productivity as well as the relative size of the labour force.[5] In short: a healthy population is a prerequisite for a healthy and competitive economy. From this perspective, health is the foundation for the economic and social development of developing countries and is also an important factor to sustain the living standard of developed countries.

Thus, protecting and improving its population's health should inevitably become a primary goal of any nation state. The best way to do so is to adopt a "Health in all Policies (HiaP)"[6] approach and understand health as a shared value which spans all societal sectors. This insight led the Council of the European Union (EU) – under the Finnish Presidency in the second half of 2006 – to develop a "Health in all Policies" initiative which invites the European Commission, the European Parliament, as well as the EU member states to set out a plan for work on HiaP.[7]

It is increasingly realized that it would be short-sighted to conceptualize the influence on health as determined merely by policies pertaining to a state's internal affairs. Rather, in an interdependent world, health and health policy are increasingly influenced by an external dimension.

The external dimension of public health: The globalization of health

Bacteria, viruses and parasites ignore national boundaries and migrate from one country to another regardless of political and diplomatic situations. A country cannot hope to enjoy health if its neighbours continue to cling to outdated ideas of sanitation and disease control – a fact recognized as early as 1926 by Dr. René Sand, Secretary General of the League of

Red Cross Societies in Paris.[8] This is also why the first embassies were established in medieval Italy as a means of providing city states with information of outbreaks occurring in their neighbouring states. If a country is to prosper (especially with respect to health), its neighbouring countries have to prosper as well.

This fact has become even more important in today's globalized and still globalizing world where there is no such place as abroad and where the whole world has become our neighbourhood: "Problems and solutions reach across national borders resulting in the need for international collaboration and abolishing the distinction between internal and external national responses".[9] As we have seen with the outbreak of Avian flu or SARS, but as we can also see with non-infectious diseases such as obesity, health risks are international.[10] Globalization, the process of reducing the barriers of time, space and ideas between people, has a significant influence on the health of a given population and no country can isolate itself from cross-border risks and threats to their national health. In our global world health is becoming increasingly interdependent. As a consequence of this globalization of health, national health problems can no longer – if ever – be dealt with in "splendid isolation" but rather call for coordinated and cooperative international health efforts. We must begin to understand health as a global public good (GPG)[11] which all countries are responsible for producing, sustaining, and protecting from material harm. The state of global health has a fundamental effect on all countries – developed as well as developing. It is thus in the best interest and to the benefit of all countries to secure global health in an internationally concerted way. Global health action is not only just a development issue that falls in the purview of the WHO or a prescription of moral duty or a form of public diplomacy – it is also an investment in self-protection and national security which coincides with the need for concerted regional and global action. The way to national health security leads through global health security which, in return, depends on critical capacity in all countries, combined with a commitment to collaborate.

Health foreign policy and health diplomacy

What has been established so far is that health policy can no longer remain purely national – interdependence has created its own dynamic and health is a key element. Foreign policy and diplomacy offer important tools to deal with interdependence and thus are complementary to, as well as extensions of, national policy efforts. Utilizing these tools and reorienting health and foreign policies in ways that align the national interest with the diplomatic, epidemiological and ethical realities of a globalized world could thus make a tangible contribution to protecting and promoting global health. The problem is that, so far, health "has not been at the heart of foreign policy theory or practice and perhaps not even at the margins"[12] – although today the degree of foreign policy attention devoted to health is historically unprecedented. What is thus needed is a political revolution that "reflects a transformation of foreign policy for the benefits of health, or a transformation of health for the benefits of foreign policy."[13] To be more precise: What is needed is what has come to be termed as "health foreign policy" and "health diplomacy", i.e. new developments bringing together diplomatic negotiating skills with expertise as regards content in order to secure global public goods by means of collective action. Such alignment also requires governments to overcome "fragmented policy competencies in national governance systems"[14] and to widen the content and concept of diplomacy to include issues such as health but also environment and energy. Foreign policy and diplomacy no longer reside solely with the traditional diplomats but also include a wide range of other state and non-state actors.[15] Diplomats no longer just have to talk to other diplomats – they need to interact with the private sector, non-governmental organizations, scientists, activists and the media, to name but a few interlocutors, since all these actors are part and parcel of the negotiating process.[16]

A first step to broaden the scope of foreign policy, to integrate national policies and create coherence between them, as well as to enhance global cooperation, has been made by the Oslo Ministerial Declaration[17] signed by the Ministers of Foreign Affairs of Brazil, France, Indonesia, Norway, Senegal, South Africa, and Thailand on 20 March 2007. The signatories hold that foreign policy and the involvement of foreign ministers and diplomats can make a difference when it comes to global health, and that the "impact on health" should be a starting point and overall rationale for developing foreign policy strategies. Closing with an agenda for action in the field of public health, this Declaration thus is a prominent example of a shared awareness and appreciation of the value of the global public good, which is health, as well as a will for bilateral, regional and multilateral cooperation.

Since the signing of the above-mentioned document, the number of countries taking the initiative and moving their global health agendas forward has been constantly increasing. More and more are undertaking steps to generate more policy coherence at the national level, bringing together the concerns of sectors, such as health and foreign policy, as well as development and trade. In an attempt to integrate health and foreign policy Switzerland has developed a "Swiss Health Foreign Policy".[18] Last year, the UK issued a report "Health is Global: Proposals for a UK Government-Wide Strategy"[19] which makes the case for developing a global health strategy bringing together all UK international health activities that influence global health. In doing so, the UK wants to protect the health of its population and contribute to safeguarding their domestic investment in health, as well as the economy, but also recognizes the fact that such endeavours benefit the rest of the world and help to harness the opportunities of globalization. Following their obligation to protect human health (Art. 152 EC Treaty) the European Commission has recently adopted a health strategy[20] which for the first time included a section on global health. With the white paper, the Commission is committing the EU and its member states to sustained collective leadership in global health aiming at improving the safety and security of the EU's citizens and protecting them against health threats. It thus focuses on the interface between European health challenges and global developments and the responsibilities Europe has towards the health of the rest of the world. Other countries such as Brazil[21] have also embarked on a process of developing a Health Foreign Policy strategy; others such as the US and Canada have started a debate about the relevance of health as foreign policy.[22]

Conclusion

The challenges of global health security have to be taken seriously and can only be tackled by strengthening global health diplomacy and coherence as well as cooperation between global health players. We are well aware of the fact that global health diplomacy faces a crucial challenge: The art of diplomacy juggles the science of public health and concrete national interest with the abstract collective concern of the larger international community.

But this challenge should not hinder us from defining health as a global public good, in order to ensure its value, understand it as a key dimension of global citizenship, and keep it high on the global political agenda. The road ahead must lead to commonly defined agendas and global health treaties translated by means of a new interface between foreign and domestic policies, as well as an increasing pooling of sovereignty by nation states in the area of health.[23]

1   Consequently, a human right to health has been recognized by a significant number of human rights instruments governing the conduct of states, organizations and individuals, the most prominent examples being the first two paragraphs of the WHO Constitution (1946), Art. 25(1) of the Universal Declaration of Human Rights (1948), Art. 11 of the Revised European Social Charter (1996), Art. 12 of the International Covenant on Economics, Social and Cultural Rights (1966), the Declaration of Alma-Ata (1978), Art. 16 of the African Charter on Human and Peoples' Rights (1981), Art. 10 of the Additional Protocol to the American Convention on Human Rights in the Area of Economic, Social and Cultural Rights (1988), Art. 24 of the UN Convention on the Rights of the Child (1989), American Declaration of the Rights and Duties of Man, the UN Convention against Torture and Other Cruel, Inhuman or Degrading Treatment or Punishment as well as the UN Convention on Elimination of all Forms of Discrimination Against Women. For an overview of different accounts to ground such right philosophically cf. Á. Castaño and L. Stella, 'El derecho a la salud en Colombia: Una propuesta para su fundamentación moral' 18(2) Revista Panamericana de Salud Pública/Pan American Journal of Public Health (2005) at 129–135, and P. McCarrick, A Right to Health Care (Washington, DC: Georgetown University, Kennedy Institute of Ethics, National Reference Center for Bioethics Literature, 1992. (Scope Note 20)), available at http:/bioethics.geo rgetown.edu/publications/scopenotes/sn20.pdf.

2   Preamble to the Constitution of the World Health Organization as adopted by the International Health Conference, New York, 19–22 June, 1946, entered into force on 7 April 1948.

3   Cf. G. Dahlgren and M. Whitehead, Policies and strategies to promote social equity in health (Stockholm: Institute of Futures Studies, 1991); H. Barton and M. Grant, 'A health map for the local human habitat' 126(6) Journal of the Royal Society for the Promotion of Health (2006) 252–253; D. P, Keating and C. Hertzman (eds.) Developmental Health

and the Wealth of Nations: Social, Biological, and Educational Dynamics (New York: Guilford Press, 1999); Institute of Medicine (IOM). Promoting Health: Intervention Strategies from Social and Behavioral Research (Washington D.C.: National Academy Press, 2000), 43; R.G. Evans and G.L. Stoddart, 'Producing health, consuming healthcare' 31 Social Science and Medicine (1990) 1347–1363; Committee on Assuring the Health of the Public in the 21st Century (Board on Health Promotion and Disease Prevention (HPDP) and Institute of Medicine (IOM)), The Future of the Public's Health in the 21st Century (Washington D.C.: National Academic Press, 2002) at 52.

4   Cf. G. Rosen, A History of Public Health (Baltimore: Johns Hopkins University Press, Expanded edition, 1993).

5   D.E. Bloom, D. Conning and D.T. Jamison, 'Health, wealth and welfare' 41(1) Finance and Development (2004) at 10–15. See also World Health Organization (WHO), Macroeconomics and Health: Investing in Health for Economic Development: Report of the Commission on Macroeconomics and Health (Geneva: World Health Organization, 2001), available at http://whqlibdoc.who.int/publications/2001/924154550X.pdf.

6   Also cf. T. Ståhl, M. Wismar, E. Ollila, E. Lahtinen and K. Leppo (eds.) Health in All Policies: Prospects and Potentials (Finland: Ministry of Social Affairs and Health, 2006), available at http://www.euro.who.int/observatory/Publications/20060915_2.

7   Cf.: Council Conclusions on Health in All Policies (HiAP), 2767th Employment, Social Policy, Health and Consumer Affairs Council meeting, Brussels, 30 November and 1 December 2006, available at http://www.eu2006.fi/news_and_documents/conclusions/vko48/en_GB/1164897086637.

8   'Germs Ignore Diplomatic Alliances' 8(270) The Science News-Letter (1926) at 7–8.

9   J.W. Owen 'Foreword' in I. Kickbusch and G. Lister, European Perspectives on Global Health: A Policy Glossary (Brussels: European Foundation Centre, 2006) at 5.

10   Cf. I. Kickbusch, 'The lesson of SARS: A wake-up call for global health', International Herald Tribune. (2003) Tuesday, 29 April 2003, available at http://www.iht.com/articles/2003/04/29/edIlona_ed3_.php.

11   I.e. a good which is non-rival in consumption and non-excludable throughout the whole world. Cf. I. Kaul, I. Grunberg and M. Stern (eds.), Global Public Goods: International Cooperation in the 21st Century (New York: Oxford University Press, 1999). See also I. Kaul, and M. Faust, 'Global public goods and health: Taking the agenda forward' 79 Bulletin of the World Health Organization (2001) at 869–74.

12   D.P. Fidler, 'Reflections on the revolution in health and foreign policy' 85(3) Bulletin of the World Health Organization (2007) at 243–244.

13   D. Fidler, 'Health as Foreign Power: Between Principle and Power', Maloy Lecture, Washington, Georgetown University, 5 October 2004.

14   Cf. N. Drager, and D.P. Fidler, 'Foreign Policy, trade and health: At the cutting edge of global health diplomacy' 85(3) Bulletin of the World Health Organization (2007) at 162.

15   R.P. Barston, Modern Diplomacy, (Harlow, New York: Pearson Longman, 2006).

16   I. Kickbusch, G. Silberschmidt and P. Buss, 'Global health diplomacy: The need for new perspectives, strategic approaches and skills in global health' 85(3) Bulletin of the World Health Organization (2007) at 230–232.

17   Ministers of Foreign Affairs of Brazil, France, Indonesia, Norway, Senegal, South Africa, and Thailand, 'Oslo Ministerial Declaration – Global Health: A pressing foreign policy issue of our time', 369.9570 The Lancet (21 April 2007 – 27 April 2007) 1373–1378, also available at http://www.regjeringen.no/en/dep/ud/About-the-Ministry/Minister-of-Foreign-Affairs-Jonas-Gahr-S/Speeches-and-articles/2007/lancet.html?id=466469).

18   Federal Department of Home Affairs (FDHA) and Federal Department of Foreign Affairs (FDFA), Swiss Health Foreign Policy. Agreement on Health Foreign Policy Objectives, Bern, 2007.

19 Department of Health, *Health is Global: Proposals for UK Government-Wide Strategy* (London: Department of Health Publications, 2007), available at http://www.dh.gov.uk/en/Publicationsand statistics/Publications/PublicationsPolicyAnd Guidance/DH_072697.

20 Commission of the European Union, 'Together for Health: A Strategic Approach for the EU 2008–2013', *White Paper* 630 COM (2007) (Brussels, 23 October 2007), available at http://ec.europa.eu/health/ph_overview/strategy/health_strategy_en.htm.

21 Cf. I. Kickbusch, G. Silberschmidt and P. Buss, *supra* note 16.

22 Cf. Institute of Medicine, *America's Vital Interest in Global Health – Protecting Our People, Enhancing Our Economy, and Advancing Our International Interests,* (Washington D. C.: National Academy Press, 1997). See also M. F. Strong, J. Austin, T. Brodhead et al., *Connecting with the World: Priorities for Canadian Internationalism in the 21st Century* (Ottawa, Ontario, Canada: International Development Research Centre, 1996).

23 Cf. I. Kickbusch, 'From Charity to Rights: Proposal for Five Action Areas of Global Health – Towards a Global Social Contract on Health' 58 *Journal of Epidemiology and Community Health* (2004) at 630–631.

Enforcing the Right to Health: Innovative Lessons from Domestic Courts

Iain Byrne

The United Nations Committee on Economic, Social and Cultural Rights, in its General Comment No. 9, has emphasized that it is up to states how they give effect to the rights contained in the International Covenant on Economic, Social and Cultural Rights (ICESCR), including the right to health, but whatever arrangements they choose they must be effective: "The Covenant norms must be recognized in appropriate ways within the domestic legal order, appropriate means of redress, or remedies, must be available to any aggrieved individual or group, and appropriate means of ensuring governmental accountability must be put in place."[1]

This chapter highlights some significant right to health cases in a non-exhaustive survey of decisions from domestic courts from both civil and common law jurisdictions. In so doing it seeks to show that (a) even where the right to health is explicitly guaranteed under the constitution, courts will still have to wrestle with challenging issues, such as resource allocation and (b) by adopting innovative approaches, the lack of express constitutional entrenchment of the right to health in domestic law is not necessarily a bar to both consideration, and enforcement, by the courts. In the latter case, courts have attempted to give practical meaning to notions of indivisibility and interdependence of rights recognizing that the right to health has clear links to many other rights, not just economic and social but also civil and political rights – e.g. the right to life and, the right not to be subjected to torture or cruel, inhuman or degrading treatment, and the right to information[2] – an unhealthy citizen is not able to play a full and active part in society either economically or politically.

Constitutional entrenchment: Addressing systemic violations whilst considering resource implications

Since Chile provided the first constitutional recognition of the right to health in 1925, nearly 70% of countries have some form of explicit guarantee regarding health, although this may take a variety of forms.[3] In South Africa the guarantee is part of a provision requiring access to health care services, food and water and social security.[4] Since the new Constitution came into force in 1994, health rights, together with housing rights, have provided the most significant constitutional economic, social and cultural rights cases considered by the courts to date. Two cases seek to highlight how the Constitutional Court sought to address issues of widespread violations affecting thousands of people and limited resources.

Arguably the most widely known case to be decided by the Constitutional Court to date, due not just to the issues involved, but also because of the successful campaign surrounding it (a frequently critical factor in ensuring enforcement), is *Minister of Health v. Treatment Action Campaign (TAC) (2002)* 5 SA 721 (CC), or the *TAC case*, where it was held that the state's failure to provide comprehensive anti-retroviral drugs to prevent mother-child HIV transmission breached their right to health. An important factor for the court was the fact that the drug was costless to the government and therefore arguments centred on lack of resources did not carry any weight. However, by requiring that the programme should include reasonable measures for counselling and testing, the court did make orders, with some (albeit limited) financial implications. Beyond this, and unlike the approach often taken by the Indian Supreme Court and the Inter-American Court of Human Rights, the court refrained from discussing detailed modes of implementation. Arguably, this created subsequent problems since it took several months of campaigning and lobbying by TAC and others to force the authorities to act and start supplying the drugs.

In *Soobramoney v. Minister of Health KwaZulu Natal* 1997 (12) BCLR 1696, the Constitutional Court set out its approach to examining right to health claims within the context of limited resources. The court, in considering a terminally ill patient's claim to access medical services to obtain costly dialysis treatment, which had been refused by the local health authority on the grounds of lack of resources, held that the health authority had acted reasonably and applied its guidelines rationally and fairly. In so doing the court (as it has done in subsequent cases) asked the crucial question: Has the state done all it could reasonably do in the circumstances?[5] By adopting this approach, similar to judicial review, although extending beyond the decision-making process to consider all the actions taken, the court has recognized that it is not in a position to assume the role of the state in making decisions about resource allocation, but is, instead, there to act as an impartial arbiter. Indeed in *Soobramoney* the court was very explicit about the large margin of discretion it would give to the state to set budgetary priorities stating that the court "will be slow to interfere with rational decisions taken in good faith by the political organs and medical authorities."[6] Justice Sachs went further, stating that: "In open and democratic societies based upon dignity, freedom and equality, the rationing of access to life-prolonging resources is regarded as integral to, rather than incompatible with, a human rights approach to health care."[7]

A region where the courts have been extremely proactive in addressing systemic violations, even where there are significant resource implications for their decisions, has been Latin America. In a number of decisions from different jurisdictions – e.g. Peru,[8] Venezuela,[9] Argentina,[10] Brazil[11] and Ecuador[12] – courts, frequently responding to *amparo*[13] actions, have handed down landmark decisions guaranteeing access to medicines and/or treatment, affecting thousands of victims, and requiring states to take concrete and immediate action, rather than a progressive realization approach. One of the leading decisions is *Mariela Viceconte v. Ministry of Health and Social Welfare* Case No 31.777/96 (1998) from Argentina in 1998.[14] The claim was brought by a number of community groups to ensure that the state would manufacture a vaccine against Argentine hemorrhagic fever, then threatening the lives of 3.5 million people, most of whom did not have adequate access to preventive medical services in certain affected areas. Whilst the state had been able to obtain 200 000 doses of a vaccine from the United States, and had been able to vaccinate 140 000 people between 1991 to 1995, it was unable to carry out a massive immunization campaign due to the lack of an adequate quantity of vaccine. A judicial writ of amparo was filed requiring the health ministry to manufacture and distribute further supplies of the vaccine to persons living in the affected areas. Following initial rejection, the Court of Appeals ruled favourably, establishing the state's obligation to manufacture the vaccine[15]. Significantly (and unlike in South Africa) the court also set a legally binding deadline for the obligation to be met. However, as in the South African *TAC* case, it required further action by the groups, including litigation, to secure enforcement.

Ultimately cases such as *Mariela Viceconte* can have a political, as well as legal impact, far beyond that perhaps envisaged when the original petition was submitted. Within five years, Argentina had developed a social plan to deliver basic medicines. The roots of this plan can be directly traced to the *Viceconte* case.

Lack of constitutional entrenchment: The need to adopt innovate approaches

The lack of express constitutional protection for health rights presents courts with significant but not insurmountable challenges for enforcement. Techniques include:

1.   Adopting expansive definitions of civil rights, some of which tend to be widely, if not universally, guaranteed under national law, e.g. rights to life or not be subjected to cruel, inhuman or degrading treatment. This approach has been sanctioned to differing degrees by both the UN Human Rights Committee[16] and the European Court of Human Rights;[17]
2.   Considering the due process issues by exercising some form of judicial review;[18]
3.   The use of cross-cutting provisions such as equality and non-discrimination, which, again, may not allow for consideration of the substantial economic or social right, but at least afford some measure of indirect protection.

The Indian story: Activism and innovation

Although South Africa has tended to attract much of the attention, at least among common law jurisdictions, for its protection of economic and social rights, Indian courts have been at the forefront of economic, social and cultural rights litigation for over three decades. The Indian Constitution, promulgated in 1947, is a creature of its age and on its face is far less progressive than its South African counterpart operating from the mid 1990s. Economic and social rights, including the right to health contained in Article 47 of the India Constitution[19] are consigned to the Directive Principles of State Policy (DPSP) section which, according to Article 37 of the Constitution, "shall not be enforceable by any court, but the principles therein laid down are nevertheless fundamental in the governance of the country and it shall be the duty of the state to apply these principles in making laws."

Therefore on its face, the Supreme Court of India is barred from considering and enforcing individual health rights claims; but rather it is concerned with offering non-binding guidelines on how health policies should be implemented, whilst leaving the final decision to the state. However, the early 1970s witnessed a watershed in Indian human rights litigation with the *Fundamental Rights Case*.[20] This case ushered in an unprecedented period of progressive jurisprudence, following the recognition by the court that DPSP should enjoy the same status as "traditional" fundamental rights. At the same time, rules on standing were relaxed in order to promote public interest litigation and access to justice. Suddenly writ petitions could be submitted on a postcard.[21]

The main means by which the Supreme Court has achieved equivalence between civil rights and their economic and social counterparts has been through the application of an expansive definition of the right to life. Unsurprisingly the right to health was one of the guarantees to first benefit from this approach.[22] In the public interest litigation case of *Paschim Banag Khet Samity v. State of West Bengal* (1996) 4 SCC 37 the Supreme Court used the right to life to secure the right to emergency medical care, concluding that such an essential obligation could not be avoided by pleading financial constraints.[23] The court, in holding that there had been a violation of the right to life under Article 21, and awarding compensation, stated that the right to emergency medical care formed a core component of the right to health which in turn was recognized as forming an integral part of the right to life. It did this by reconceptualizing the right to life as imposing a positive obligation on the state to safeguard the life of every person, stating that *"preservation of human life was of utmost importance"* and that: "The Constitution envisages the establishment of a welfare state ... Providing adequate medical facilities for the people is an essential part of the obligations undertaken by the government in this respect [and it] discharges this obligation by running hospitals and health centres."[24]

In line with its general approach of frequently offering comprehensive remedies that go beyond merely providing redress for the victim, but also laying down the necessary policy and administrative steps to be taken by the state in the wider public interest, the court not only ordered compensation, but also directed the type of facilities that the state government had to provide.[25] The court also ruled that its orders should apply to other states, together with the national government, and that these other states should be sent a copy of the judgment.

However, the court has also recognized that state resources are not unlimited:

> "No State or country can have unlimited resources to spend on any of its projects. That is why it only approves its projects to the extent it is feasible. The same holds good for providing medical facilities to its citizens including its employees. Provision for facilities cannot be unlimited. It has to be to the extent finances permit. If no scale or rate is fixed then in case private clinics or hospitals increase their rate to exorbitant scales, the State would be bound to reimburse the same."[26]

How the court reconciles this general pragmatic approach with its recourse, on occasion, to orders with clearly significant cost implications, is not clear, and has certainly led to the Indian approach not being adopted in other common law jurisdictions beyond the South Asian region.

Another important line of public interest litigation cases impacting on rights to health have been those concerning protection of the environment, not only reinforcing the links between environmental rights and rights to health and to life, but also exemplifying the judicial activism for which the Indian courts have become well known. However, in so doing the courts have had to contend with the frequent charge that their orders are inconsistent with existing statutes, and that they have illegitimately extended their jurisdiction into an area of competence normally reserved for the executive. The Supreme Court has responded to such charges by stating that such directions are necessary to safeguard people's right to health and therefore should trump statutory provisions. On this basis the court has justified taking major policy decisions rather than a stricter adherence to the separation of powers' doctrine.[27]

This activist approach has had an impact beyond India's own borders to other countries in the South Asian region with similar constitutional arrangements to India. The result is that courts in Bangladesh and Pakistan have adopted equally progressive interpretations on the fundamental nature of economic, social and cultural rights.[28] At the same time other countries, such as New Zealand, with a restrictive Bill of Rights, have also utilized the right to life principle to indirectly protect health rights.[29]

Pushing the envelope so far: Further creative approaches from other jurisdictions

Canada has no express provision protecting the right to health in its Charter of Rights and Fundamental Freedoms. Yet this has not prevented the Supreme Court from indirectly offering protection to the right by using other provisions. In particular, the equality provision under Article 15 has been used to protect economic, social and cultural rights on the basis that similar treatment may not always guarantee substantive equality, so that one achieves, according to one of its leading proponents, former Supreme Court Justice L'Heureux-Dubé, a contextual and empathetic approach to ensuring each person's human dignity.[30] In this context the court has ruled that, whilst section 15 does not impose upon the government the obligation to take positive action to remedy the symptoms of systematic inequality, it does require that the government should not be a further source of inequality.[31] In particular, the government should ensure that, in providing general benefits to the population, they should guarantee that disadvantaged members of society have the resources to take full advantage of these benefits and, in this context, effective communication was an indispensable component of the delivery of medical services. To hold otherwise was, for the Supreme Court, a "thin and impoverished view ... of equality."[32]

The UK courts, in the absence of any express right to health or any other economic and social rights guarantees incorporated into national law (with some limited exceptions),[33] can only apply the limited set of fundamental civil and political guarantees contained in the European Convention on Human Rights (ECHR) and incorporated through the Human Rights Act 1998.[34] In particular, in relation to the right to health this has involved the protection against cruel and inhuman treatment and respect for private and family life (but not right to life[35]). However, it is important to recognize that in the United Kingdom (UK), as in other jurisdictions where health rights are not entrenched, this is still very much an emerging area of law, and that recent cases provide a mixed record at best.

Cases have included the question of the extent of the state's positive obligations to provide healthcare regarding a claim for reimbursement of costs following treatment abroad. Here the High Court recognized that the jurisprudence of the European Centre of Human Rights demonstrates that Articles 3 and 8 of the European Convention on Human Rights not only impose negative obligations not to act in a particular way, but also, in certain circumstances, impose positive obligations to take measures designed to ensure that those rights are effectively protected.[36] The courts have addressed the failure of a local authority to sufficiently consider a patient's right to private life under Article 8 of the ECHR when deciding to transfer her to a nursing home.[37] And a number of cases have dealt with the health of asylum-seekers.

Asylum-seekers, clearly a particularly vulnerable segment of any population, have been the subject of both positive and negative decisions. In a landmark judgment, the House of Lords in *Secretary of State for the Home Department v. Limbuela & Ors* [2005] UKHL 66[38] held that asylum-seekers should not be thrown into destitution by denying them access to welfare benefits. In this respect the state has a duty under Article 3 of the ECHR to prevent homeless asylum-seekers from suffering destitution even where they had failed to make an asylum claim as soon as was reasonably practicable.[39]

Whilst *Limbuela* could be successfully argued using the right to protection against cruel, degrading or inhuman treatment, other decisions illustrate the difficulties presented by the high threshold required to engage this safeguard. In *N v. Secretary of State for the Home Department*[40] the House of Lords found that that the UK had not breached Article 3 of the ECHR by deporting a failed asylum-seeker with terminal HIV/AIDS back to her country of origin, despite the fact that Uganda's medical facilities were clearly significantly less advanced than the UK.[41] For their Lordships, a claim would only succeed where "the applicant's medical condition has reached such a critical state, that there are compelling humanitarian grounds for not removing him or her to a place which lacks the medical and social services which he or she would need to prevent acute suffering."[42]

Therefore Article 3 did not require contracting states to undertake the obligation of providing aliens with indefinite medical treatment lacking in their home countries. To hold otherwise, they maintained, would be to open the floodgates to a myriad of claims placing an unreasonable burden on the state. Whilst expressing sympathy for the appellant's plight, and reminding the Home Secretary that he was not bound to deport her, but could exercise his discretion, their Lordships concluded that she should not be allowed to remain in the host state to enjoy decades of healthy life at the expense of [the] state."[43] Yet their Lordships admitted themselves, that, without the necessary medication she had been receiving in the UK, the appellant's life expectancy could be two years at best, and in Uganda treatment was available only at considerable cost.

In May 2008 the European Court of Human Rights upheld the Lords' decision finding that:

> "The fact that the applicant's circumstances, including his life expectancy, would be significantly reduced if he were to be removed from the Contracting State is not sufficient in itself to give rise to breach of Article 3. The decision to remove an alien who is suffering from a serious mental or physical illness to a country where the facilities for the treatment of that illness are inferior to those available in the Contracting State may raise an issue under Article 3, but only in a very exceptional case, where the humanitarian grounds against the removal are compelling."[44]

Indeed, to date, the court has only concluded on one occasion that such exceptional circumstances have merited a stay of deportation – where the applicant was critically ill and appeared to be close to death, could not be guaranteed any nursing or medical care in his country of origin and had no family there willing or able to care for him or provide him with even a basic level of food, shelter or social support.[45] It is clear that both the House of Lords, as they themselves recognized, and the European Court of Human Rights faced difficult moral choices in the case. Yet, whilst acknowledging that a line must be drawn somewhere to prevent the state (even one as wealthy as the UK) from becoming overburdened, the scope of the protection offered to desperately ill people in the wake of the decision appears too narrow.[46]

Conclusions

This limited survey of right to health jurisprudence has demonstrated that express codification is not a bar to enforcement of issues impacting on the right to health by courts. However, such judicial enforcement will often require a creative approach and a generous interpretation of existing guarantees, by both lawyers and judges, in order to give true meaning to the principles of the indivisibility and interdependence of rights.

1   Committee on Economic, Social and Cultural Rights, *General Comment No. 9 on the domestic application of the Covenant*, 3 December 1998, UN Doc. E/C.12/1998/24, at paras. 1 and 2.

2   See, for example, the decision of the European Court of Human Rights in *Guerra v. Italy* (1998) 26 EHRR 357 with respect to the lack of available information on a facility which threatened the health of the applicants.

3   See Eleanor Kinney and Brian Clark, 'Provisions for Health and Health Care in the Constitutions of the Countries of the World' 37 *Cornell International Law Journal* (2004) 285 in which they calculate that 67.5% of constitutions have provisions regarding health and health care. Examples include a right to free medical services (Guyana); a right to a healthy environment (Hungary); a right to enjoy the highest possible level of physical and mental health (Hungary again) and a direct relationship to the right to life (Haiti).

4   Article 27(1) of the Constitution of the Republic of South Africa provides: '(1) Everyone has the right to have access to (a) health care services, including reproductive health care; (b) sufficient food and water; and (c) social security, including, if they are unable to support themselves and their dependants, appropriate social assistance. (2) The state must take reasonable legislative and other measures, within its available resources, to achieve the progressive realization of each of these rights. (3) No one may be refused emergency medical treatment.'

5   See the landmark decision of *Government of RSA v. Grootboom* 2000 (11) BCLR 1169 (CC).

6   *Soobramoney*, para. 29.

7   Ibid., para. 52.

8   *Azanca Alhelí Meza García*, Expediente No. 2945-2003-AA/TC: *Amparo* action seeking drugs needed to treat HIV/AIDS upheld by the Constitutional Court which ordered full treatment to be provided regardless of resource implications and subject to immediate and concrete state action. Consequently, the case is seen as a key precedent for the enforceability of social rights in the country.

9   *Cruz del Valle Bermúdez y otros v. MSAS s/amparo*, Expediente No. 15.789, Sentencia N° 196: *Amparo* action to obtain supply of the drugs needed to treat persons living with HIV/AIDS upheld by the Supreme Court which urged the Health and Assistance Ministry to deliver the drugs on a regular and reliable basis. The order also required appropriate budgetary allocation and to develop preventive policies including information, awareness, education and full assistance programmes. See also *López, Glenda y otros c. Instituto Venezolano de los Seguros Sociales (IVSS) s/ acción de amparo*, Expediente No. 00-1343, Sentencia No. 487, where it was also affirmed that a group of HIV infected people could petition the court on behalf of those similarly affected. In another landmark case, *Programa Venezolano de Educación-Acción en Derechos Humanos (PROVEA) y otros c. Gobernación del Distrito Federal s/ Acción de Protección*. Expediente No. 3174, the Caracas City Juvenile Court ordered that the state must provide timely and adequate surgical treatment in order to protect young people's rights to life and to health. Accordingly, the state was under a duty to guarantee sufficient budgetary allocations in order to fully equip a surgery room, together with the creation of a dialogue table aimed at identifying and addressing problems with hospital facilities.

10 *Menores Comunidad Paynemil s/acción de amparo* (2/03/1999): The Appeals Court upheld amparo action seeking protection for the health of indigenous children and youth due to consumption of water contaminated with lead and mercury. The state was found to have arbitrarily failed to diligently protect the right to health and was ordered to provide drinking water to the victims, to determine the existence of damages and, if required, to ensure adequate medical treatment. The case is considered to be one of the most important Argentinian precedents regarding enforceability. See also *Quevedo Miguel Angel y otros c. Aguas Cordobesas S.A. Amparo* (8/04/2002) where the Civil and Commercial Court of First

Instance of the City of Cordoba held that a water services company had the right to reduce, but not completely cut, the water supply to a group of low-income and indigent families due to non-payment. The right to have access to the provision of drinking water concerned the individual right to health and physical integrity.

11 *Estado do Rio de Janeiro* AgR No. 486.816-11: Duty of the state to supply medication to patients without the resources to afford the necessary medications. See also *Bill of Review* 0208625-3 (August 2002) in which the Special Jurisdiction Court of Parana held that an individual's disconnected water supply should be immediately reconnected to safeguard his constitutional rights particularly in light of the vulnerability of one of the residents due to sickness.

12 *Mendoza & Ors v. Ministry of Public Health* Resolution No. 0749-2003-RA (28 Jan 2004): The Constitutional Court held that the Ministry of Health had failed in its obligation under Article 42 of the Constitution to protect the right to health by suspending a HIV treatment programme. The court also held that although the right to health is an autonomous right, it also forms part of the right to life. In so doing it envisaged that a right to health entitled citizens not only to take legal action for the adoption of policies and plans related to general health protection, but also to demand that appropriate laws be enacted and that the Government provide the necessary resources.

13 A constitutional remedy providing individual relief.

14 For a further discussion of the case see Victor Abramovich, 'Argentina: The Right to Medicines' in *Litigating Economic, Social and Cultural Rights: Achievements, Challenges and Strategies* (Geneva: COHRE, 2003). Abramovich states that the case is seen as important for a number of reasons. It reaffirmed the judicial process as a method for enabling ordinary citizens to challenge state agencies regarding the merit of health policies; it saw the direct application by a domestic court of international standards on the right to health,

thereby expanding the scope for further realization of economic, social and cultural rights; it imposed personal responsibility on two ministers for the manufacture of the vaccine with a specific deadline, thereby demonstrating that the obligations arising from economic, social and cultural rights are legal in nature, and entail legal liabilities; and it affirmed the role of the state as guarantor of the right to health in the event that the private sector is unable or (more likely) unwilling to provide the necessary services.

15 In reaching its judgment the court drew on regional and international human rights standards, including the American Declaration on the Rights and Duties of Man, and the Universal Declaration of Human Rights, but particularly the right to health under Article 12 of the International Covenant on Economic, Social and Cultural Rights (ICESCR), all of the instruments having been incorporated into domestic law in Argentina and considered to form part of the Constitution. This was in direct response to the petitioners' assertion that where a state is facing a major health problem threatening a significant numbers of lives, the legal obligation under Article 12 of the ICESCR is particularly strong.

16 See the Human Rights Committee's General Comment No. 6, para. 5 on the right to life: "The right to life has been too often narrowly interpreted. The expression 'inherent right to life' cannot properly be understood in a restrictive manner, and the protection of this right requires that states adopt positive measures. In this connection, the Committee considers that it would be desirable for states parties to take all possible measures to reduce infant mortality and to increase life expectancy, especially in adopting measures to eliminate malnutrition and epidemics." Human Rights Committee, *General Comment No. 6 on the right to life*, 30 April 1982, UN Doc. HRI/GEN/1/Rev.6, at 127 (2003).

17 In the case of *Osman v. UK* 29 EHRR 245 (2000) the Court recognized the positive obligations on the state to protect the right to life (in this case for the police in relation to threats to the victim made by another individual).

18 This has tended to be the approach adopted by the British courts in the absence of any express constitutional protection, but suffers from the fact that only the reasonableness of the decision-making process itself is considered, rather than the substance of the right, although it may still allow for some indirect protection of economic, social and cultural rights (see further below).

19 Article 47 provides: 'The State shall regard the raising of the level of nutrition and the standard of living of its people and the improvement of public health as among its primary duties and, in particular, the State shall endeavour to bring about prohibition of the consumption except for medicinal purpose of intoxicating drinks and of drugs which are injurious to health.'

20 Keshavananda Bharati v. State of Kerala (1973) 4 SCC 225.

21 For a good overview of the Indian courts' approach to economic, social and cultural rights see S. Muralidhar, 'Justiciability of Economic and Social Rights: The Indian Experience' in Circle of Rights (Washington D. C.: International Human Rights Internship Program, 2000).

22 See Francis Coralie Mullin v. The Administrator, Union Territory of Delhi 2 SCR 516 (1981) concerning detention conditions and Parmanand Katara v. Union of India 4 SCC 286 (1989) regarding the obligation of the state to provide emergency medical treatment.

23 The petitioner had been taken to a succession of eight state medical institutions ranging from a local health centre to two medical colleges and was refused treatment at each, either due to lack of beds or lack of technical capacity. Eventually he was admitted to a private hospital where he had to pay for treatment. See also State of Punjab & Ors v. Mohinder Singh Chawla Etc [1996] INSC 1666 in which the Supreme Court held that where certain medical treatment is not available in some states, and the patient is being treated at government expense outside his state, the latter should bear the costs of renting the room.

24 Paschim & Ors v. State of West Bengal & Anor (1996) AIR SC 2426 at 2429.

25 This included hospitals and emergency provision (ambulances and communications) by formulating a blueprint for primary health care with particular reference to treatment of patients under an emergency as part of the state's public health obligation under Article 47.

26 Consumer Education and Research Centre v. Union of India 3 SCC 42 (1995) finding that no breach of the Constitution was incurred by reducing some employees' entitlements to medical benefits.

27 See in particular Mehta v. Union of India 6 SCC 9 (1999) where the Supreme Court, after appointing an expert committee to formulate a detailed policy on conversion from petrol to cleaner fuels for vehicles in heavily polluted Delhi and incorporating its recommendations, issued several time-bound directions for conversion.

28 For example, in Dr Mohiuddin Farooque v. Bangladesh & Ors (No. 1) 48 DLR (1996) HCD 438 the Bangladeshi Supreme Court, upon finding that a consignment of powdered milk, imported by a company, exhibited in some cases a radiation level above the acceptable limit, upheld the claim that the actions of government officers in not compelling the importer to send the consignment back to the exporter had violated the constitutional right to life of people who were potential consumers. Where lives were threatened by a man-made hazard then the state could be compelled by the court to remove the threat (unless justified by law) even where its primary DPSP obligation under Art 18 to raise the level of nutrition and improve public health could not be enforced. See also Zima v. WAPDA PLD 1994 SC 693 in which the Supreme Court of Pakistan, relying on the rights to life and dignity, which included the right to live in a clean environment, held that the local power authority, prior to constructing a potentially health threatening electricity grid station had to carry out a full consultation process with the affected community.

29 In Shortland v. Northland Health Ltd [1998] 1 NZLR 433 the Court of Appeal, generously inter-

preting the right to life as protected by Article 8 of the Bill of Rights, and drawing on the equivalent international provision – Article 6 of the International Covenant on Civil and Political Rights (ICCPR) ratified by New Zealand – was able to assess whether a clinical decision to withdraw dialysis treatment amounted to a breach of the Bill of Rights. In so doing the court recognized that section 151 of the *Crimes Act 1961* placed a legal duty on the local health authority to supply the patient with "the necessaries of life" and that a failure to perform that duty "without lawful excuse" could lead to criminal responsibility. The Court noted that this positive duty was related to the right to life as guaranteed by Article 6(1) of the ICCPR and the understanding of that provision as elaborated by the United Nations Human Rights Committee in its General Comment 6. On the facts, the Court held that the consideration of a patient's condition by the clinical team which had knowledge of his condition and his ability to benefit from dialysis, meant that there was a bona fide decision that the cessation of treatment was in the patient's best interests. Consequently, Northland Health could not be said to be in breach of its duty to provide the necessaries of life, and therefore the decision to withdraw dialysis was not objectionable and would not deprive the patient of his right to life. In so doing it recognized that judges were concerned with the lawfulness of the decision to discontinue dialysis, and not with the likelihood of the effectiveness of the treatment (cf. South African decision of *Soobramoney* discussed above).

30 See for example decisions such as *Corbiere v. Canada* [1999] 2 SCR 203 and *M v. H* 2 SCR 203 [1999]. This approach has been criticized by the leading Canadian constitutional commentator Peter Hogg as "vague, confusing and burdensome to claimants": Peter Hogg, *Constitutional Law of Canada* (Toronto: Carswell, Student Edition, 2002) at 1059.

31 *Eldridge v. British Columbia* 3 SCR 624 [1997] where deaf individuals successfully challenged the failure of a provincial government to provide sign-language interpreters as part of its publicly funded healthcare system.

32 Ibid., para. 73.

33 The rights to education (Article 2 Protocol 1) and property (Article 1 Protocol 1) are the only economic and social rights explicitly protected under the European Convention on Human Rights and thus under the Human Rights Act 1998.

34 Although the UK has ratified the ICESCR, together with a number of other major UN human rights treaties, it has yet to incorporate this treaty into national law.

35 One arguable exception was the holding by the Court of Appeal that given the decision to refuse the breast cancer drug Herceptin to the applicant was a life or death decision (without confirming whether Article 2 of the ECHR was engaged or not) the decision should be subject to rigorous scrutiny (*Rogers, R (on the application of) v. Swindon NHS Primary Care Trust & Anor* [2006] EWCA Civ 392, at para. 56). Both the European Commission and Court of Human Rights have held that Article 2 ECHR can be engaged in healthcare cases (see *X v. Ireland* 7 DR 78 (1976); *Association X v. UK* 14 DR 31 (1978) and *LCB v. UK* 27 EHRR 212 (1998)).

36 *Watts, R (on the application of) v. Bedford Primary Care Trust & Ors* [2003] EWHC 2228 para 45. However, the Court went on to hold that in the light of the Court of Appeal decision *R v. North West Lancashire Health Authority ex p A* [2000] 1 WLR 977, Article 8 imposes no positive obligations to provide medical treatment and that the pain and suffering endured by the applicant in not receiving treatment was not sufficiently serious to engage Article 3. Although the applicant was not able to succeed using human rights law he was able to on the basis of European Community law. Nevertheless, it appears unlikely until *R v. North West Lancashire Health Authority ex p A* is overruled that claims for meeting medical treatment costs based solely on human rights arguments will succeed.

37 *Goldsmith, R (on the application of) v. London Borough of Wandsworth* [2004] EWCA Civ 1170. The Court concluded inter alia that the decision-making process had not acted in the best interests

of the patient in securing her health, together with a complete failure to take into account her Article 8 rights, thereby recognizing that a patient's right to respect for her private life does not cease upon her entering a healthcare institution.

38 Two other cases were joined in the hearing: *R v. Secretary of State for the Home Department ex p Tesema* and *R v. Secretary of State for the Home Department ex p Adam (FC)*.

39 Applying *R (Q) v. Secretary of State for the Home Department* [2004] QB 36 the House of Lords held it was not necessary for the claimant to show the actual onset of severe illness or suffering for a claim to be established. If the evidence established clearly that charitable support in practice was not available, and that he had no other means of fending for himself, the presumption would be that severe suffering would imminently follow. The majority of the court recognized that the correct approach was one of prevention rather than "wait and see" which could result in the victim having to endure unnecessary suffering before upholding a claim.

40 [2005] UKHL 31.

41 The Lords distinguished the European Court of Human Rights decision of *D v. UK* 24 EHRR 423 (1997), relied on by the appellant, on the grounds that the situation in the receiving state was not as extreme as that faced by a terminally ill patient

in that case, where there was no prospect of any medical care or family support.

42 At para. 94. The high threshold approach has also been confirmed in relation to the right to private and family life under Article 8 ECHR. In *Dbeis and Ors v. Secretary of State for the Home Department* [2005] EWCA Civ 584 the Court of Appeal ruled that a failed asylum-seeker and her son suffering from cerebral palsy did not meet the exceptional test under Article 8 to prevent her being returned to her country of origin where there were adequate medical and education facilities.

43 At para. 92.

44 *N v. UK* (26565/05) para 42.

45 *Supra* n.41.

46 See also *ZT v. Secretary of State for the Home Department* [2005] EWCA Civ 1421 where the Court of Appeal adopted a similar approach in refusing an HIV positive Zimbabwean leave to remain. ZT's lawyers unsuccessfully sought to distinguish N on the grounds that the Zimbabwe regime had deliberately destroyed much of the medical infrastructure of the country through its economic policies. In *Razgar, R (on the Application of) v. Secretary of State for the Home Department* [2004] UKHL 27 the House of Lords recognized that Article 8, safeguarding respect for private and family life, could also be engaged by such cases but rejected the claim on the facts.

Public-Private Partnership to Promote Health: The GAVI Alliance Experience

Geoff Adlide, Alison Rowe and Julian Lob-Levyt

The mission of the Global Alliance for Vaccines and Immunization (GAVI) is to save children's lives and protect people's health by increasing access to immunization in poor countries. It is a mission that directly supports the right of individuals to enjoy the highest attainable standard of health. Established in 2000 as a public-private partnership, GAVI has attracted long-term commitments of over USD 7.5 billion from governments and philanthropists. It has already had an impact on the shape and dynamic of the global vaccine market and, through helping to strengthen health services and immunization programmes, has delivered direct benefits to millions of people.

The World Health Organization projects that, by the end of 2008, GAVI support to more than 70 of the poorest countries in the world will have protected an additional 213 million children, using new and under-used vaccines, and averted 3.4 million premature deaths.[1] By the end of 2007, GAVI had made long-term commitments to countries through to 2015 totaling over USD 3.5 billion. These commitments focus strongly on provision of vaccines (74% of funds committed) but also illustrate the essential concomitant support to improving the delivery systems through which mothers and children not only get immunized, but also contact other vital health services.

Immunization coverage with DTP3, hepatitis B and Hib vaccines in GAVI-supported countries, 2000–2009

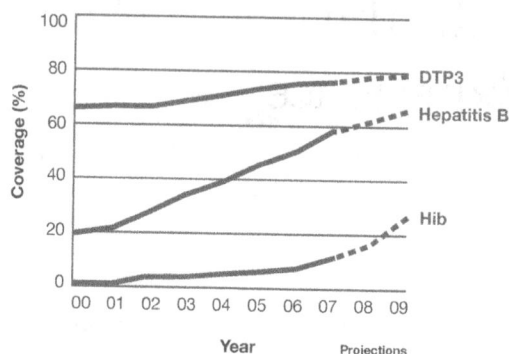

Source: WHO-UNICEF coverage estimates for 1980–2007, as at August 2008; WHO ICE-T coverage projections for 2008–2010, as at September 2008.

A key enabler of GAVI's success is its approach to public-private partnership, which has leveraged the skills and attributes of individuals and organizations from across the spectrum, and brought them together in a united mission. The last 10 years have seen a proliferation of public-private partnerships (PPPs) in global health. PPPs captured attention as an exciting new way of approaching international development. But just how valuable are PPPs in ensuring the right to health and what does it really mean to speak of a public-private partnership?

In the early days, the PPP label was readily attached to any organization that had some engagement with public and private sectors. For example, a representative of industry on a governing board lent the organization the legitimacy of a partnership. Indeed one part of GAVI – the GAVI Alliance Board – was established on this premise and, from the start, included representatives of the pharmaceutical companies that produce vaccines. But GAVI's evolution as a PPP runs much deeper than industry representation on the Alliance Board, and offers to others in the health sector and beyond some examples and lessons learned on the potential of public-private partnership.

In January 2000, the Global Alliance for Vaccines and Immunization was launched in Davos, Switzerland at the World Economic Forum, by governments, multilateral agencies and private philanthropists. An initial substantial grant of USD 750 million over five years from the Bill & Melinda Gates Foundation was soon supplemented by a number of other donors – mostly governments – and in 2005 the Bill & Melinda Gates Foundation expanded its contribution.

The GAVI Alliance Board's first Chair, Dr. Gro Harlem Bruntland, Director-General of WHO, described the partnership and its purpose as being, "to deliver more than each of us can do if we go it alone. An alliance where the glue is the commitment we bring. The merger of our comparative advantages."[2] Almost a decade later, that description holds true and is evidenced by the results that GAVI has achieved – a significant and growing number of boys and girls in developing countries with access to immunization, and a vaccine market that increasingly takes into account the demand for old and new vaccines from the poorest countries of the world.

For the first eight years, GAVI had two Boards – the Alliance Board and the Fund Board. The Alliance Board brought together all of the main actors engaged in immunization: The World Health Organization, the United Nations Children's Fund (UNICEF), the World Bank, the Bill & Melinda Gates Foundation, developing and donor governments, research and technical institutes, vaccine manufacturers, and civil society. The Fund Board

GAVI long-term commitments to countries 2000–2015 (as at 2007)

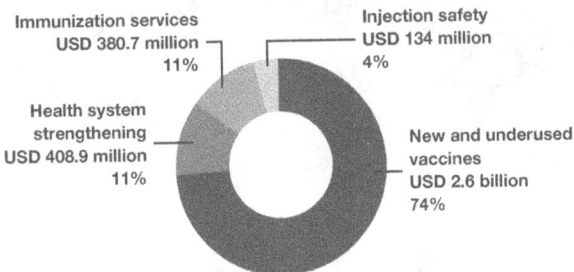

Immunization services
USD 380.7 million
11%

Injection safety
USD 134 million
4%

Health system
strengthening
USD 408.9 million
11%

New and underused
vaccines
USD 2.6 billion
74%

Source: GAVI Alliance Progress Report 2007.

comprised individuals from a range of private sector and civil society back-grounds, including a number of internationally prominent figures and business people from the financial sector. The bringing together of these two Boards in 2008 embedded in GAVI's governance structure a new form of public-private partnership; one that combines the best of multilateral and public sector values and experience with the added value of private sector dynamics and challenge.

GAVI's starting premise is simple: It is wrong that people in the developing world should be denied access to health technologies and services that can save their lives and prevent debilitating illness. Of the over 9 million children who die in the developing world each year, over 2 million die from diseases for which the world has available vaccines. These inequities amount to a denial of the rights to life and health of those affected, and exact a heavy toll on their families and communities.

Recent history tells us that the availability of vaccines in low-income countries can lag up to 15 years behind their introduction in middle and upper-income countries. In addition, developing and producing vaccines is a costly business, and the incentives to invest in vaccines appropriate to the

Leading causes of vaccine-preventable deaths in children under five years old

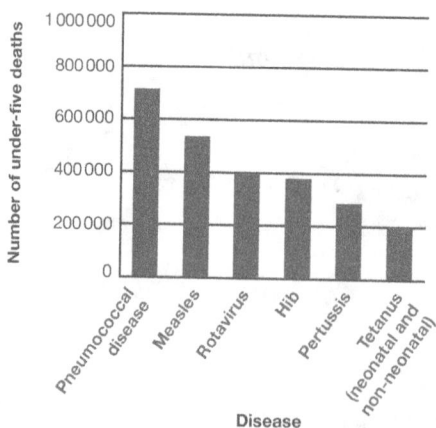

Source: WHO Global Immunization Data, January 2008 (WHO data for 2002).

Decrease in price of auto-disable syringes procured globally by UNICEF, 1997–2007

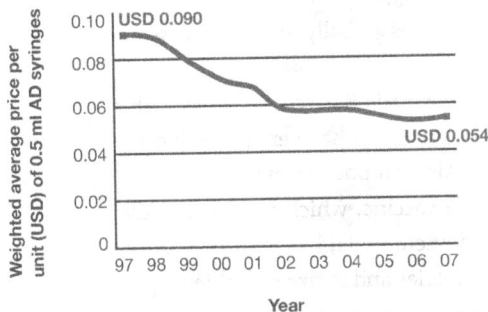

Source: UNICEF Supply Division, Copenhagen 2008.

disease profiles of the developing world are not sufficient. It is what economists call a "market failure". GAVI seeks to address the vaccine market failure and the inequity that results.

GAVI works in the 72 poorest countries of the world – those with a gross national income per capita of less than USD 1000. They are not the traditional view of a promising market, especially not for a product which requires enormous up-front investment in research, development and testing. By offering to support the financing of vaccines in poor countries, GAVI potentially consolidates these populations into one giant market, and in the process changes the incentives that motivate vaccine producers. GAVI creates new dynamics of supply and demand and plays a market-shaping role. Prices decline as the volume of demand, consolidated through GAVI, makes production investment worthwhile. More manufacturers enter the market with better demand forecasts and greater security of long-term, predictable financing. The long-term security of vaccine supplies is strengthened.

GAVI's first big success story was with hepatitis B vaccine. By 2008, all but two countries eligible for GAVI support had been approved for hepatitis B vaccine support. The weighted average price for the vaccine had dropped, from 33 cents per dose to 26 cents per dose since 2001.[3] Over the same period the weighted average price of combination diphtheria-tetanus-pertussis-hepatitis B vaccine has dropped from USD 1.11 per dose to 71 cents.[4]

And WHO projects that by the end of 2008, GAVI will have supported the immunization of 192 million children against hepatitis B – thus protecting them against possible fatal liver cancer as an adult.[5] Similarly, as part of the support for immunization safety, GAVI has supported the distribution and use of more than 2 billion auto-disable syringes globally. In the process, we have seen prices almost halve since 1997.[6]

GAVI is now looking to build on the hepatitis B vaccine success with a range of other underused and new vaccines, which have enormous potential to save lives and ease the disease burden on poor families and economies. *Haemophilus influenzae* type b (Hib) vaccine, which is very effective in protecting against Hib meningitis and pneumonia, has been introduced with GAVI support into more than 50 countries and is already achieving excellent results. For example, an independent WHO study in Uganda showed that in five years, vaccination had virtually eliminated Hib meningitis in children under five nationwide, preventing almost 30 000 cases of severe disease and 5000 deaths annually.[7] New vaccines against pneumococcal disease and rotavirus are also being introduced into routine immunization programmes, and a range of other new and underused vaccines are being considered for support.

Success is not just to be found in the technology of vaccines. The vaccines have to reach the people and this means having health service delivery capacity. In 2006, GAVI initiated a new programme of support, providing flexible cash-based grants to countries to help them address systems constraints that are inhibiting the delivery of immunization and other health services.

In addition to market-shaping through demand creation, GAVI has attracted substantial new resources to immunization and, again reflecting the PPP dynamic, has introduced innovative ways of raising development finance.

In November 2006, the International Finance Facility for Immunization (IFFIm) piloted a completely new way of using the capital markets for financing development. In the same way that GAVI is able to consolidate the vaccine demand from developing countries and present it as a coherent market, IFFIm takes the aid commitments of sovereign governments over up to 20 years, consolidates them, and sells bonds against that combined commitment, producing immediate, up-front funds. The first bond issuance – designed to put IFFIm's stamp on the capital markets – raised USD 1 billion for GAVI programmes. The structure and size of subsequent IFFIm

GAVI Alliance Board (28 members)

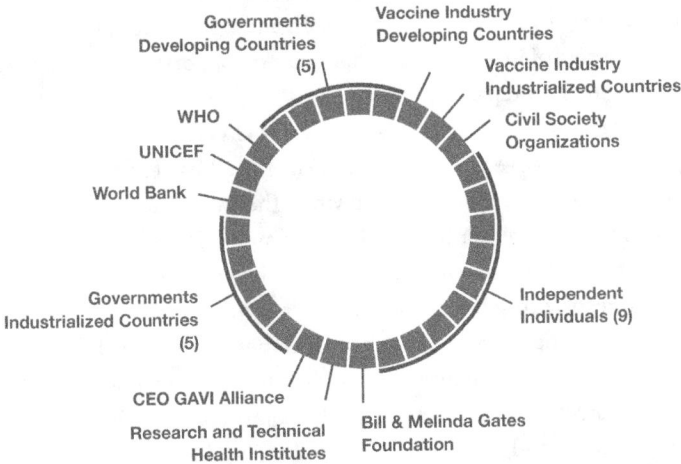

Governments Developing Countries (5)

Vaccine Industry Developing Countries

Vaccine Industry Industrialized Countries

WHO

Civil Society Organizations

UNICEF

World Bank

Governments Industrialized Countries (5)

Independent Individuals (9)

CEO GAVI Alliance

Research and Technical Health Institutes

Bill & Melinda Gates Foundation

bond issuances reflect GAVI's programme funding needs and the knowledge of financial market experts. IFFIm represents a unique example of private-public partnership: Using public donor commitments to harness the strength of the world's private capital markets and manage the cash flows to shape vaccine markets and ultimately save lives and protect the health of people in the developing world.

Another example of combining market-based thinking with public good is the pilot Advance Market Commitment (AMC) designed to speed up the availability of a vaccine against pneumococcal disease, which kills 1.6 million people (half of them children) every year. In February 2007, GAVI announced the support of key donors to a USD 1.5 billion programme to pilot the AMC, which aims to accelerate the development of new vaccines and speed up their availability and uptake through structured financial incentives that guarantee long-term, low and sustainable prices for developing country vaccines. It is a bold new experiment with the potential to avert 7 million deaths by 2030.[8]

GAVI is demonstrating that public commitment can spur private investment and that understanding market forces and incentive structures is a key to leveraging the full potential of public donor funds. There has been some early success in accelerating the uptake and use of new and under-used vaccines in the world's poorest countries, and early evidence of the scale of GAVI operations driving down vaccine prices. In addition, there is a new preparedness on the part of industry to consider market opportunities where previously they were not prepared to invest.

Public-private partnership has been a key enabler of GAVI's success. This is not simply the comparative strength of each in the Alliance, it is also the special space and dynamic that is created when the two value systems and cultures are brought together in pursuit of a common mission. It makes for a space where there is a risk-taking mindset, the generation of new ideas, and a shared resolve to achieve results.

The strength of commitment to public-private partnership in GAVI was tested in 2008 when the GAVI Alliance and Fund Boards were merged and in the process decisions had to be taken as to the composition of the new single GAVI Board. In the end, the Boards agreed that, in order to preserve the public-private dynamic that had served GAVI so well in its formative years, one third of the new Board's members would be independent individual men and women with personal skills and qualifications to contribute to the GAVI mission. The basis for this decision was that a true public-private partnership went beyond simply including industry representatives. The added value of the "private" was best captured by ensuring a significant voice in strategic decisions was given to those who could speak without potential conflict with the interests of their organization or company. It was a model borrowed in part from the private sector, where corporate board membership is not based on representation but on individual qualifications.

The representatives of the main stakeholders in immunization and public health, including multilateral agencies, governments and industry, continue to contribute important knowledge and skills to the GAVI partnership. The public sector, particularly the central, critical role of developing country governments, represents the foundation of GAVI's capacity to deliver on the mission. What distinguishes the new GAVI governance model is the significant presence of independent individuals. These key individuals contribute their particular specialized knowledge and governance skills, and provide a challenge function that contributes to driving the partnership to even greater ambition and achievement.

1   WHO ICE-T coverage projections for 2008–2010, as at September 2008; *World Population Prospects, The 2006 Revision'* (New York: United Nations, 2007).

2   Minutes, First GAVI Alliance Board Meeting, Davos, Switzerland, January 2000 (on file with authors).

3   UNICEF Supply Division, Copenhagen 2008.

4   Ibid.

5   WHO, *supra* note 1.

6   UNICEF, *supra* note 3.

7   R. Lewis et al., 'Action for child survival: Elimination of Meningitis Due to *Haemophilus Influenza* Type b following Introduction of Hib Vaccine in Uganda', *WHO Bulletin*, April 2008.

8   See AMC, 'Saving Lives with New Vaccines: Advance Market Commitments', Fact Sheet available at http://www.vaccineamc.org/files/AMC_FactSheet_v2.pdf.

Torture by Worms

Nicholas D. Kristof

JIMMA, Ethiopia – Presidents are supposed to be strong, and on his latest visit to Africa, Jimmy Carter proved himself strong enough to weep.

The first stop of Mr. Carter's four-nation African trip was Ghana, where he visited his projects to wipe out the Guinea worm, a horrendous two-foot-long parasite that lives inside the body and finally pops out, causing excruciating pain.

Mr. Carter was shaken by the victims he met, including a 57-year-old woman with a Guinea worm coming out of her nipple.

"She and her medical attendants said she had another coming out her genitals between her legs, and one each coming out of both feet," Mr. Carter added. "And so she had four Guinea worms emerging simultaneously."

"Little 3, 4 and 5-year-old children were screaming uncontrollably with pain" because of the worms emerging from their flesh, Mr. Carter said. "I cried, along with the children."

We tend to think of human rights in terms of a right to vote, a right to free speech, a right to assembly. But a child should also have a right not to suffer agony because of a worm that is easily preventable, as well as a right not to go blind because of a lack of medication that costs a dollar or two, even a right not to die for lack of a USD 5 mosquito net.

As president, Mr. Carter put the issue of human rights squarely on the national agenda. Now Mr. Carter argues – and he's dead right – that we conceive of human rights too narrowly as political and civil rights, and that we also need to fight for the human right of children to live healthy lives.

He has led the way in waging that battle. Because of Mr. Carter's two-decade battle against Guinea worm disease, it is expected to be eradicated worldwide within the next five years. It will be the first ailment to be eliminated since smallpox in 1977, and it has become a race between the worm and the ex-president to see who outlasts the other.

"I'm determined to live long enough to see no cases of Guinea worm any-where in the world," Mr. Carter said as he walked in blue jeans through a couple of villages in a remote corner of southwestern Ethiopia, the third country of his African tour.

After leaving the White House, Mr. Carter ended up "adopting" dis-eases like Guinea worm disease, river blindness, elephantiasis, trachoma and schistosomiasis that afflict the world's most voiceless people. These are horrific diseases that cause unimaginable suffering, yet they rarely get at-tention, treatment or research funding because their victims are impover-ished and invisible.

When Mr. Carter met with Mohammad Zia ul-Haq, then Pakistan's president, President Zia had never heard of Guinea worm and didn't know it existed in Pakistan. Nor did his health minister. But after Mr. Carter put the issue on the agenda, Pakistan worked energetically with the Carter Center to eliminate the parasite in that country.

The villages here in Ethiopia that Mr. Carter visited cradle a fast-moving creek, making a lovely image of thatch huts and bubbling water. But the creek is home to the black flies whose bites spread the parasite that causes river blindness, leading to unbearable itching and often eventually to blindness.

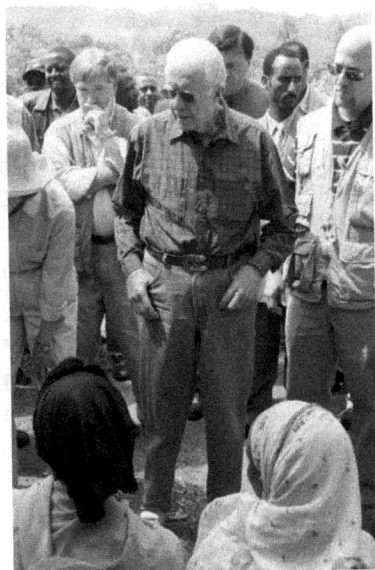

01
Former US-President Carter visiting a river blindness area in Ethiopia.
(Photograph by Nicholas D. Kristof)

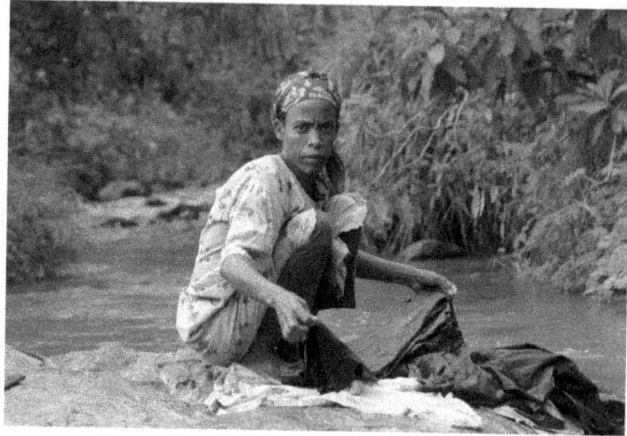

02

"It's almost impossible to imagine the suffering of people with river blindness," Mr. Carter said as he traipsed through the village beside his wife, Rosalynn.

Already, Mr. Carter's campaign is making huge progress against the disease.

Kemeru Befita, a woman washing her clothes in the creek near Mr. Carter, told me that two of her children had caught river blindness in the last couple of months. After a visit to the witch doctor didn't help, she took them to a clinic where – thanks to Mr. Carter's program – they received medicine that killed the baby worms. They are two of the nearly 10 million people to whom the Carter Center gave medication last year alone, who won't go blind.

At the end of the day, this one-term president who left office a pariah in his own party will transform the lives of more people in more places over a longer period of time than any other recent president. And I hope that he can also transform our conception of human rights, so that we show an interest not only in the human rights of people suffering from the oppression of dictators, but also from the even more brutal tyranny of blindness, malaria and worms.

02
Ethiopian woman washing clothes in a stream
that still is a source of river blindness.
(Photograph by Nicholas D. Kristof)

Editors

Andrew Clapham is a Professor of International Law at the Graduate Institute of International and Development Studies in Geneva, and the Director of the Geneva Academy of International Humanitarian Law and Human Rights. He teaches international human rights law and public international law. Prior to joining the Graduate Institute in 1997, he was the Representative of Amnesty International at the United Nations in New York. He has worked as Special Adviser on Corporate Responsibility to High Commissioner for Human Rights Mary Robinson, and Adviser on International Humanitarian Law to Sergio Vieira de Mello, Special Representative of the UN Secretary-General in Iraq. His publications include *Human Rights: A Very Short Introduction* (2007), *Human Rights Obligations of Non-State Actors* (2006), and *International Human Rights Lexicon* (2005), with Susan Marks.

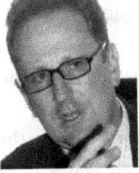

Mary Robinson is the founder of Realizing Rights: The Ethical Globalization Initiative, an organization whose mission is to put human rights standards at the heart of global governance and policy-making and to ensure that the needs of the poorest and most vulnerable are addressed on the global stage. She was the first woman President of Ireland (1990–1997) and more recently the United Nations High Commissioner for Human Rights (1997–2002). She has spent most of her life as a human rights advocate, and has served, for example, on the International Commission of Jurists, the International Council on Human Rights Policy, and on expert European Community and Irish parliamentary committees. The recipient of numerous honours and awards throughout the world, Mary Robinson is a member of The Elders and, since 2002, has been Honorary President of Oxfam International. She is Chair of the Council of Women World Leaders, Vice President of the Club of Madrid and serves on several boards including the GAVI Alliance Board.

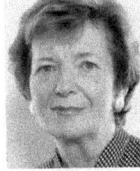

Co-Editors

Claire Mahon is the joint Coordinator of the Project on Economic, Social and Cultural Rights at the Geneva Academy of International Humanitarian Law and Human Rights, and Adjunct Clinical Professor of Law at the University of Michigan Law School. She has previously worked for Amnesty International, the International Commission of Jurists, the International Service for Human Rights, the Centre on Housing Rights and Evictions, and the UN Office of the High Commissioner for Human Rights. She has authored and edited numerous publications on economic, social and cultural rights, and has trained human rights advocates in many countries around the world. Claire holds a Diplôme d'études approfondies (Masters) in International Law from the Graduate Institute of International Studies; an LL. B. (Hons.) from the Australian National University (ANU); a BA (International Relations and Development Studies) from ANU; and is currently completing her PhD on the Optional Protocol to the International Covenant on Economic, Social and Cultural Rights.

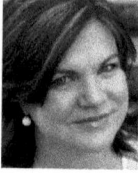

Scott Jerbi is Senior Adviser, Realizing Rights: The Ethical Globalization Initiative. Previously he worked as a human rights officer in the Office of the UN High Commissioner for Human Rights. Before joining the United Nations, Scott was a Program Coordinator with the Amherst Wilder Foundation, a non-profit health and human services organization serving low-income individuals and families in central neighbourhoods and communities in Saint Paul, Minnesota, USA. He received his BA from the University of Wisconsin-Eau Claire, USA; MBA from the University of Miami, USA; and Master's in International Relations from the University of Cambridge, UK.

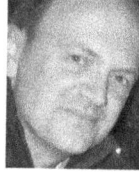

Authors

Geoff Adlide joined GAVI in July 2007 as Head of the Advocacy and Public Policy team. His previous position was Counsellor (Development) at the Australian Permanent Mission to the United Nations in Geneva. Prior to this, he held several posts in the Australian Agency for International Development (AusAID), managing aid programmes in various countries in Asia and the Pacific Islands. Originally a radio journalist and producer, Geoff worked for six years for the Australian Broadcasting Corporation before moving into advocacy and policy work with Aboriginal Land Rights organizations in remote areas of Australia. He holds a Bachelor of Arts (Communications) and has undertaken further studies in development and anthropology. Geoff formerly represented the Australian Government on the Board of the Global Fund to Fight AIDS, TB and Malaria and the UNAIDS Programme Coordinating Board. He was born in Sydney in 1959.

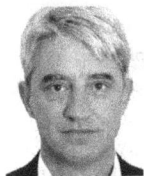

Obijiofor Aginam is on leave of absence from his tenured position as Professor of Law at Carleton University, Ottawa, Canada, and is currently Director of Studies in the Peace and Governance Program, United Nations University headquarters, Tokyo. He holds law degrees from Nigeria, Master of Laws from Queen's University at Kingston, Canada, and a PhD in Law from the University of British Columbia. He was Global Health Leadership Fellow and Legal Officer at the World Health Organization from 1999–2001. Professor Aginam has held numerous fellowships including the Social Science Research Council (SSRC) of New York Fellow on Global Security and Cooperation, and Fellow of the 21st Century Trust, U.K. He has been a visiting professor at universities in Costa Rica,

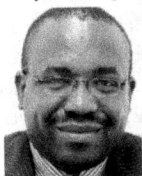

Italy, and South Africa. He has served as international law consultant for a number of national and international agencies. He is the author of numerous academic publications including *Global Health Governance: International Law and Public Health in a Divided World* (Toronto: University of Toronto Press, 2005).

George J. Annas holds degrees in economics, law, and public health from Harvard University. He is the Edward R. Utley Professor and Chair, Department of Health Law, Bioethics and Human Rights, Boston University School of Public Health, School of Law, and School of Medicine, Boston, MA, USA. He is the co-founder of Global Lawyers and Physicians, a transnational professional NGO dedicated to promoting human rights and health. His most recent book is *American Bioethics: Crossing Human Rights and Health Law Boundaries*, published by Oxford University Press, 2005.

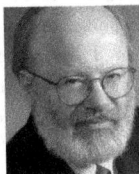

Gunilla Backman, BA, MSc, MA, Gunilla was a Senior Research Officer to Paul Hunt, the UN Special Rapporteur on the right to the highest attainable standard of health, based at the Human Rights Centre, University of Essex. She is presently working as a right to health consultant to the Global Alliance for Vaccine Initiative on Health System Strengthening. She is also the project coordinator of the postgraduate course, Theory and Practice of Health and Human Rights, part of the LL. M. in Health Care Law at the University of Essex. She is sitting on the Advisory Group on Human Rights in Healthcare Advisory Group for the Department of Health of England. She is a public health practitioner with academic qualifications in both health service management, which she obtained from the Lon-

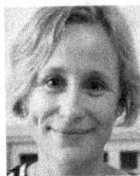

don School of Hygiene and Tropical Medicine, and human rights, which she studied at the University of Essex. She has extensive field experience in conflict, post-conflict and developing countries. She has held health management positions with WHO, UNDP, MSF and IOM. She is fluent in Swedish, English, Spanish and French. Her particular area of focus is health systems, HIV/AIDS, reproductive and sexual health and violence prevention.

Kumariah Balasubramaniam, born on 12 September 1926 in Jaffna, Sri Lanka, studied medicine at the University of Ceylon and Clinical Pharmacology in the University of Manchester (UK) where he obtained a PhD. He taught pharmacology in University Medical School in Peradeniya, Sri Lanka 1964–1977. In 1978 he joined the Technology Division of the United Nationals Conference on Trade and Development (UNCTAD), Geneva as a Senior Pharmaceutical Adviser. His responsibilities included working with Ministry officials in developing countries in Africa, Asia and Latin America who required technical assistance in formulating, developing and implementing national drug policies. In 1983 he relocated to the Caribbean Community (CARICOM) Secretariat, Georgetown, Guyana, South America to work with officials in the Ministries of Health of the 13 member states in developing Caribbean regional pharmaceuticals policy. In 1987 he became the Adviser and Co-ordinator of Health Action International Asia – Pacific (HAIAP), then in Malaysia and now based in Colombo, Sri Lanka, and during the last 20 years he has been working with network partners of HAIAP to achieve their mission objective – to build a just and equitable society where there will be, among others, regular access to essential medicines for all who need them, irrespective of their ability to pay. He has been consultant to Essential Medicines and Drug Policy, WHO Geneva and to the South East Asian Regional Organization WHO, New Delhi. He is a member of the Editorial Committee of PLoS Medicine, a member of the International Advisory Board of Southern Medical Review and a member of the Steering Committee of the People's Health Movement.

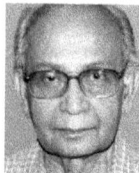

Manmeet K. Bindra is a policy researcher with the Service Employees International Union and a research affiliate with the Technological Change Lab at Columbia University where she examines enforcement of labour laws in urban India. Previously, she worked with economic development and public health organizations in South Africa and India through the Third Millennium Human Rights Fellowship. In South Africa, she served as a coordinator with Mamelani Projects. In India, she worked with LabourNet, a Bangalore-based economic development initiative that connects informal sector workers to employment opportunities. Manmeet K. Bindra holds a BA from Barnard College, Columbia University in Anthropology and History.

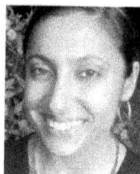

Rahel Bösch studied philosophy and languages at the University of Munich (Germany) and social anthropology and social sciences at the Universities of Freiburg i. Brsg. (Germany) and Zurich (Switzerland). She did post graduate studies in international law and minority rights. She has worked in the fields of political analysis, migration, crisis prevention and development cooperation with various non-governmental and governmental institutions. Since 2001, Rahel Bösch has worked for the Swiss Development Cooperation. In her function as a human rights and governance adviser for Swiss development programmes, she acted also as the first chair of the Human Rights Task Team of the OECD/DAC Govnet and played an instrumental role in coming up with the first DAC policy paper on integrating human rights in development. Currently, she is deputy country director of the Swiss Cooperation Office in Tirana, Albania with a focus on decentralization, private sector develop-

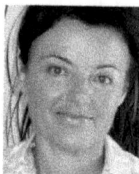

ment and basic service delivery, where support to the health sector reform is included. Rahel is married with two (adult) children.

Gian Luca Burci is the Legal Counsel of the World Health Organization. He has served in WHO since June 1998, dealing mostly with international as well as constitutional and procedural issues. Between 1989 and 1998, Mr. Burci was legal officer in the Office of the Legal Counsel of the United Nations, where he dealt with international law issues related to the activities of the UN, particularly of a political nature. Before joining the United Nations, Mr Burci served in the Division of International Affairs of the Italian Agency for Nuclear and Alternative Energies and in the Department of Technical Cooperation of the International Atomic Energy Agency. Mr Burci is the author of a book on the World Health Organization and of numerous articles on topics ranging from UN economic sanctions and peace-keeping operations to succession of states and the law and practice of the World Health Organization.

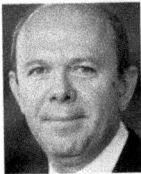

Iain Byrne is a Senior Lawyer with lead responsibility for litigation work on economic and social rights at INTERIGHTS, the international centre for the legal protection of human rights, based in London. Since 2000 he has been a Fellow of the Human Rights Centre, University of Essex from where he graduated with an MA (distinction) in 1994 after obtaining a LL.B. (Hons) degree from the University of Manchester. From 2001 until 2008 he led INTERIGHTS' work in the Commonwealth, including editorship of the *Commonwealth Human Rights Law Digest*. He has litigated widely in domestic fora across the Commonwealth and beyond and before the European Committee of Social Rights and the UN Human Rights Committee. He has taught for many years at the University of Essex, and has also taught in Brazil and Costa Rica. He is a member of the Executive Committee of the EuroMed Human Rights Network. He has authored numerous articles, papers and books on human rights and democracy issues and is currently co-authoring *The Judicial Protection of ESR in South Asia* which is due to be published by OUP in 2009.

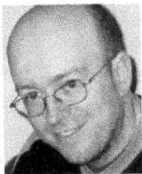

Luisa Cabal is the Director of the International Legal Program at the Center for Reproductive Rights, where she leads the Center's international litigation and legal advocacy efforts in Africa, Asia, Latin America and Europe. In her nine years at the Center, Luisa has pioneered the Center's international litigation efforts, filing cases before the Inter-American Commission of Human Rights and the United Nations Human Rights Committee. She also designed and co-coordinated the first comparative study in Latin America on women's rights jurisprudence of the region's highest level courts. She is co-founder of Red Alas, a network of Latin American law professors who are integrating a gender perspective and women's rights into law school curricula in the region. Luisa received her law degree from the Universidad de los Andes in Colombia, and her Master of Laws from Columbia University School of Law.

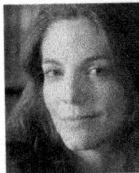

Raymond G. Chambers is the Special Envoy of the Secretary-General for Malaria. Mr. Chambers is a philanthropist and humanitarian who has directed most of his efforts towards children. He is the Founding Chairman of the Points of Light Foundation and co-founded, with Colin Powell, America's Promise Alliance. Mr. Chambers is Co-Founder of the National Mentoring Partnership, and Founding Chairman of both The Millennium Promise Alliance and Malaria No More. Mr. Chambers is also the Founding Chairman of the New Jersey

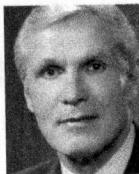

Performing Arts Center and is a member of the President's Council on Service and Civic Participation. His board memberships include The National Mentoring Partnership, The Points of Light Foundation/Hands on Network, America's Promise Alliance, Communities in Schools, University of Notre Dame, and American Museum of Natural History. He is the former Chairman of Wesray Capital Corporation, which he co-founded with William E. Simon. In February 2008, the Secretary-General of the United Nations appointed Mr. Chambers as the first Special Envoy of the Secretary-General for Malaria.

Vincent Chetail is Associate Professor in Public International Law at the Graduate Institute of International and Development Studies, Research Director at the Geneva Academy of International Humanitarian Law and Human Rights and Research Director in International Migration Law at the Programme for the Study of Global Migration. He is also Editor-in-Chief of *Refugee Survey Quarterly* (Oxford University Press) and Visiting Professor at the universities of Cotonou, Paris XI, Lyon III and Tunis. He has published several books and articles on international refugee law, international migration law, international humanitarian law, human rights law and international criminal law.

Mary Crewe studied at the Universities of Natal (Pietermaritzburg South Africa) and the Witwatersrand (South Africa) specializing in education and social and political theory. She has taught at the University of the Witwatersrand. She has worked in HIV and AIDS since 1989 – first in the Greater Johannesburg Metropolitican Council AIDS programme, in the National Department of Health (1996/1997) and is currently the Director of the Centre for the Study of AIDS, based at the University of Pretoria (South Africa). Her research areas are focused on creating new ways of understanding the HIV and AIDS epidemic in South Africa through social, cultural and political theory.

Christian Erk studied political theory (MSc) at the London School of Economics and Political Science (LSE) (United Kingdom) as well as management, economics and international relations (BA) at the University of St. Gallen (Switzerland) and the Copenhagen Business School (Denmark). He currently is a PhD student at the Institute of Political Science and the Philosophical Seminar of the University of Zurich (Switzerland). His research areas are health, rights/duties, human rights, natural rights philosophy, health diplomacy, public and global health ethics, global health governance as well as social determinants of health.

Lynn P. Freedman is the Director of the Averting Maternal Death and Disability (AMDD) Program and Professor of Clinical Population and Family Health at the Mailman School of Public Health at Columbia University. She holds a graduate law degree (JD) from Harvard University, a Masters in Public Health (MPH) from Columbia University, and a bachelor's degree (BA) from Yale University. Before joining the faculty at Columbia University in 1990, Prof. Freedman worked as a practicing attorney in New York City. As Director of the Law & Policy Project at Columbia's Mailman School of Public Health since 1997, she has been a leading figure in the field of health and human rights, working extensively with women's groups, health groups and human rights NGOs internationally. Prof. Freedman has published widely on issues of maternal mortality and on health and human rights, with a particular focus on gender and women's health. She served as a Senior Adviser to the UN Millennium Project Task Force on Child Health and Maternal Health and was the lead author for the Task Force's report, *Who's Got the Power? Transforming Health Systems for Women and Children.*

Julio Frenk, MD, MPH, PhD, is the Dean of the Harvard School of Public Health, since January 1, 2009. Prior to his appointment, he was Senior Fellow at the Global Health Program of the Bill and Melinda Gates Foundation, as well as President of the CARSO Health Institute, a new foundation focusing on health-systems innovations in Latin America. He also chairs the Board of the Institute for Health Metrics and Evaluation at the University of Washington. Dr. Frenk served as Minister of Health of Mexico from 2000 to 2006. Frenk's career has also included executive positions at the World Health Organization and the Mexican Health Foundation. He was the founding Director-General of the National Institute of Public Health of Mexico, was a Visiting Professor at Harvard University, and was awarded the position of National Researcher in his country. Among the 29 books and monographs he has authored are two best-selling novels for youth explaining the functions of the human body. Dr. Frenk holds a medical degree from the National University of Mexico, as well as a Master's of Public Health and a joint doctorate in Medical Care Organization and in Sociology from the University of Michigan.

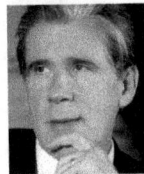

Eric A. Friedman studied psychology at Yale College (USA) and received a law degree from Yale Law School (USA). He is the Senior Global Health Policy Advisor at Physicians for Human Rights (Washington, DC, USA) and chairs the Health Workforce Advocacy Initiative, an international civil society-led network affiliated with the Global Health Workforce Alliance. He has authored or co-authored several publications on Africa's health workforce crisis and the right to health.

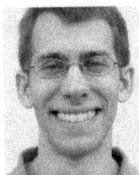

Lance Gable, JD, MPH, is an Assistant Professor of Law at Wayne State University Law School and a Scholar at the Centers for Law and the Public's Health: A Collaborative at Johns Hopkins and Georgetown Universities, a Collaborating Center of the World Health Organization and the Centers for Disease Control and Prevention. Professor Gable has worked extensively on international human rights issues, and has focused on the human rights of persons with mental disabilities and the right to health, authoring or co-authoring several recent publications on these topics. He has helped develop course materials for the new WHO Diploma in International Human Rights and Mental Health and has worked as a human rights consultant for the Pan American Health Organization. Prior to joining the Wayne State law faculty, Professor Gable previously served as a Senior Fellow at the Center for Law and the Public's Health; as the Project Director for the Emergency System for Advance Registration of Volunteer Health Professionals (ESAR-VHP) Legal and Regulatory Issues project, administered by the Health Resources and Services Administration (HRSA); as the Alfred P. Sloan Fellow in Bioterrorism Law and Policy at the Center for Law and the Public's Health; and as a health care law attorney at a major international law firm in Washington, D.C. Professor Gable received a Juris Doctor from Georgetown University Law Center and a Master's of Public Health from the Johns Hopkins Bloomberg School of Public Health.

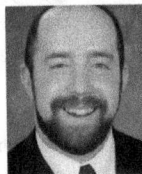

Gilles Giaccia is a Research Assistant at the Geneva Academy of International Humanitarian Law and Human Rights. He holds a Master's Degree in International Relations from the Graduate Institute of International Studies in Geneva and a Master of Law (LL. M.) in International Law from the University of Essex. He has worked in the research and evaluation unit of the UN Office of the High Commissioner for Refugees (UNHCR), for the Interna-

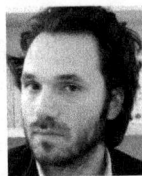

tional Commission of Jurists and as a journalist in the written and audiovisual press. He is also assistant Editor for the *Refugee Survey Quarterly* (published by Oxford University Press).

Octavio Gómez-Dantés, MD, MPH, is currently Director of Analysis and Evaluation at the CARSO Health Institute, a new foundation based in Mexico City focusing on health-systems innovations in Latin America. Between 2001 and 2006 he was Director General for Performance Evaluation at the Ministry of Health of Mexico. Before that he was a researcher at the National Institute of Public Health of Mexico. His areas of research were health policy and international health. Dr. Gómez-Dantés holds a medical degree from the Autonomous Metropolitan University (Mexico), as well as a Master's in Public Health from Harvard University.

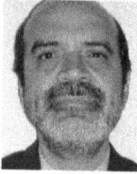

Lawrence O. Gostin is Associate Dean and the Linda D. and Timothy J. O'Neill Professor of Global Health Law at the Georgetown University Law Center, where he directs the O'Neill Institute for National and Global Health Law. Dean Gostin is also Professor of Public Health at the Johns Hopkins University and Director of the Center for Law & the Public's Health at Johns Hopkins and Georgetown Universities – a Collaborating Center of the World Health Organization and the Centers for Disease Control and Prevention. Dean Gostin is Visiting Professor of Public Health (Faculty of Medical Sciences) and Research Fellow (Centre for Socio-Legal Studies) at Oxford University. He is the Health Law and Ethics Editor, Contributing Writer, and Columnist for the Journal of the American Medical Association. He is a member of the WHO International Health Regulations (IHR) Roster of Experts and the Expert Advisory Panel on Mental Health, and is leading a drafting team on developing a WHO Model Public Health Law.

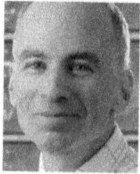

He is an elected lifetime Member of the Institute of Medicine/National Academy of Sciences. He currently chairs the IOM Committee on Health Informational Privacy, and has chaired committees on genomics and on prisoner research. Dean Gostin has been awarded many honours, including the Public Health Law Association's Distinguished Lifetime Achievement Award. Previously, Lawrence Gostin was the Legal Director of the UK National Association for Mental Health, and Director of the UK National Council of Civil Liberties. Dean Gostin's latest books include: *Public Health Law: Power, Duty, Restraint* (2008); *Public Health Ethics: Theory, Policy and Practice* (2007); *The AIDS Pandemic: Complacency, Injustice, and Unfulfilled Expectations* (2004); and *The Human Rights of Persons with Intellectual Disabilities: Different But Equal* (2003).

Thomas Greminger, Head of Political Affairs Division IV, Human Security (Peace, Human Rights, Humanitarian Policy) since August 2004. Ambassador Thomas Greminger joined the diplomatic service of the Swiss Federal Department of Foreign Affairs in 1990 after completing his studies in history, economics and political science at the University of Zurich (PhD). He started his diplomatic career as an attaché at the Swiss Embassy in Tel Aviv. In 1992 he became diplomatic adviser for development policy at the Swiss Agency for Development and Cooperation ("SDC"). He was a co-author of the Federal Council's Guidelines North-South and deputy-head of the division in charge of their implementation in the SDC. In 1996, he was promoted to head of the Development Policy and Research Division of the SDC and Secretary of the Federal Council's Consultative Commission for International Cooperation. From 1999 to 2001, he was chargé d'affaires of the Swiss Embassy in Maputo and country-director of Swiss Development Cooperation in Mozambique. On his return to headquarters, he became deputy-head of

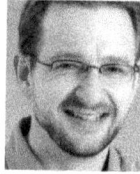

Political Affairs Division IV, in charge of the Peace Policy and Human Security Section.

Monika Hauser, MD, born in 1959 and a gynaecologist by profession, planned, set up and later served as head of *Medica Zenica*, a women's therapy centre, together with Bosnian women experts from 1992 to 1994. In connection with these activities, *medica mondiale* gradually evolved into an international advocate for the rights and interests of women who have survived sexualized violence in war situations. For the next six years, Monika Hauser continued to further the development of *medica mondiale* in her capacity as a board member. In 1999, she initiated the project *medica mondiale Kosova*, involving numerous project visits to Albania and Kosova. In 2000, Monika Hauser assumed the professional and political management of *medica mondiale*. In addition to founding *medica mondiale* as a professional and human rights organization, Monika Hauser's most important task is public relations and awareness rising. Also, since 2002, Monika Hauser has been active as a trainer for the *medica mondiale* Qualification Programme for Afghan women doctors, nurses and midwives in Kabul. Monika Hauser has received numerous esteemed awards for her work. Monika Hauser was among the 1000 women selected as a member of the '1000 Women for Peace' initiative, which was nominated for the Nobel Peace Prize in 2005. She was awarded the Right Livelihood Award in 2008.

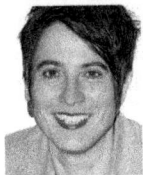

Paul Hunt, a national of New Zealand, was elected in 1998 by the UN to serve as an independent expert on the UN Committee on Economic, Social and Cultural Rights (1999–2002). Between 2001–2002, at the request of Mary Robinson, then UN High Commissioner for Human Rights, he co-authored draft Guidelines on Human Rights Approaches to Poverty Reduction. In 2002, he was appointed as the first UN Special Rapporteur on the right to the highest attainable standard of health. In his work as Special Rapporteur (2002–2008), he chose to focus in particular on poverty, discrimination and the right to health. He submitted some 30 country and thematic reports to the UN General Assembly, UN Commission on Human Rights and UN Human Rights Council. Paul has lived, and undertaken human rights work, in Europe, Africa, the Middle East and South Pacific. In addition to his numerous UN reports on the right to health, he has written extensively on economic, social and cultural rights, including *Reclaiming Social Rights: International and Comparative Perspectives* (1996), *Culture, Rights and Cultural Rights: Perspectives from the South Pacific* (co-ed, 2000), and *World Bank, IMF and Human Rights* (co-ed, 2003). He is a Professor in Law, and member of the Human Rights Centre, at the University of Essex (England) and Adjunct Professor at the University of Waikato (New Zealand). In 2008, Paul Hunt was awarded an honorary doctorate by the Nordic School of Public Health, Gothenburg, Sweden.

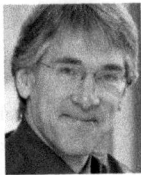

Douglas A. Johnson, M. P. P. M., is the Executive Director, Center for Victims of Torture. Mr. Johnson has been a committed advocate of human rights since the 1970s, when he chaired the Infant Formula Action Coalition (INFACT). As CVT's executive director since 1988, he has led the organization through an important period of growth, as offices and treatment centres opened in St. Paul, Washington, D. C., Guinea and Sierra Leone. He has also pioneered the New Tactics in Human Rights project and the Tactical Mapping methodology. Prior to joining CVT, Mr. Johnson also served as a consultant on strategic planning to human rights organizations in Latin America, as a consultant to UNICEF and the World Health Organization on an international marketing code for breast milk substitutes, and as director of the Third World Institute of the Newman Center. He was an

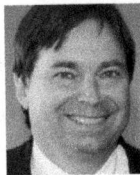

original member of the OSCE Advisory Panel on the Prevention of Torture and has served on the panel since 1998. Mr. Johnson holds a Master's in Public and Private Management (M. P. P. M.) from Yale University. He has also been an Associate Fellow of the Institute for Policy Studies, Washington D. C. and Fellow of Albert Einstein Institute, Cambridge, Mass. He has received the David W. Preus Leadership Award (2003), the Twin Cities International Citizen Award (1999), the Letelier-Moffitt Human Rights Award (1982) and the Archbishop John Ireland Award for Distinguished Service to Justice (1981).

Sarah Joseph is a Professor of Human Rights Law and the Director of the Castan Centre for Human Rights Law at Monash University, Melbourne. She is the lead investigator on an Australian Research Council grant on the World Trade Organization and Human Rights, and has written on various aspects of that issue, including the issue of intellectual property protection and access to medicines. She has also published in many areas of human rights, on topics such as corporations and human rights, the International Covenant on Civil and Political Rights, and self determination. She has also co-authored a book on Australian constitutional law.

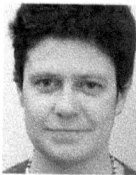

Sarah Kalloch currently serves as Outreach and Constituency Organizing Director at Physicians for Human Rights. Part of her work includes managing PHR's collaboration with the Action Group for Health, Human Rights and HIV/AIDS Uganda (AGHA) and the Kenya Health Rights Advocacy Forum (HERAF). PHR, AGHA and HERAF work together to engage Ugandan and Kenyan health professionals in human rights and AIDS advocacy networks, which bring their powerful voice to decision makers, create positive change around AIDS and help build civil society capacity in East Afri-

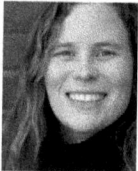

ca. Prior to coming to PHR, Ms. Kalloch worked in philanthropy and eco-tourism, and spent over a year doing research on gender, economics and community management in fishing communities around Lake Victoria in East Africa. Ms. Kalloch received a BA, magna cum laude, in Social Studies from Harvard University in 2000.

Ilona Kickbusch received her PhD from the University of Konstanz (Germany) and has had a distinguished career with the World Health Organization (WHO) and Yale University (USA). She currently heads the new Global Health Programme at the Graduate Institute of International and Development Studies, Geneva (Switzerland) and serves as senior health policy adviser to the Swiss Federal Office for Public Health as well as a range of national and international organizations. She also is an adjunct professor at Deakin University, Melbourne (Australia). Her most recent book is *Health and Modernity* (2007). Further information can be found on her website at www.ilonakickbusch.com.

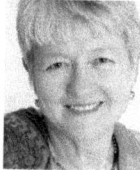

Georg Kohler, born in 1945, studied philosophy and law in Zurich and Basel. After his habilitation in philosophy, he lectured in Munich. Since 1994, he has held the professorial chair for political philosophy at Zurich University.

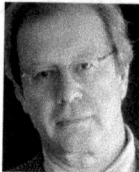

Riikka Koskenmäki, LL. M. (Univ. Helsinki), DEA (IUHEI, Geneva), is a Technical Officer (Legal) at the World Health Organization in Geneva. Prior to this position, she was a Legal Officer with the International Labour Organization and the International Health Organization, and a Legal Adviser with the Iran-United States Claims Tribunal. Ms. Koskenmäki has also worked as a Special Assistant for the Ministry for Foreign Affairs of Finland, as

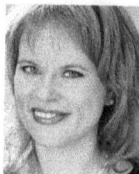

an Associate Researcher for the Finnish Institute of International Affairs, and as a Research and Teaching Assistant for l'Institut universitaire de hautes études internationales (IUHEI, Geneva). She serves as associate editor of the *Finnish Yearbook of International Law*. Her research interests and publications are in the field of public international law, in particular, international health and institutional law.

Nicholas D. Kristof, a columnist for *The New York Times* since November 2001, is a two-time Pulitzer Prize winner who writes op-ed columns that appear twice a week. Mr. Kristof grew up on a sheep and cherry farm near Yamhill, Oregon. He graduated from Harvard College and then won a Rhodes Scholarship to Oxford, where he studied law and graduated with first class honours. He later studied Arabic in Cairo and Chinese in Taipei. After working in France, he caught the travel bug and began backpacking around Africa and Asia, writing articles to cover his expenses. Mr. Kristof has lived on four continents, reported on six, and traveled to 140 countries, plus all 50 states, every Chinese province and every main Japanese island. He's also one of the very few Americans to be at least a two-time visitor to every member of the Axis of Evil. During his travels, he has been arrested or detained in more countries than most career criminals and has had unpleasant experiences with malaria, mobs and an African airplane crash. After joining *The New York Times* in 1984, initially covering economics, he served as a correspondent in Los Angeles and as bureau chief in Hong Kong, Beijing, and Tokyo, and later was appointed Associate Managing Editor. In 1990 Mr. Kristof and his wife, Sheryl WuDunn, won a Pulitzer Prize for their coverage of China's Tiananmen Square democracy movement. Mr. Kristof won a second Pulitzer in 2006, for his work on Darfur. Mr. Kristof has also won other prizes including the George Polk award, the Overseas Press Club award, the Michael Kelly award, the Online News Association award, and the American Society of Newspaper Editors award. Mr. Kristof and Ms. WuDunn are authors of *China Wakes: The Struggle for the Soul of a Rising Power* and *Thunder from the East: Portrait of a Rising Asia* and they are now writing a book about women in the developing world.

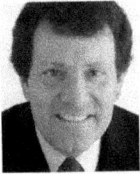

Virginia A. Leary is a former Vice-President of the American Society of International Law. She earned her J. D. degree from the University of Chicago, a doctoral degree from the Graduate Institute of International Studies in Geneva, and the diploma of the Hague Academy of International Law. After working for an international women's organization in Geneva, the Intercultural Cooperation Association, she worked for the International Labour Organization until joining the faculty of the State University of Buffalo and then the University of California-Hastings. She now serves on the Advisory Board of the Program for the Study of International Organizations at the Graduate Institute of International and Development Studies, where she recently directed a project on the social aspects of trade liberalization. Virginia Leary was a founding member of the Geneva-based International Council for Human Rights Policy. She has undertaken human rights missions on behalf of Amnesty International, the International Commission of Jurists, and Human Rights Watch, and has been a consultant to the WHO and the Office of the UN High Commissioner for Human Rights. She serves on the boards of several organizations, including the Centre on Housing and Evictions (COHRE), Human Rights Advocates, and the International Labor Rights Forum. She has written books, book chapters and articles on international labour law, workers' rights, the right to health, child labour issues, and international trade and human rights. She recently co-edited the book *Social Issues, Globalization and International Institutions: Labour Rights and the EU, ILO, OECD and WTO*.

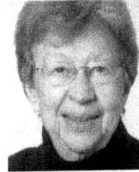

Julian Lob-Levyt joined GAVI in January 2005 as the Executive Secretary of the GAVI Alliance and CEO and President of the GAVI Fund. Prior to taking up the leadership of GAVI, Dr. Lob-Levyt worked with UNAIDS as Senior Policy Adviser to the Executive Director. Dr. Lob-Levyt's career in global health has included work with both bilateral and multilateral organizations. Under the leadership of the UK Secretary of State for International Development Clare Short, Dr. Lob-Levyt was Chief Health Adviser at the UK Department for International Development (DFID) from 2000–2004. Other key posts have included serving as Regional Health Adviser for the European Commission (EC) in Zimbabwe (1998–1999) and health sector reform coordinator for WHO in Cambodia (1994–1997). Dr. Lob-Levyt formerly represented the UK Government and donor constituencies as a member of the GAVI Board, and represented the United Kingdom as a founding board member of the Global Fund to Fight AIDS, TB and Malaria. He is currently a board member of the International AIDS Vaccine Initiative (IAVI).

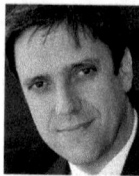

Louis Loutan, MD, MPH, is the Head of the Division of International and Humanitarian Medicine, Department of Community Medicine and Primary Care, Geneva University Hospitals, Geneva, Switzerland. He is also Associate Professor in International Health at the University of Geneva and Assistant Professor in Community Health at Tufts University, School of Medicine, Boston, USA. In addition to his MPH from Harvard School of Public Health, Professor Loutan is specialized in internal medicine, tropical medicine and migrant health. His initial clinical practice as an MD and in coordinating community-based projects was carried out in Geneva, Nepal, Bosnia and Herzegovina, and – for five years in nomadic communities – in Niger. He was formerly president of the Swiss Society for Tropical Medicine and Parasitology, the International Society of Travel Medicine, and the Geneva University Hospitals Committee of Humanitarian and International Cooperation Activities. Since 2006, he is the president of the Organizing Committee of the Geneva Health Forum, an international forum on Access to Health.

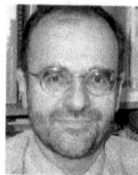

Stephen P. Marks is the François-Xavier Bagnoud Professor of Health and Human Rights at the Harvard School of Public Health, where he directs the Human Rights in Development Program. He also teaches human rights in the Faculty of Arts and Sciences at Harvard University. He holds academic degrees from Stanford University, the Universities of Paris, Strasbourg, Besançon and Nice, France, as well as the University of Damascus, Syria. He has also held teaching positions at Columbia University, Princeton University, the University of Phnom Penh Faculty of Law; Cardozo School of Law; the New School for Social Research; Rutgers University School of Law, City University of Hong Kong School of Law and University of Hong Kong Law School. He spent 12 years in the service of the United Nations, working for UNESCO in Paris and in various peacekeeping operations. He is currently chair of the UN High Level Task Force on the Implementation of the Right to Development. His latest publications relate to human reproductive cloning, universal jurisdiction, cultural rights, human rights education, human rights in development, human rights and bioethics, and the war on terrorism.

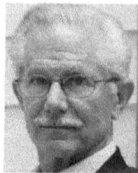

Steven H. Miles, MD, is Professor of Medicine at the University of Minnesota Medical School in Minneapolis and is on the faculty of the University's Center for Bioethics. His latest book, *Oath Betrayed: Torture, Medical Complicity, and the War on Terror,* Random House, 2006 examines military medicine in the war on terror prisons.

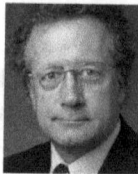

Nelson Musoba serves as Executive Director of the Action Group for Health Human Rights and HIV/AIDS (AGHA) Uganda and also holds the post of senior health planner at the Ministry of Health. In his Ministry capacity, Dr. Musoba coordinates and supervises groundbreaking health research and policy formulation across Uganda. He has also worked at the district and sub-district levels both as manager and operational level worker. In addition to this work, Dr. Musoba specializes in HIV/AIDS management and advocacy. He is the founder and currently serves as Executive Director of the Action Group for Health, Human Rights and HIV/AIDS (AGHA) and as Chair of AIDS Information Center (AIC) Advisory Committee, Western region, and has formerly served as Rakai district HIV/AIDS coordinator. Dr. Musoba received his MB. Ch. B. from Mbarara University of Science and Technology, and earned a Postgraduate Diploma in Anesthesiology and a Master's Degree in Public Health, both from Makerere University. In 2000, Dr. Musoba was awarded 'Best Health Worker of the Year in Uganda' by the Uganda Medical Association and the Ministry of Health.

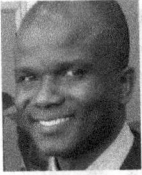

Sisule F. Musungu, a Kenyan national currently living in Switzerland, studied law at the University of Nairobi (Kenya) and University of Pretoria (South Africa) and is currently working on his PhD thesis at the University of Bern (Switzerland). He is currently the President of IQsensato and has previously worked at the South Centre (Geneva) and at the law firm Hamilton, Harrison and Mathews (Kenya). He has also advised many international organizations including UNDP, WHO, UNCTAD, UNITAID, the International Development Research Centre (IDRC), the Ford Foundation, the Open Society Institute (OSI), and GTZ. Mr. Musungu's research specialization and expertise are in intellectual property (IP) law and policy, innovation for development; and international human rights law, particularly the implementation of economic, social and cultural rights. He also has an interest, and has participated, in a number of scenario building processes. His most recent publication is 'The TRIPS Agreement and Public Health' in Correa, C. and A. Yusuf (eds.) *Intellectual Property and International Trade: The TRIPS Agreement,* 2nd Edition, Kluwer Law International, The Netherlands, 2008.

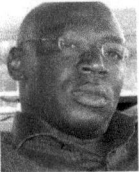

Helena Nygren-Krug is the World Health Organization's Health and Human Rights Adviser, a post that she has held since late 1999. She is based in Geneva, Switzerland. Her current responsibilities include coordinating and further developing WHO's activities on health and human rights. Before joining the WHO, she worked at the UN Centre for Human Rights as part of the Secretariat for the UN World Conference on Human Rights (1992–1993) and later with the UN High Commissioner for Human Rights (1998–1999). She has had field assignments in Haiti as a UN Human Rights Observer and with the Red Cross in Tanzania dealing with the humanitarian crisis following the genocide in Rwanda in 1994. She worked at The Carter Center, Atlanta (1995–1998) and as Adjunct Professor at Emory Law School, Atlanta, USA. She is a Swedish national and has masters' degrees in International Law (LL. M.) from Harvard Law School and the London School of Economics as well as a bachelor's degree in law (LL. B.). She has authored numerous articles and publications on health and human rights.

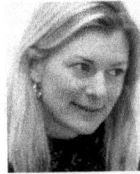

Lisa Oldring is Special Adviser to Mary Robinson, Chair of the GAVI Alliance Board. She is currently on secondment from the UN Office of the High Commissioner for Human Rights, where she has served as adviser on human rights and security (2006–2007), and as assistant to the UN Special Rapporteur on the right to health (2002–2006). Pre-

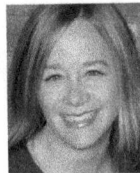

viously she has worked as human rights officer with the UN Human Rights Field Operation in Rwanda (1995–1996), and with the international commissions of inquiry on Darfur (2004) and on Lebanon (2006). Lisa holds degrees in criminology (1992) and in law (1995) from the University of Alberta, Canada, and has been a member of the Law Society of Alberta since 1997. She received her Diplôme d'Etudes Supérieures in International Law from the Graduate Institute of International Studies in Geneva in 1999.

Francis Omaswa is the Executive Director of the African Centre for Global Health and Social Transformation (CHEST), an independent "think-tank and network" initiative promoted by a network of African and International leaders in health and development. Until May 2008, he was the founding Executive Director of the Global Health Workforce Alliance (GHWA). This work culminated in the first ever global forum on human resources for health and the Kampala Declaration and Agenda for Global Action that now guides the global response on health workforce development. Before joining GHWA, he was the Director General for Health Services in the Ministry of Health in Uganda, during which time he was responsible for coordinating major reforms in the health sector in Uganda. At the global level he was Vice-Chairman of the Global Stop TB Partnership, Chair of the Portfolio and Procurement Committee of the Global Fund Board and a member of the steering committee of the High Level Forum on health-related MDGs and has served as an adviser to governments in developing and developed countries. Dr. Omaswa is a graduate of Makerere Medical School, Kampala, Uganda, a Fellow of the Royal College of Surgeons of Edinburgh, founding President of the College of Surgeons of East, Central and Southern Africa and is a Senior Associate at the Johns Hopkins Bloomberg School of Public Health.

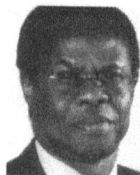

Pierre Perrin, MD, MPH, is an Associate Professor at the University Medical Centre, Geneva, Switzerland. He has been an Associate Professor at the Institut de Médecine Sociale et Préventive since 1998. Dr. Perrin is a graduate of the Medical Faculty of Rennes. He obtained a Master of Public Health from Johns Hopkins University (Baltimore, USA). From 1975 to 1979, he carried out several missions on behalf of Médecins Sans Frontières in refugee camps in Africa and Asia. In 1980, he joined the staff of the International Committee of the Red Cross, working in the field and in Geneva. In 1996, he was nominated Physician in Chief of the ICRC, a position he held until leaving the ICRC at the end of 2006. In 1986, on behalf of the ICRC and in cooperation with the WHO and the University of Geneva, he created the course HELP (Health Emergencies in Large Populations) to train health professionals for missions. Initially, the course was given annually in Geneva, in English, but currently the three week training course is offered seven times per year: In Switzerland, the USA (2×), Japan, Benin (French), South Africa, and Mexico (Spanish). He holds numerous academic positions: Associate at the Johns Hopkins School of Public Health; Associate Professor at the Faculty of Law and Political Sciences of Aix-Marseille; Guest Professor at the Université Libre of Brussels (2007–2008). He has been granted The Distinguished Alumnus Award 2004 from the Alumni Association of Johns Hopkins University.

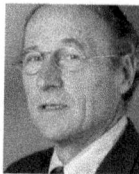

Helen de Pinho is from South Africa where she trained as a physician, specialized in public health, and completed an MBA focusing on management education and systems thinking. She has worked as a health service manager in the areas of reproductive health, HIV/AIDS and health service delivery in both rural and urban areas of South Africa. In addition, she was a senior lecturer in the School of

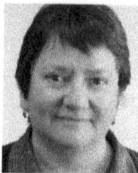

Public Health and Family Medicine at the University of Cape Town, where she worked in the Women's Health Research Unit and was also responsible for health management development programmes for senior health systems managers. Dr. de Pinho currently holds the title of Assistant Professor of Clinical Population and Family Health at the Mailman School of Public Health, Columbia University, where she is a member of the Averting Maternal Death and Disability Program (AMDD). Prior to joining AMDD, Dr. de Pinho worked as policy adviser to the UN Millennium Project Task Force on Child Health and Maternal Health, and was one of the authors of the task force's final report: *Who's got the power? Transforming health systems for women and children.*

Peter Piot is Professor and Director of the Institute of Global Health, Imperial College, London UK. From 1994 to 2008, he was Executive Director of UN-AIDS and Under Secretary-General of the United Nations. Dr. Peter Piot comes from a distinguished academic and scientific career focusing on AIDS and women's health in the developing world. Drawing on his skills as a scientist, manager and activist, Dr. Piot has challenged world leaders to view AIDS in the context of social and economic development and human rights. He earned a medical degree from the University of Ghent, a PhD in Microbiology from the University of Antwerp, Belgium, and was a Senior Fellow at the University of Washington in Seattle. After graduating from medical school, Dr. Piot co-discovered the Ebola virus in Zaire in 1976. He is the author of 16 books and more than 500 scientific articles. He is a member of the Institute of Medicine of the National Academy of Sciences of the United States and the Royal Academy of Medicine of Belgium, and a Fellow of the Royal College of Physicians of London, UK.

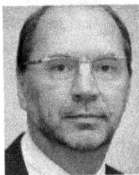

Eibe Riedel, Professor Dr., LL. B., A. K. C., Chair of German and Comparative Public Law, European and International Law (em.) at the University of Mannheim, Germany, and a member of the UN Committee on Economic, Social and Cultural Rights, Geneva. He studied law and theology at King's College London, and law at the University of Kiel/Germany. He obtained his Dr. iuris in 1974 and Dr. iur. habil. in 1983. He has been a Professor of Public Law and International Law at the University of Mainz, then at the University of Marburg, then at Mannheim. Prof. Riedel has recently been appointed a Judge at the Hague Court of Arbitration. He is a Director of the Inland Navigation Law Institute, and the Director of the Institute of Medical Law, Bioethics and Public Health. He was Pro-Vice Chancellor of the University of Mannheim from 1996–2000. Prof. Riedel is currently a member of the Scientific Advisory Council at the German Foreign Office; member of the German UNESCO Commission; Chairperson, Advisory Council on Students' Fees, Baden-Württemberg; Honorary Adjunct Professor, University of Adelaide; and Visiting Professor, University of Kingston.

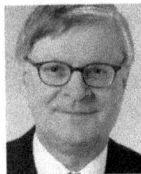

Alison Rowe joined the GAVI Alliance in December 2006 in the area of strategic communications, following two decades of work in policy analysis and creative communications in both the public and private sectors, in Asia and Europe, with particular focus in later years on public health in development. Her previous roles in each sector include: Analyst and speech-writer for the Director-General of the World Health Organization, Dr. J. W. Lee, and Director of the Financial Services Group for Shandwick plc in Thailand.

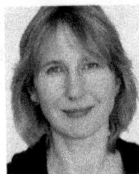

Leonard Rubenstein is President of Physicians for Human Rights and during the 2008–2009 academic year a Fellow at the United States Institute of Peace. He has a JD degree from Harvard Law School and an LL. M. from Georgetown University Law Center. A human rights researcher and advocate for 25 years, he has also written and lectured extensively about the right to health; torture and interrogation; and the role of physicians in human rights. He led the International Working Group on Dual Loyalty and Human Rights, which recommended standards of conduct for health professionals based on human rights. He is a member of the Board of Directors of the International Federation of Health and Human Rights Organizations and the Committee on Scientific Freedom and Responsibility of the American Association for the Advancement of Science.

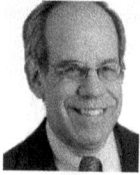

Jeffrey D. Sachs is the Director of The Earth Institute, Quetelet Professor of Sustainable Development, and Professor of Health Policy and Management at Columbia University. He is also Special Adviser to United Nations Secretary-General Ban Ki-moon. From 2002 to 2006, he was Director of the UN Millennium Project and Special Adviser to United Nations Secretary-General Kofi Annan on the Millennium Development Goals, the internationally agreed goals to reduce extreme poverty, disease, and hunger by the year 2015. Sachs is also President and Co-Founder of Millennium Promise Alliance, a nonprofit organization aimed at ending extreme global poverty. He is widely considered to be the leading international economic adviser of his generation. For more than 20 years, Professor Sachs has been at the forefront of the challenges of economic development, poverty alleviation, and enlightened globalization, promoting policies to help all parts of the world to benefit from expanding economic opportunities and well-being.

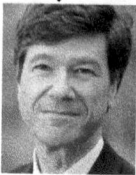

He is the author of hundreds of scholarly articles and many books, including the New York Times bestsellers *Common Wealth: Economics for a Crowded Planet* (Penguin, 2008) and *The End of Poverty* (Penguin, 2005).

Tido von Schön-Angerer was born 1966 in Germany and studied medicine in Mainz (Germany) and Uppsala (Sweden). He completed specialty training in pediatrics at the Albert Einstein College of Medicine (Bronx, N. Y., USA) and has worked with Médecins Sans Frontières (MSF) in different field and headquarter positions. He is currently the Executive Director of MSF's Campaign for Access to Essential Medicines, based in Geneva (Switzerland). He publishes and advocates on the problems of access to medicines and lack of innovation for diseases that primarily affect people in poor countries.

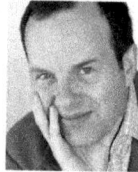

Claudio Schuftan, MD (pediatrics and international health), was born in Chile and is currently based in Ho Chi Minh City, Vietnam, where he works as a freelance consultant in public health and nutrition. He is an Adjunct Associate Professor in the Department of International Health, Tulane School of Public Health, New Orleans, LA. He received his medical degree from the Universidad de Chile, Santiago, in 1970. He also studied nutrition and nutrition planning at the Massachusetts Institute of Technology (MIT) in Cambridge, MA, in 1975. Dr. Schuftan is the author of two books, several book chapters and over fifty scholarly papers published in refereed journals plus over two hundred other assorted publications. Since 1976, Dr. Schuftan has carried out over one hundred consulting assignments in 45 countries in Africa, Asia, Latin America and the Caribbean, for organizations such as the World Health Organization, USAID, UNICEF, World Food Program, the Euro-

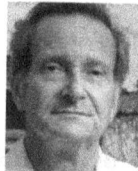

pean Union, the World Bank, the Asian Development Bank, the UNU, the FAO, and several international NGOs. He is currently an active member of the Steering Group of the People's Health Movement.

Dr. Abhay Shukla, MD, is a medical graduate with a postgraduate degree in Community Medicine from the All India Institute of Medical Sciences, New Delhi. For the last one and a half decades, he has been working on health issues in association with people's organizations. As a Senior Programme Coordinator in SATHI-CEHAT, he has been involved in training health workers, developing health training material and advocacy on Health rights and primary health care issues in Western India. He is one of the National Joint Convenors of Jan Swasthya Abhiyan (People's Health Movement-India) and has been involved in hosting the National Secretariat of PHM-India during 2003 to 2008. He has authored a number of publications including *A Compiled Review of the Rights Approach to Health and Health Care* and is the co-editor of the books *Review of Health Care in India* and *A Report on Health Inequities in Maharashtra.*

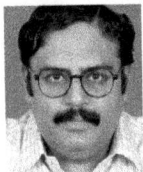

Jason Sigurdson is currently a human rights and law programme officer with the Joint United Nations Programme on HIV/AIDS (UNAIDS) in Geneva. In 1999, he received his joint honours in sociology and political science from McGill University (Montreal, Canada), and in 2004 a Master of Public Administration and Bachelor of Laws (MPA/LL. B.) from Dalhousie University (Halifax, Canada), where he also worked as a research assistant in the Bioethics Department of the Faculty of Medicine. His graduate studies included course work at Lund University and the Raoul Wallenberg Institute of Human Rights (Lund, Sweden). Prior to joining UNAIDS in March 2005, Jason was a research assistant in the economic and social issues unit of the Office of the United Nations High Commissioner for Human Rights, focusing on the rights to adequate housing and the highest attainable standard of health. Since February 2006, he has served as an external member of the Research Ethics Review Committee of the World Health Organization.

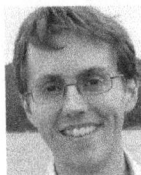

Slim Slama, MD, is Chief Resident, Division of International and Humanitarian Medicine Department of Community Medicine and Primary Care, Geneva University Hospitals, Geneva, Switzerland. Slim Slama graduated from the University of Geneva in 1998 and subsequently specialized in Internal Medicine. After eight years in the Department of Internal Medicine, Dr. Slama joined the Department of Community Medicine and Primary Care, Geneva University Hospitals, Switzerland. He is part-time attending physician in the Primary Care Division and dedicates the rest of his time to the development of international cooperation activities, including research and teaching in the field of global health, in the recently established Division of International and Humanitarian Medicine. Dr. Slama is also the programme manager of the Geneva Health Forum, an international forum on Access to Health.

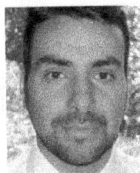

Carly Tanur is the Director and co-founder of Mamelani projects, a community health organization based in Cape Town, South Africa. She graduated from the University of South Africa (UNISA) with a Bachelor of Social Work (BSW) Degree. She is also an active member of the People´s Health Movement-South Africa (PHM-SA), who are focussed on a Right to Health for ALL Campaign. She is passionate about people-centred community health initiatives.

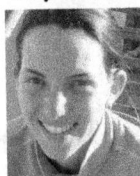

Susan Timberlake received a Bachelors of Arts in anthropology from Stanford University in 1976. In 1982, she graduated cum laude from the University of Georgia School of Law, and in 1984 received an LL. M. in international law from Cambridge University in England. Since then, she has worked in and for the UN system. She was a staff member of the United Nations High Commissioner for Refugees for 19 years where she functioned as a UNHCR Protection Officer in Thailand, as the UNHCR Legal Officer in the United States, as the UNHCR Senior Legal Adviser for Asia and the Pacific, and as Executive Assistant to the Deputy High Commissioner for Refugees. Seconded from UNHCR, she served as the Human Rights Adviser for the WHO Global Programme on AIDS (1994–1996) and as Senior Human Rights and Policy Adviser for UNAIDS (1996–2000). From 2000–2004, she worked as an independent consultant for UNAIDS, WHO, UNFPA and UNIFEM. In November 2004, Susan rejoined UNAIDS as the Senior Human Rights and Law Adviser. She and her team work to promote human rights and gender equality within the Secretariat, with cosponsors, with governments and with civil society, in particular with regard to HIV-related law reform and a rights-based, ethical and gendered approach to the epidemic.

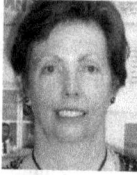

Jaime M. Todd-Gher, JD, LL. M., is the Global Research and Advocacy Fellow for the Center for Reproductive Rights. She engages in reproductive rights advocacy before United Nations human rights bodies and in conjunction with local partner organizations worldwide. She also conducts research regarding issues of gender, sexuality, reproductive health, gender-based violence and human rights. Ms. Todd-Gher holds an LL. M. specializing in gender and human rights from American University – Washington College of Law (WCL). Through WCL's International Legal Studies Program, she developed advocacy strategies to eradicate female genital mutilation, in collaboration with an NGO based in Sierra Leone, and sought immigration relief on behalf of women fleeing gender-based violence. Prior to obtaining her LL. M., Ms. Todd-Gher practiced labour and employment law with a prominent firm in San Francisco, California, served on the Executive Board and Program Planning and Grants Committee for the AIDS Legal Referral Panel, and helped battered women to obtain restraining orders with the Cooperative Restraining Order Clinic.

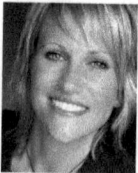

Laura Turiano, MS, PA-C, is a family practice physician assistant who studied anthropology at the State University of New York at Potsdam and Temple University, and health sciences at the George Washington University Physician Assistant Program. Prior to entering the programme, she lived in El Salvador where she provided primary care services and supported local health systems development in communities of demobilized combatants of the Frente Farabundo Martí para la Liberación Nacional and their families. She has worked in a community health centre and an addiction treatment programme in Oakland, California. Currently, she serves on the global coordination group of the People's Health Movement Right to Health and Health Care Campaign and on the coordination committee of the PHM USA.

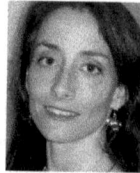

Barbara Wilson studied law and obtained her doctorate in law at the University of Lausanne, Switzerland. She is at present Professor of Public International Law at Lausanne University. She has also taught as guest professor at the University Centre for International Humanitarian Law, Geneva (now called the Geneva Academy of International Humanitarian Law and Human Rights). On several

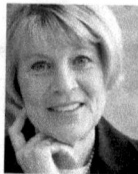

occasions, she has taught in the UNIDEM programme on the protection of minorities, organized in Trieste (Italy) by the Council of Europe.
For the past seven years, she has given courses
on Swiss Constitutional Law and Fundamental
Rights at the University of Savoie (Chambéry,
France). She is also a member of the Committee on Economic, Social and Cultural Rights of
the United Nations and member of the Advisory
Committee of the Framework Convention on the
Protection of National Minorities of the Council
of Europe. Her research areas are human rights
and, in particular, minority rights.

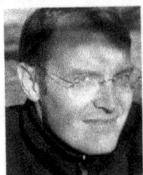

Hans Wolff, MD, MPH, is the Head of the Unit of
Penitentiary Medicine, Depart-
ment of Community Medicine
and Primary Care, Geneva University Hospitals, Geneva, Switzerland. Trained as a medical doctor
at Marburg University (Germany),
he completed his advanced training in Internal
Medicine in 1998. From 1999 to 2007, Dr. Wolff
was responsible for a Health Care Unit for vulnerable populations (homeless, undocumented migrants). Dr. Wolff holds a Master in Public Health
from the University of Geneva, where he now
teaches Clinical Epidemiology. One of his main
research interests is social epidemiology with an
emphasis on access to health care for vulnerable
populations.

Acknowledgements

This book was a collaborative project among a number of different organizations and some very hardworking individuals. The Human Rights Policy Section in the Swiss Federal Department of Foreign Affairs, initially under Wolfgang Amadeus Brülhart, and then under Ralf Heckner, conceived and supported the idea of having such a book. Vincent Chetail from the Graduate Institute of International and Development Studies suggested health as an appropriate topic for the forthcoming Swiss Human Rights Book and then helped to design the project. When Mary Robinson accepted to co-edit the book, her organization, Realizing Rights: The Ethical Globalization Initiative, geared up to shape the table of contents, select the contributors, and help edit the chapters. Special thanks are due to Scott Jerbi and Lisa Oldring who brought their considerable knowledge and experience to bear on this project, going through each chapter with care and consideration. Claire Mahon from the newly created Geneva Academy of International Humanitarian Law and Human Rights took on the delicate task of cajoling contributors to deliver what they had promised, and reworking the chapters to present the reader with cross-references, consistency, coherence, and clarity; all this without losing the diversity and the distinctive style of each chapter. The institutional support given to the Academy by the Faculty of Law of the University of Geneva and the Graduate Institute is gratefully acknowledged.

Natalie Erard from the Human Rights Policy Section and Andrea Keller from the publisher rüffer & rub worked tirelessly to ensure the success of this publication. Their hard work, together with the unstinting support of Georg Kohler and Anne Rüffer, was essential to bring this multi-authored, multi-dimensional project to conclusion. Lastly, we would also like to acknowledge the work of the translator Salomé Hangartner and the contribution from Nils Rosemann, Daniela Kohler, and Stephanie Grillet from the Human Rights Policy Section.

Realizing the Right to Health confronts disciplines, professions, sectors, and differences in approach. Thank you to everyone who contributed to this ambitious project.

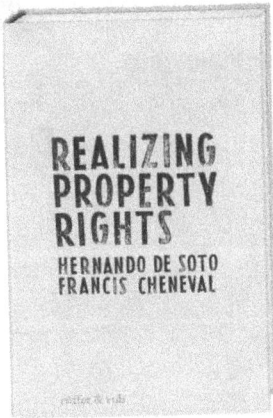

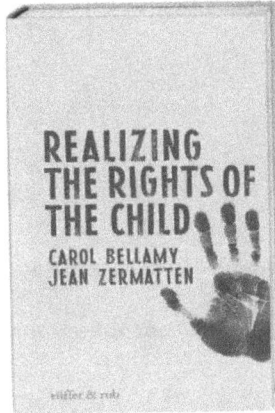

Realizing Property Rights
Swiss Human Rights Book Vol. 1

Hernando de Soto, Francis Cheneval

Property rights are human rights. They protect an external sphere of freedom of humans as such and of their free associations. A working property system is an indispensable vehicle of ethical, economic, and political progress. In this book, leading experts deal with the manifold problems of the realization of property rights in different cultural, historical, and thematic contexts. Additionally, property rights are put into the context of a more comprehensive system of human rights protection.

Realizing the Rights of the Child
Swiss Human Rights Book Vol. 2

Carol Bellamy, Jean Zermatten

The rights of the child protect children and ensure that every child gets the chance to live a worthy and dignified life. Most violations against the rights of the child come from regarding children as things that can be owned, bought and sold, and used and abused as one wishes. In this book, leading experts discuss problems of implementing children's rights. Their contributions deal with various cultural and historical contexts and explore different perspectives on this pressing issue.

www.swisshumanrightsbook.com